Aggressive B-Cell Lymphoma

Editor

LAURIE H. SEHN

HEMATOLOGY/ONCOLOGY CLINICS OF NORTH AMERICA

www.hemonc.theclinics.com

Consulting Editors
GEORGE P. CANELLOS
H. FRANKLIN BUNN

December 2016 • Volume 30 • Number 6

ELSEVIER

1600 John F. Kennedy Boulevard • Suite 1800 • Philadelphia, Pennsylvania, 19103-2899

http://www.theclinics.com

HEMATOLOGY/ONCOLOGY CLINICS OF NORTH AMERICA Volume 30, Number 6
December 2016 ISSN 0889-8588, ISBN 13: 978-0-323-47741-3

Editor: Stacy Eastman
Developmental Editor: Kristen Helm

Hematology/Oncology Clinics (ISSN 0889-8588) is published bimonthly by Elsevier Inc., 360 Park Avenue South, New York, NY 10010-1710. Months of Issue are February, April, June, August, October, and December. Business and Editorial Offices: 1600 John F. Kennedy Blvd., Ste. 1800, Philadelphia, PA 19103–2899. Customer Service Office: 3251 Riverport Lane, Maryland Heights, MO 63043. Periodicals postage paid at New York, NY and at additional mailing offices. Subscription prices are $385.00 per year (domestic individuals), $707.00 per year (domestic institutions), $100.00 per year (domestic students/residents), $440.00 per year (Canadian individuals), $875.00 per year (Canadian institutions) $520.00 per year (international individuals), $875.00 per year (international institutions), and $255.00 per year (international and Canadian students/residents). International air speed delivery is included in all *Clinics* subscription prices. All prices are subject to change without notice. **POSTMASTER:** Send address changes to *Hematology/Oncology Clinics of North America*, Elsevier Health Sciences Division, Subscription Customer Service, 3251 Riverport Lane, Maryland Heights, MO 63043. Customer Service (orders, claims, online, change of address): Elsevier Health Sciences Division, Subscription **Customer Service, 3251 Riverport Lane, Maryland Heights, MO 63043. Tel: 1-800-654-2452 (U.S. and Canada); 314-447-8871 (outside U.S. and Canada). Fax: 314-447-8029. E-mail: journalscustomerservice-usa@elsevier.com (for print support); journalsonlinesupport-usa@elsevier.com (for online support)**.

Reprints. For copies of 100 or more, of articles in this publication, please contact the Commercial Reprints Department, Elsevier Inc., 360 Park Avenue South, New York, New York 10010-1710; Tel.: 212-633-3874, Fax: 212-633-3820, E-mail: reprints@elsevier.com.

Hematology/Oncology Clinics of North America is covered in *MEDLINE/PubMed (Index Medicus), EMBASE/ Excerpta Medica, and BIOSIS.*

Contributors

CONSULTING EDITORS

GEORGE P. CANELLOS, MD
William Rosenberg Professor of Medicine, Department of Medical Oncology, Dana-Farber Cancer Institute, Boston, Massachusetts

H. FRANKLIN BUNN, MD
Professor of Medicine, Division of Hematology, Brigham and Women's Hospital, Harvard Medical School, Boston, Massachusetts

EDITOR

LAURIE H. SEHN, MD, MPH
Chair, Lymphoma Tumour Group, British Columbia Cancer Agency and the Centre for Lymphoid Cancer; Clinical Professor, University of British Columbia, Vancouver, British Columbia, Canada

AUTHORS

JEREMY S. ABRAMSON, MD
Director, Center for Lymphoma, Massachusetts General Hospital Cancer Center; Assistant Professor of Medicine, Harvard Medical School, Boston, Massachusetts

MARY ANN ANDERSON, MBBS, FRACP, FRCPA
Cancer and Haematology Division, Walter and Eliza Hall Institute of Medical Research; Department of Clinical Hematology and Bone Marrow Transplantation, The Royal Melbourne Hospital, Parkville, Australia

EMMANUEL BACHY, MD, PhD
Assistant Professor, Université Claude Bernard Lyon1, Université de Lyon; Centre de Recherche en Cancérologie de Lyon, Lyon, France; Department of Hematology, Hospices Civils de Lyon, Hôpital Lyon Sud, Pierre-Bénite, France

PIERS BLOMBERY, MBBS, FRACP, FRCPA
Department of Haematology, Peter MacCallum Cancer Centre, Parkville, Australia

ALESSANDRO BROCCOLI, MD
Institute of Hematology L. e A. Seràgnoli, University of Bologna, Bologna, Italy

JULIA CARNEVALE, MD
Division of Hematology/Oncology, University of California, San Francisco, San Francisco, California

ALESSIA CASTELLINO, MD
Hematology, Città della Salute e della Scienza Hospital and University, Torino, Italy

ANNALISA CHIAPPELLA, MD
Hematology, Città della Salute e della Scienza Hospital and University, Torino, Italy

MICHAEL CRUMP, MD, FRCPC
Professor of Medicine, University of Toronto; Division of Medical Oncology and Hematology, Princess Margaret Cancer Centre, Toronto, Ontario, Canada

KIERON DUNLEAVY, MD
Clinical Director, Lymphoid Malignancies Branch, Center for Cancer Research, National Cancer Institute, Bethesda, Maryland

ANDREW M. EVENS, DO, MSc, FACP
Professor of Medicine and Chief, Division of Hematology/Oncology, Tufts Medical Center, Boston, Massachusetts

EVA GINÉ, MD
Hospital Clínic of Barcelona and Institut d'Investigacions Biomèdiques August Pi i Sunyer (IDIBAPS), Barcelona, Spain

ANDRE GOY, MD
John Theurer Cancer Center, Hackensack University Medical Center, Hackensack, New Jersey

ATHENA KRITHARIS, MD
Division of Hematology/Oncology, Tufts Medical Center, Boston, Massachusetts

RICHARD F. LITTLE, MD
Head of Hematologic, HIV and Stem Cell Therapeutics, Cancer Therapeutic Evaluation Program (CTEP), National Cancer Institute, Bethesda, Maryland

CRAIG H. MOSKOWITZ, MD
Steven A. Greenberg Chair in Lymphoma Research; Clinical Director, Division of Hematologic Oncology; Attending Physician; Lymphoma and Adult BMT Services Member, Memorial Sloan Kettering Cancer Center; Professor of Medicine, Weill Medical College of Cornell University, New York, New York

MAIKE NICKELSEN, MD
Department of Hematology, Oncology and Stem Cell Transplantation, Asklepios Hospital St. Georg, Hamburg, Germany

MONIKA PILICHOWSKA, MD
Department of Pathology and Laboratory Medicine, Tufts Medical Center, Boston, Massachusetts

JAMES L. RUBENSTEIN, MD, PhD
Division of Hematology/Oncology, Helen Diller Family Comprehensive Cancer Center, University of California, San Francisco, San Francisco, California

GILLES SALLES, MD, PhD
Professor, Université Claude Bernard Lyon1, Université de Lyon; Centre de Recherche en Cancérologie de Lyon, Lyon, France; Department of Hematology, Hospices Civils de Lyon, Hôpital Lyon Sud, Pierre-Bénite, France

KERRY J. SAVAGE, MD, MSc
Department of Medical Oncology, British Columbia Cancer Agency, Vancouver, British Columbia, Canada

NORBERT SCHMITZ, MD, PhD
Department of Hematology, Oncology and Stem Cell Transplantation, Asklepios Hospital St. Georg, Hamburg, Germany

LAURIE H. SEHN, MD, MPH
Chair, Lymphoma Tumour Group, British Columbia Cancer Agency and the Centre for Lymphoid Cancer, Clinical Professor, University of British Columbia, Vancouver, British Columbia, Canada

JOHN F. SEYMOUR, MBBS, FRACP, PhD
Professor, Department of Haematology, Peter MacCallum Cancer Centre, Parkville, Australia; Faculty of Medicine, Dentistry and Health Sciences, The University of Melbourne, Parkville, Australia

GUNJAN L. SHAH, MD, MS
Assistant Member, Adult BMT Service, Memorial Sloan Kettering Cancer Center; Instructor of Medicine, Weill Medical College of Cornell University, New York, New York

PIERRE SUJOBERT, MD, PhD
Laboratory of Hematology, Hospices Civils de Lyon, Hôpital Lyon Sud, Pierre-Bénite, France; Université Claude Bernard Lyon1, Université de Lyon; Centre de Recherche en Cancérologie de Lyon, Lyon, France

UMBERTO VITOLO, MD
Hematology, Città della Salute e della Scienza Hospital and University, Torino, Italy

WYNDHAM H. WILSON, MD, PhD
Deputy Branch Chief, Lymphoid Malignancies Branch, Center for Cancer Research, National Cancer Institute, Bethesda, Maryland

ANAS YOUNES, MD
Lymphoma Service, Memorial Sloan Kettering Cancer Center, New York, New York

PIER LUIGI ZINZANI, MD, PhD
Professor, Institute of Hematology L. e A. Seràgnoli, University of Bologna, Bologna, Italy

Contents

methotrexate-based induction programs may contribute to improved outcomes. An accumulation of insights into the molecular and cellular basis of disease pathogenesis is providing a foundation for the generation of molecular tools to facilitate diagnosis as well as a roadmap for integration of targeted therapy within the developing therapeutic armamentarium for this challenging brain tumor.

HEMATOLOGY/ONCOLOGY
CLINICS OF NORTH AMERICA

Preface

The Increasing Complexity of Aggressive B-cell Lymphoma

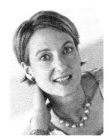

Laurie H. Sehn, MD, MPH
Editor

Aggressive B-cell lymphoma is a descriptive term that has been applied to histologic subtypes of B-cell lymphoma that exhibit a rapid growth rate with disease evolving over weeks to months of time, typically requiring immediate intervention. Historically, these entities were often grouped within the context of clinical trials leading to a collective management strategy. Gradual refinement of lymphoma classification has distinguished an increasing number of unique clinicopathologic entities, which now must be recognized when considering treatment. This issue of *Hematology/Oncology Clinics of North America* provides an update on the biology and state-of-the-art management of the most common subtypes of aggressive B-cell lymphoma.

Improved biological insight has unveiled the complexity of aggressive B-cell lymphoma. In particular, diffuse large B-cell lymphoma (DLBCL) has been dissected into a variety of subtypes, such as primary central nervous system lymphoma, which require unique approaches. In addition, histologic subtypes previously considered clinical variants of DLBCL have been recognized as unique entities, such as primary mediastinal B-cell lymphoma, which exhibits a characteristic gene expression signature. DLBCL, NOS remains the most commonly encountered histologic subtype of aggressive B-cell lymphoma, but is itself largely heterogeneous. In addition to the molecular subtypes (activated B cell and germinal center B cell) identified by gene expression profiling, a large number of genetic aberrations have been identified and found to be variably present. The presence of dual translocation of *MYC* and *BCL2* (or *BCL6*), commonly referred to as double-hit lymphoma, portends a poor prognosis and has been declared a separate entity within the most recent version of the WHO classification. Gray zone lymphomas exhibit pathologic characteristics that overlap different lymphoma subtypes (such as DLBCL and Hodgkin lymphoma) and represent a poorly understood category. Similarly, transformed lymphoma frequently resembles DLBCL morphologically, but is biologically diverse reflecting its varied pathogenesis. Finally,

Hematol Oncol Clin N Am 30 (2016) xiii–xiv
http://dx.doi.org/10.1016/j.hoc.2016.10.001
0889-8588/16/© 2016 Published by Elsevier Inc.

both Burkitt lymphoma and mantle cell lymphoma represent subtypes with pathogno-monic genetic features, yet are molecularly and clinically heterogeneous.

While many patients with aggressive B-cell lymphoma (with the exception of mantle cell lymphoma) can be cured with immunochemotherapy, those who fall frontline management continue to have a dismal outcome. Recognizing the molecular diversity between subtypes and individual patients, at both diagnosis and relapse, will be essential to allow for a more rational and tailored therapeutic strategy. Importantly, a greater understanding of the underlying oncogenic mechanisms that drive these lymphomas has led to the discovery of potential therapeutic targets and to the development of novel agents that may exploit these processes. Future progress will rely on well-designed clinical trials employing validated biological predictive markers that enable patient enrichment such that promising agents can be evaluated in patients who are most likely to benefit.

Laurie H. Sehn, MD, MPH
Lymphoma Tumour Group
British Columbia Cancer Agency and
the Centre for Lymphoid Cancer
University of British Columbia
600 West 10th Avenue
Vancouver, BC V5Z 4E6, Canada

E-mail address:
lsehn@bccancer.bc.ca

State-of-the-art Therapy for Advanced-stage Diffuse Large B-cell Lymphoma

 CrossMark

Annalisa Chiappella, MD, Alessia Castellino, MD, Umberto Vitolo, MD*

KEYWORDS

- Diffuse large B-cell lymphoma • Advanced stage • Rituximab-CHOP
- High-dose therapy • Novel biologic drugs

KEY POINTS

- Identification of prognostic diffuse large B-cell lymphoma (DLBCL) subgroups, standard treatment with rituximab plus cyclophosphamide, vincristine, doxorubicin, and prednisone (R-CHOP), role of high-dose chemotherapy followed by autologous stem cell transplant, addition of novel biologic drugs to R-CHOP therapy.
- R-CHOP 21 is still the standard treatment in both low-risk and high-risk advanced-stage DLBCL.
- Approximately 30% to 40% of patients fail R-CHOP, mainly not achieving complete response (CR) or with early relapse.
- An essential step to improve the outcomes of these patients is to increase the CR rate.
- A better recognition of unfavorable DLBCL subtypes is necessary, in order to personalize the treatment with targeted and tailored approaches.

INTRODUCTION

Diffuse large B-cell lymphoma (DLBCL) is the most common lymphoid malignancy in adults, representing almost 35% to 40% of lymphomas in Western countries. The estimated incidence is 7 to 8 cases per 100,000 per year and has doubled in recent decades.[1,2] The peak incidence of DLBCL is in the sixth decade.

DLBCL shows a diffuse pattern of proliferation, with high proliferation rate of atypical large cells with vesicular nuclei. There are different histologic subtypes of DLBCL with peculiar features, including immunoblastic lymphoma,[3] T-cell/histiocyte rich, primary cutaneous DLBCL leg-type, and Epstein-Barr virus–positive DLBCL of the elderly.

Disclosure: Lecture fee/educational activities for Amgen, Celgene, Janssen, Pfizer, Roche, Teva (A. Chiappella); nothing to declare (A. Castellino); advisory board for Roche and Janssen, lecture fee/educational activities for Roche, Celgene, Janssen, Gilead (U. Vitolo).
Hematology, Città della Salute e della Scienza Hospital and University, corso Bramante 88, Torino 10126, Italy
* Corresponding author.
E-mail address: uvitolo@cittadellasalute.to.it

Hematol Oncol Clin N Am 30 (2016) 1147–1162
http://dx.doi.org/10.1016/j.hoc.2016.07.002
0889-8588/16/© 2016 Elsevier Inc. All rights reserved.

hemonc.theclinics.com

PATIENT EVALUATION OVERVIEW

Surgical excision or incision tumor biopsy is required for histology definition and DLBCL diagnosis; in some cases (deep mass, mediastinal mass, unacceptable surgical risk), a core needle biopsy is advisable.

Standard staging includes physical examination, evaluation of performance status (PS), and assessment of B symptoms (fever>38°C, night sweats, body weight loss >10% during the 6 months before the diagnosis). Laboratory examinations should include complete blood cell counts; assessment of renal and hepatic function; lactate dehydrogenase (LDH); and screening tests for human immunodeficiency virus, hepatitis B (HB) virus (HBs antigen, anti-HBs and anti-HBc antibodies), and hepatitis C virus.

A complete radiological assessment with a computed tomography (CT) scan and an [18]flourodeoxyglucose (FDG) positron emission tomography (PET) scan, in addition to a bone marrow aspirate and biopsy evaluation, are required for the staging of the disease, based on the Ann Arbor Classification.[4]

Based on the Lugano Classification,[5] PET-CT is now considered the standard imaging examination, both for staging and for response evaluation,[6] because it is more sensitive to detect nodal and extranodal sites compared with CT scan. However, CT scan is often performed and it is useful to show vessel compression or thrombosis, to differentiate abdominal lymphadenopathy from bowel involvement, to delineate radiation sites, and to measure nodal sites. On this basis, both CT scan and PET are recommended at diagnosis, whereas for evaluation of response only PET could be sufficient. In contrast, in the follow-up setting, PET should not be used, because of a high incidence of false-positive results. Furthermore, recent publications suggest that focal bone marrow FDG uptake, even in the absence of diffuse uptake, is highly specific and more sensitive than bone marrow biopsy for detection of DLBCL involvement, with less than 10% of cases of positive biopsy and false-negative PET imaging.[7,8] On this basis, bone marrow biopsy has been claimed to no longer be necessary for patients with PET scan positive for bone or marrow involvement. However low-volume (<20%) involvement or the presence in marrow of discordant lymphoma, such as low-grade lymphomas, may be missed by PET scan and this could suggest that bone marrow biopsy should be performed in all cases regardless of PET findings.

In patients with high risk of central nervous system (CNS) recurrence, including patients with high-intermediate and high-risk International Prognostic Index (IPI), especially with more than 1 extranodal site or increased LDH level; or with testicular, renal, or adrenal involvements; or cases with MYC gene rearrangements, a cerebral spinal fluid (CSF) examination with flow cytometry and cytology is recommended.[9,10] Brain nuclear MRI is recommended in patients with clinical signs of CNS involvement.

A cardiac function evaluation may be useful in all patients with a new diagnosis of DLBCL in case they are candidates for an anthracycline-containing regimen; in particular, a cardiac evaluation is mandatory in elderly patients or patients with known cardiac risk factors.

The Comprehensive Geriatric Assessment (CGA), based on age, comorbidities, and functional abilities of daily living, is an important tool in the elderly, in order to personalize the treatment and discriminate between fit, unfit, and frail patients.[11]

The risk of infertility secondary to chemotherapy and the fertility preservation options should be discussed with women of childbearing potential and men who are sexually active.

Moreover, DLBCLs localized in particular extranodal sites require specific further examinations for a complete staging. In primary CNS lymphoma,[12] besides diagnostic brain MRI, cytologic evaluation and flow cytometry of the CSF are mandatory and slit-lamp examination should be performed to investigate possible ocular involvement; in DLBCL with gastrointestinal or Waldeyer ring involvement,[13] an endoscopic evaluation should be performed in staging and at the moment of response assessment. In primary testicular lymphoma (PTL), orchiectomy is mandatory for the diagnosis, and ultrasonography of the contralateral testis, a brain MRI, and a cytologic and flow cytometric analysis of CSF are mandatory for a complete staging.[13,14] In primary breast lymphoma, contralateral breast examination should be performed, whereas the role of a complete CNS work-up remains unclear with the exception of patients with bilateral breast involvement, who are at high risk of CNS progression.

PROGNOSTIC INDEX

Prognostic indices are important tools for clinicians to predict the outcome of patients affected by DLBCL.

The standard prognostic score for DLBCL is the IPI published in 1993; based on age, stage, LDH level, PS, and number of extranodal sites, patients are stratified into 4 classes of risk at different prognosis: low, low-intermediate, intermediate-high, and high risk. In patients younger than 61 years, the abbreviate age-adjusted IPI (aa-IPI) should be applied.[15] In the elderly, a prognostic index with an age cutoff point of 70 years has been proposed; the elderly IPI.[16]

With the introduction of rituximab in the clinical practice, a revised version has been developed (rituximab-IPI [R-IPI]).[17] Moreover, the IPI has been reevaluated in a series of 1062 patients with DLBCL treated in clinical trials with the combination of immunotherapy with the anti-CD20 monoclonal antibody rituximab with a chemotherapy regimen of cyclophosphamide, vincristine, doxorubicin and prednisone (R-CHOP), showing that the IPI is still valid in the rituximab era.[18]

Recently, using raw clinical data from the National Comprehensive Cancer Network (NCCN) database collected during the rituximab era, a novel prognostic score, NCCN-IPI, was developed, with the goal of improving risk stratification. Compared with the IPI, the NCCN-IPI introduces as negative parameters 2 levels of increased LDH and the involvement of at least 1 of bone marrow, CNS, liver/gastrointestinal, or lung instead of the number of extranodal sites, and it is able to better discriminate the high-risk subgroup.[19] The new NCCN-IPI was also subsequently validated in a cohort of 1660 patients with DLBCL treated with R-CHOP between 2001 and 2013 at the British Columbia Cancer Agency (**Table 1**).

This article discusses the state of the art for the treatment of advanced-stage DLBCL.

PHARMACOLOGIC TREATMENT OPTIONS

The best frontline treatment of patients affected by DLBCL should be tailored by age, PS, stage, and prognostic score risk.

R-CHOP administered every 21 days represents the standard treatment of patients with DLBCL.[20,21]

YOUNG PATIENTS WITH LOW-RISK INTERNATIONAL PROGNOSTIC INDEX DISEASE

The role of R-CHOP chemoimmunotherapy in young patients with low-risk IPI was investigated in an important trial conducted by the Mabthera International Trial (MInT) Group.[22] In the multicentric phase III MInT, 824 patients with DLBCL, aged 18 to 60 years, with no risk factors or only 1 risk factor (aaIPI, stage II–IV

Table 1
Comparison between IPI, revised IPI, and NCCN-IPI score

Risk Group	IPI Factors (N)	Patients (%)	5-y PFS (%)	5-y OS (%)
Standard IPI[15]				
Low	0, 1	28	85	90
Low-intermediate	2	27	66	77
Intermediate-high	3	21	52	62
High	4, 5	24	39	54
Revised IPI[17]				
Very good	0	10	94	94
Good	1, 2	45	80	79
Poor	3, 4, 5	45	53	55
NCCN-IPI[19]				
Low	0, 1	19	91	96
Low-intermediate	2, 3	42	74	82
Intermediate-high	4, 5	31	51	64
High	≥6	8	30	33

disease, or stage I disease with bulk) were enrolled. They were randomized to receive 6 cycles of cyclophosphamide, vincristine, doxorubicin and prednisone (CHOP)–like chemotherapy alone or in association with rituximab. Additional radiotherapy was planned to bulky localization and extranodal sites. Patients assigned to the rituximab chemotherapy arm achieved a significantly better complete response (CR) rate (86% [82%–89%] vs 68% [63%–73%]) in the arm without rituximab, with 3-year event-free survival (EFS) of 79% (95% confidence interval [CI], 75%–83% versus 59% [54%–64%], respectively) and with 3-year overall survival (OS) of 93% (90%–95%) versus 84% (80%–88%), respectively. The MInT also showed that there is no difference between CHOP21 chemotherapy and more intensive CHOP-like regimens (such as CHOEP21 or MACOP-B) in association with rituximab, underlining that rituximab equalizes chemotherapy regimens with different intensity. Moreover, in this study, 2 different prognostic groups were identified within young patients with low IPI risk, with significantly different 3-year EFS: a favorable one, IPI 0, without bulky disease; and a less favorable one, with IPI 1 or bulky mass or both. The recently updated MInT data, at a 6-year follow-up, suggested a central role of radiotherapy on bulky disease in this less favorable group of young patients.[23]

The management of a similar subgroup of patients, with an age-adjusted IPI equal to 1, was investigated in a phase III randomized study by the Gruope d'Etude des Lymphomes de l'Adulte (GELA), which compared the standard R-CHOP21 regimen with an experimental arm with a dose-dense rituximab plus doxorubicin, cyclophosphamide, vindesine, bleomycin, prednisone (R-ACVBP) scheme. This trial was conducted in 379 patients, aged 18 to 59 years, affected by previously untreated DLBCL, with an age-adjusted IPI equal to 1. At a median follow-up of 3 years, the dose-dense R-ACVBP arm seemed to achieve a significant better 3-year EFS and 3-year OS compared with R-CHOP21 (3-year OS, 92% vs 84%; $P = .007$), even if it was associated with an increased incidence of mucositis and hematological toxicities.[24] Note that the R-CHOP21 regimen was given without any radiation therapy. **Table 2** summarizes the principal results of studies.

Table 2
Characteristics and outcome of an IPI 1 patient in the MInT trial treated with R-CHOP compared with the GELA LNH03-2B trial

	MInT[22]	LNH03-2B[24]	
	6 R-CHOP21 IPI 1 N 118	R-ACVBP N 196	8 R-CHOP21 N 183
Age (y)	50 (19–60)	47 (18–59)	48 (19–59)
Stage III–IV	58 (49%)	115 (59%)	93 (51%)
Increased LDH level	58 (49%)	77 (39%)	89 (49%)
Bulky (>10 cm)	47 (40%)	38 (19%)	45 (25%)
3-y PFS (%)	86 (78–91)	87 (81–91)	73 (66–79)
3-y OS (%)	92 (85–96)	92 (87–95)	84 (77–89)
Radiotherapy	58 (49%)	—	—

Data are median (range) or n (%); data for survival are estimate (95% CI).

In patients with more favorable features, a reduction of a full course of chemoimmunotherapy treatment could be taken into account and a randomized phase III trial of The German High-Grade Non-Hodgkin Lymphoma Study Group (DSHNHL) is ongoing (the FLYER trial) randomizing 4 R-CHOP versus 6 R-CHOP.[25]

STANDARD TREATMENT OF ADVANCED STAGE

Based on the result of the GELA trial, R-CHOP21 represents the standard treatment of patients with DLBCL[20]; the results showed a CR rate of 76%, an 2-year EFS of 66%, and a 2-year OS of 70%.[20] A long-term analysis performed at a follow-up at 10 years showed a 10-year progression-free survival (PFS) of 37% and 10-year OS of 44%, but these data are affected by deaths from other causes.[21] These data were validated and confirmed in a large retrospective population-based analysis of the British Columbia University that showed a dramatic improvement in the outcomes of patients with the introduction of rituximab to chemotherapy CHOP in the clinical practice setting.[26]

Another trial was conducted by DSHNHL in elderly patients (>60 years old), to investigate the role of dose-dense regimens. In this RICOVER60 trial[27]; 1222 patients were randomized to receive 6 or 8 cycles of R-CHOP14 administered every 2 weeks with or without rituximab plus radiotherapy on bulky mass. The addition of rituximab to the CHOP chemotherapy regimen significantly improved EFS and OS compared with CHOP alone (3-year EFS after 6 courses of R-CHOP + 2 R was 66.5% (95% CI, 60.9%–702.0%) versus 47.2% (41.2%–53.3%) after 6 cycles of CHOP alone and 63.1% (57.4%–68.8%) after 8 courses of R-CHOP versus 53% (47%–59.1%) of 8 cycles of CHOP alone), but no differences were observed with the addition of 2 further courses of chemotherapy.

In the past few years there was a long debate, indirectly comparing the results of R-CHOP21 with the more dose-dense R-CHOP14 regimen. This debate prompted the design of 2 large randomized phase III trials comparing R-CHOP21 with R-CHOP14 in patients with untreated DLBCL. One trial conducted by the GELA group was restricted to elderly patients,[28] and the second was run by the British National Lymphoma Investigation in patients of all ages and IPI risks.[29] The results of both studies, conducted in more than 1000 cases, failed to show a significant benefit for the dose-dense therapy arm (**Table 3**).

Table 3
Survival results of 2 phase III randomized trial comparing R-CHOP14 with R-CHOP21

	Cunningham et al,[29] 2011 N 1080Cunningham			Delarue et al,[28] 2009 N 602	
	R-CHOP14	R-CHOP21		R-CHOP14	R-CHOP21
2-y PFS (%)	75	75	3-y EFS (%)	56	60
2-y OS (%)	83	81	3-y OS (%)	69	72

YOUNG PATIENTS WITH HIGH-RISK INTERNATIONAL PROGNOSTIC INDEX

Young patients with intermediate-high/high-risk IPI treated with standard chemoimmunotherapy experience a worse prognosis, and at least 40% still relapse. In order to improve the poor prognosis of these patients, the use of dose-dense regimens of chemotherapy has been investigated in several phase II[30] and III trials, but the benefit remains unclear.

Designed to ameliorate the prognosis of young poor-risk patients with DLBCL, a consolidation with high-dose chemotherapy (HDC) followed by autologous stem cell transplant (ASCT) was investigated.

In the prerituximab era, the results of several studies with HDC-ASCT remained controversial[31–34]; a meta-analysis on several phase III trials conducted by Greb and colleagues[35] failed to show the superiority of high-dose chemotherapy compared with the standard chemotherapy regimen. On this basis, HDC-ASCT was not recommended as standard frontline therapy in high-risk DLBCL.

With the advent of rituximab in clinical practice, some phase II[36–39] trials were conducted in order to investigate the role of intensification with HDC-ASCT in young patients with poor-prognosis DLCL, with promising results.

Tarella and colleagues[37] published the results of a phase II study on 112 young patients diagnosed with high-risk DLBCL, with a median age of 48 years (range, 18–65 years), treated with a rituximab-based chemotherapy followed by HDC-ASCT, showing a 4-year PFS of 73% and 4-year OS of 76%.

Vitolo and colleagues[38] conducted a phase II study on 97 patients with analogous unfavorable clinical features; the patients underwent a dose-intensified regimen of chemotherapy with R-Mega-CEOP scheme, followed by HDC-ASCT, obtaining analogous promising results (4-year PFS 73% [95% CI, 63–82] and 4-year OS 76% [95% CI, 68%–85%]).

On these bases, the major cooperative international lymphoma study groups designed phase III randomized trials in order to clarify the role of an intensification with HDC-ASCT compared with standard chemoimmunotherapy in poor-prognosis, patients with untreated DLBCL eligible for transplant.

Le Gouill and colleagues[40] randomized 340 patients with newly diagnosed DLBCL in a prospective multicenter study, comparing R-CHOP14 treatment versus HDC-ASCT; preliminary results showed no differences either in terms of 3-year EFS or 3-year OS.

The Italian phase III trial DLCL04, conducted by the Fondazione Italiana Linfomi (FIL),[41] was designed with a 2 × 2 factorial approach to evaluate the benefit of a full course of rituximab dose–dense chemotherapy at 2 different levels of intensification (R-CHOP14 or R-Mega-CHOP14) compared with a brief program of the same dose-dense chemoimmunotherapy followed by HDC-ASCT (R-HDC-ASCT) in young patients with DLBCL at aa-IPI 2 to 3 at diagnosis. The results of the DLCL04 trial showed a significant improvement in PFS in favor of the intensification with R-HDC plus autologous stem cell transplant, but no differences in terms of OS were observed: CRs were 76% in the R-HDC-ASCT arm versus 72% in the rituximab dose–dense arm, 3-year PFS was 70% (95% CI, 63%–76%) versus 59% (95% CI, 51%–66%) respectively, and 3-year OS was 79% in both arms.

In another randomized phase III trial conducted by the German group,[42] high-risk young patients with DLBCL were randomly assigned at diagnosis to receive R-CHOP14 plus etoposide (R-CHOEP14) and R-MegaCHOEP14. The study showed that the R-MegaCHOEP14 regimen was associated with a significant increase in toxicity, without an improvement of the outcome, compared with conventional R-CHOEP14: 3-year PFS was 61% in R-MegaCHOEP14 versus 70% in R-CHOEP14, and 3-year OS was 77% versus 85%, respectively.

The phase III trial SWOG (Southwest Oncology Group) S9704 conducted by the US/Canadian Intergroup,[43] investigated the benefit of HDC-ASCT in first-line therapy for DLBCL; patients were not randomized up-front but only responding patients after a course of chemoimmunotherapy were randomized. Three-hundred and ninety-seven patients up to age 65 years, with intermediate-high/high-risk IPI DLBCL, stage II to IV, and bulky disease were enrolled to received 5 cycles of chemotherapy CHOP with or without rituximab (with rituximab only in 47% of patients); patients who achieved a complete or partial response (n = 253) were randomized to receive an additional 3 courses of CHOP with or without rituximab (standard arm) or 1 additional course of chemotherapy followed by HDC-ASCT (experimental arm). A significant improvement in PFS was observed in the experimental arm, but this difference did not translate into a benefit for OS. However, an exploratory analysis, conducted only in high-risk IPI patients, suggested an advantage in term of PFS and OS for the intensified arm, with 2-year PFS of 69% in the experimental arm versus 56% in the standard arm (P = .005) and 2-year OS of 74% versus 71% respectively (P = .15). Some flaws of this study that may impair the overall results included that only 47% of patients receiving rituximab and many cases with histotypes other than DLBCL, such as T-cell lymphoma, were included in the analysis.

In addition, another Italian phase III randomized study, conducted by Cortelazzo and colleagues,[44] was performed, showing comparable results (**Table 4**).

In conclusion, from the results of these phase III randomized trials, consolidation of HDC-ASCT should not be routinely used in frontline treatment in young high-risk patients with DLBCL.

Therefore, chemoimmunotherapy with R-CHOP remains, at the present time, the standard of care for young patients diagnosed with DLBCL; consolidation with intensified regimens should be an option only in very-high-risk patients or in patients not achieving complete remission after the induction chemoimmunotherapy. The identification of poor prognosis patients on the basis of clinical or biological factors remains an important tool; for example, the evaluation of MYC and BCL2 anomalies allow to identify the double-hit lymphomas that should require an alternative approaches[45–48]; the role of MYC and the treatment of double-hit lymphoma is covered in Dr. Jeremy S. Abramson's article on "The Spectrum of Double Hit Lymphomas" in this issue.

ELDERLY PATIENTS

The current standard of treatment of elderly patients with DLBCL at diagnosis, FIT according to CGA evaluation,[11] is R-CHOP, performed with the standard 3-weekly schedule.

The German group, in the NHL-B2 trial,[49] observed that the deepest and longest neutropenia and the highest rate of therapy-related death were recorded after the first course of R-CHOP14 or R-CHOP21. With the aim of reducing the toxicities in elderly patients, a

Table 4
Principal results of the phase III trial evaluating standard chemoimmunotherapy compared with HDC and ASCT

	CR HDC (%)	CR Chemotherapy Standard (%)	PFS HDC (%)	PFS Chemotherapy Standard (%)	OS HDC (%)	OS Chemotherapy Standard (%)
Vitolo et al,[41] 2012 FIL DLCL04	76	72.5	71	58	81	78
Cortelazzo et al,[44] 2012 GITIL RHDS	76.3	76.4	73.5	68	81	80
Stiff et al,[43] 2013 SWOG/US	75	71	72	62	74	71
Schmitz et al,[42] 2012 DSHNHL	78.7	71.4	69.5	61.4	85	77
Le Gouill et al,[40] 2011 GOELAMS	67	54	72	72	83	83

Abbreviations: GITIL, Gruppo Italiano Terapie Innovative nei Linfomi; GOELAMS, Groupe Ouest-Est d'études des Leucémies Aigües et autres Maladies du Sang; RHDS, Rituximab-High dose sequential therapy.

prephase with a single dose of 1 mg of vincristine and 7 days of oral prednisone before starting R-CHOP treatment was adopted, with a reduction of deaths after the first course of chemoimmunotherapy from 5% to less than 2%. Clinical practice suggests that a pre-phase with steroids with or without vincristine could reduce the risk of complications such as the tumor lysis syndrome in elderly patients with low PS and high tumor burden; however, this strategy has not been validated in a prospective or randomized trial.

For very elderly patients with DLBCL (aged >80 years), or cases with several comorbidities and in patients who have been considered unfit or frail at CGA evaluation, milder chemotherapy approaches should be considered; some retrospective analyses[50–52] showed satisfactory results in terms of outcomes with acceptable toxicities in these patients.

Peyrade and colleagues[53] conducted a single-arm phase II trial in 150 patients more than 79 years old, with DLBCL at diagnosis, treated with 6 courses, repeated every 21 days, of R-mini-CHOP (400 mg/m^2 of cyclophosphamide, 25 mg/m^2 doxorubicin, 1 mg vincristine, and 40 mg/m^2 prednisolone for 5 days, in combination with 375 mg/m^2 rituximab). At a median follow-up of 20 months, the 2-year PFS was 47% and the 2y-2-year OS was 59%. The most frequent toxicity was hematological, with greater than grade 2 neutropenia in 59 patients and febrile neutropenia in 11 cases.

Considering these promising results, R-mini-CHOP could be considered the standard of care in very elderly patients with DLBCL, representing a good compromise between efficacy and safety.

To reduce the cardiotoxicity related to doxorubicin, doxorubicin was replaced with a nonpegylated liposomal doxorubicin (Myocet) in an R-CHOP regimen (R-COMP) in several studies.[54–57]

Luminari and colleagues[55] conducted a phase II study in 75 elderly patients (median age, 72 years; range, 61–83 years), with newly diagnosed DLBCL and left ventricular ejection fraction (LVEF) greater than 50%; planned treatment was 8 courses of R-COMP. A retrospective comparison between this population and the one published by Coiffier and colleagues[20] in the randomized GELA study was performed; the investigators concluded that R-COMP is an effective regimen for elderly patients with DLBCL (overall response rate [ORR], 71%, with 57% CR, 3-year PFS 69%, and 3-year OS 72%), with an acceptable safety profile; R-COMP seems to reduce cardiotoxicity compared with standard doxorubicin (21% of cardiac event, with 4% of patients grade 3–4). An analogous study was conducted by Corazzelli and colleagues,[56] applying a dose-dense R-COMP14 regimen to elderly poor-risk patients with DLBCL. Both the trials were conducted in patients without active cardiopathy.

Fridrik and colleagues[58] conducted a phase III trial, randomizing 88 patients with DLBCL to receive R-CHOP or R-COMP regimen therapy. Patients were stratified for N-terminal pro–brain natriuretic peptide (NT-pro-BNP) serum level and for IPI score. Only 1 patient presented left-ventricular ejection fraction (LVEF) less than 50% at diagnosis, and he received R-CHOP therapy at randomization. The investigators concluded that, in patients with normal cardiac function at diagnosis, nonpegylated liposomal doxorubicin did not reduce cardiotoxicity, although cardiac safety signals were increased in R-CHOP compared with R-COMP: during treatment the LVEF measurements were less than 50% in 4.6% of patients in the R-COMP arm, compared with 15.8% in the R-CHOP arm ($P<.001$) and NT-proBNP levels were less than 400 pg/mL during and at the end of treatment in 90% patients in the R-COMP arm, but only in 66.7% in the R-CHOP arm ($P = .013$). The efficacy was similar in both R-COMP and R-CHOP arms, but this trial was not powered to detect differences in outcome between the two arms.

Another alternative regimen, investigated in older patients or patients ineligible for anthracyclines, was R-CEOP, substituting etoposide (50 mg/m^2 intravenously on day 1 and 100 mg/m^2 by mouth on days 2 and 3 in the standard regimen) for doxorubicin. Moccia and colleagues[59] reported the efficacy of the R-CEOP regimen compared with a historical cohort treated with R-CHOP, with similar 5-year time to progression (57% vs 62% respectively), but lower 5-year OS rate in patients who received R-CEOP (49% vs 64%; $P = .02$). Recent reports suggested a major activity of the etoposide-based scheme in patients with DLBCL of germinal center origin.[60]

DIFFUSE LARGE B-CELL LYMPHOMAS WITH EXTRANODAL INVOLVEMENT

DLBCL that arise primarily at some extranodal sites require specific treatment strategies; for primary mediastinal lymphoma and primary CNS lymphoma, see Drs. Zinzani and Broccoli's article on "Optimizing outcomes in primary mediastinal B-cell lymphoma" and Drs. Carnevale and Rubenstein's article on "The Challenge of Primary CNS Lymphoma", in this issue.

PTLs have poor prognosis with a high risk of CNS recurrence and contralateral testis relapse.[61] The International Extranodal Lymphoma Study Group (IELSG) and the FIL designed an international trial, IELSG10, to address the activity of conventional R-CHOP21 associated with CNS intrathecal prophylaxis and contralateral testis radiotherapy. After diagnostic orchiectomy, patients enrolled in IELSG10 study were planned to receive 6 or 8 courses of R-CHOP21 followed by prophylactic irradiation (involved-field radiotherapy) to the contralateral testis at 25 to 30 Gy. During chemotherapy, 4 lumbar punctures with 12 mg of intrathecal methotrexate were administered as CNS prophylaxis. The results of the IELSG10 trial showed an improvement in outcomes, with reduced relapse rate: 5-year PFS and 5-year OS were 74% (95% CI, 59%–84%) and 85% (95% CI, 71%–92%), respectively; 5-year cumulative incidence of CNS relapse was 6% (95% CI, 0%–12%), no contralateral testis recurrences were observed.[62] Hence, prophylactic radiotherapy (>25–30 Gy) to the contralateral testis is warranted to abrogate contralateral testicular relapse. Despite CNS prophylaxis, the risk of CNS relapse was still present and the best strategy is not yet clearly defined; based on these results, FIL and IELSG designed the ongoing international trial, IELSG30,[63] with intensified CNS prophylaxis, which includes both intrathecal chemotherapy with liposomal cytarabine, and systemic prophylaxis with an intermediate dose of intravenous methotrexate (1.5 g/m^2). In conclusion, the best known treatment of PTLs, localized or advanced, consisted of a complete standard chemoimmunotherapy approach (R-CHOP21) in association with CNS prophylaxis and radiotherapy to the contralateral testis.

In primary breast lymphomas, extranodal relapses were common; the most frequent sites of recurrence described are ipsilateral or contralateral breast, but bone marrow, lung or pleura, skin, gastrointestinal tract, and CNS relapses were also reported. Based on the experience of the IELSG15 trial, the standard approach is a standard chemoimmunotherapy R-CHOP21 for 6 courses followed by consolidation with ipsilateral breast radiotherapy at 30 to 36 Gy; CNS prophylaxis should be considered and it is recommended in high-risk patients and in women with bilateral involvement.[64]

Primary bone lymphomas at diagnosis present unique or multiple bone localization, sometimes associated with soft tissue involvement. The frontline treatment is the standard R-CHOP with or without consolidation radiotherapy. The risk of CNS relapse is low and, in the absence of additional risk factors, CNS prophylaxis is not usually a standard practice.[65]

FUTURE PROSPECTS

Standard chemoimmunotherapy represents the gold standard treatment in DLBCL, but a relevant percentage of patients still relapse or have chemorefractory disease. A better recognition of the biological bases of lymphomagenesis represents the basis for a personalized and tailored treatment. Novel drugs (such as immunomodulatory drugs, inhibitor of Bruton kinase, inhibitor of proteasome) were investigated as single agents in the relapse setting or in combination with standard chemoimmunotherapy R-CHOP as first-line treatments.[66–79]

A specific article devoted to novel therapies appears elsewhere in this issue.

SUMMARY

R-CHOP21 is still the standard treatment in both low-risk and high-risk advanced-stage DLBCL. However, approximately 30% to 40% of patients failed R-CHOP, with most not achieving CR or with early relapse. An essential step to move forward and improve the outcomes of these patients is to increase the CR rate. A better recognition of unfavorable DLBCL subtypes is necessary in order to personalized the treatment with targeted and tailored approaches.

REFERENCES

1. Sant M, Allemani C, Tereanu C, et al. Incidence of hematologic malignancies in Europe by morphologic subtype: results of the HAEMACARE project. Blood 2010;116:3724–34.
2. Fisher SG, Fisher RI. The epidemiology of non-Hodgkin's lymphoma. Oncogene 2004;23(38):6524–34.

3. Ott G, Ziepert M, Klapper W, et al. Immunoblastic morphology but not the immunohistochemical GCB/non-GCB classifier predicts outcome in diffuse large B-cell lymphoma in the RICOVER-60 trial of the DSHNHL. Blood 2010;116:4916–25.

4. Carbone PP, Kaplan HS, Musshoff K, et al. Report of the committee on Hodgkin lymphoma staging classification. Cancer Res 1971;31:1860–1.

5. Cheson BD, Fisher RI, Barrington SF, et al. Recommendations for initial evaluation, staging, and response assessment of Hodgkin and non-Hodgkin lymphoma: the Lugano classification. J Clin Oncol 2014;32:3059–68.

6. Seam P, Juweid ME, Cheson BD. The role of FDG-PET scans in patients with lymphoma. Blood 2007;110(10):3507–16.

7. Pelosi E, Penna D, Douroukas A, et al. Bone marrow disease detection with FDGPET/CT and bone marrow biopsy during the staging of malignant lymphoma: results from a large multicentre study. Q J Nucl Med Mol Imaging 2011;55: 469–75.

8. Khan AB, Barrington SF, Mikhaeel NG, et al. PET-CT staging of DLBCL accurately identifies and provides new insight into the clinical significance of bone marrow involvement. Blood 2013;122:61–7.

9. Tilly H, Gomes da Silva M, Vitolo U, et al, on behalf of the ESMO Guidelines Committee. Diffuse large B-cell lymphoma (DLBCL): ESMO Clinical practice Guidelines for diagnosis, treatment and follow-up. Ann Oncol 2015;26(Suppl 5): v116–25.

10. Benevolo G, Stacchini A, Spina M, et al. Final results of a multicenter trial addressing role of CSF flow cytometric analysis in NHL patients at high risk for CNS dissemination. Blood 2012;120:3222–8.

11. Tucci A, Martelli M, Rigacci L, et al. Comprehensive geriatric assessment is an essential tool to support treatment decisions in elderly patients with diffuse large B-cell lymphoma: a prospective multicenter evaluation in 173 patients by the Lymphoma Italian Foundation (FIL). Leuk Lymphoma 2015;56:921–6.

12. Ferreri AJ, Reni M. Primary central nervous system lymphoma. Crit Rev Oncol Hematol 2007;63(3):257–68.

13. Ferreri AJ, Montalbán C. Primary diffuse large B-cell lymphoma of the stomach. Crit Rev Oncol Hematol 2007;63:65–71.

14. Vitolo U, Ferreri AJM, Zucca E, et al. Primary testicular lymphoma. Crit Rev Oncol Hematol 2008;65:183–9.

15. A predictive model for aggressive non-Hodgkin's lymphoma. The International Non Hodgkin's Lymphoma Prognostic Factors Project. N Engl J Med 1993; 329(14):987–94.

16. Advani RH, Chen H, Habermann TM, et al. Comparison of conventional prognostic indices in patients older than 60 years with diffuse large B-cell lymphoma treated with R-CHOP in the US Intergroup Study (ECOG 4494, CALGB 9793): consideration of age greater than 70 years in an elderly prognostic index (E-IPI). Br J Haematol 2010;151(2):143–51.

17. Sehn LH, Berry B, Chhanabhai M, et al. The revised International Prognostic Index (R-IPI) is a better predictor of outcome than the standard IPI for patients with diffuse large B-cell lymphoma treated with R-CHOP. Blood 2007;109(5):1857–61.

18. Ziepert M, Hasenclever D, Kuhnt E, et al. Standard International Prognostic Index remains a valid predictor of outcome for patients with aggressive CD201 B-cell lymphoma in the rituximab era. J Clin Oncol 2010;28(14):2373–80.

19. Zhou Z, Sehn LH, Rademaker AW, et al. An enhanced International Prognostic Index (NCCN-IPI) for patients with diffuse large B-cell lymphoma treated in the rituximab era. Blood 2014;123:837–42.

20. Coiffier B, Lepage E, Briere J, et al. CHOP chemotherapy plus rituximab compared with CHOP alone in elderly patients with diffuse large-B-cell lymphoma. N Engl J Med 2002;346(4):235–42.

21. Coiffier B, Thieblemont C, Van Den Neste E, et al. Long-term outcome of patients in the LNH-98.5 trial, the first randomized study comparing rituximab-CHOP to standard CHOP chemotherapy in DLBCL patients: a study by the Groupe d'Etudes des Lymphomes de l'Adulte. Blood 2010;116(12):2040–5.

22. Pfreundschuh M, Trümper L, Osterborg A, et al. CHOP-like chemotherapy plus rituximab versus CHOP-like chemotherapy alone in young patients with good-prognosis diffuse large-B-cell lymphoma: a randomised controlled trial by the MabThera International Trial (MInT) Group. Lancet Oncol 2006;7(5):379–91.

23. Pfreundschuh M, Kuhnt E, Trümper L, et al. SCHOP-like chemotherapy with or without rituximab in young patients with good-prognosis diffuse large-B-cell lymphoma: 6-year results of an open-label randomised study of the MabThera International Trial (MInT) Group. Lancet Oncol 2011;12(11):1013–22.

24. Recher C, Coiffier B, Haioun C, et al. Intensified chemotherapy with ACVBP plus rituximab versus standard CHOP plus rituximab for the treatment of diffuse large B-cell lymphoma (LNH03-2B): an open-label randomised phase 3 trial. Lancet 2011;378:1858–67.

25. Rituximab and combination chemotherapy in treating patients with non-Hodgkin's lymphoma. (FLYER trial). Clinical trial.gov identifier NCT0027821.

26. Sehn LH, Donaldson J, Chhanabhai M, et al. Introduction of combined CHOP plus rituximab therapy dramatically improved outcome of diffuse large B-cell lymphoma in British Columbia. J Clin Oncol 2005;23(22):5027–33.

27. Pfreundschuh M, Schubert J, Ziepert M, et al. German High-Grade Non-Hodgkin Lymphoma Study Group (DSHNHL). Six versus eight cycles of bi-weekly CHOP-14 with or without rituximab in elderly patients with aggressive CD201 B-cell lymphomas: a randomised controlled trial (RICOVER-60). Lancet Oncol 2008;9(2):105–16.

28. Delarue R, Tilly H, Salles G, et al. R-CHOP14 compared to R-CHOP21 in elderly patients with diffuse large B cell lymphoma: results of the interim analysis of the LNH03-6B GELA study. Blood 2009;114:169 [abstract: 406].

29. Cunningham D, Smith P, Mouncey P, et al. CHOP14 versus R-CHOP21: result of a randomized phase III trial for the treatment of patients with newly diagnosed diffuse large B-cell non-Hodgkin lymphoma. J Clin Oncol 2011;29(Suppl) [abstract: 8000].

30. Brusamolino E, Rusconi C, Montalbetti L, et al. Dose-dense R-CHOP-14 supported by pegfilgrastim in patients with diffuse large B-cell lymphoma: a phase II study of feasibility and toxicity. Haematologica 2006;91(4):496–502.

31. Vitolo U, Liberati AM, Cabras MG, et al. High dose sequential chemotherapy with autologous transplantation versus dose-dense hemotherapy MegaCEOP as first line treatment in poor-prognosis diffuse large cell lymphoma: an "Intergruppo Italiano Linfomi" randomized trial. Haematologica 2005;90(6):793–801.

32. Martelli M, Gherlinzoni F, De Renzo A, et al. Early autologous stem-cell transplantation versus conventional chemotherapy as front-line therapy in high-risk, aggressive non-Hodgkin's lymphoma: an Italian multicenter randomized trial. J Clin Oncol 2003;21(7):1255–62.

33. Milpied N, Deconinck E, Gaillard F, et al. Initial treatment of aggressive lymphoma with high-dose chemotherapy and autologous stem-cell support. N Engl J Med 2004;350(13):1287–95.

34. Greb A, Bohlius J, Schiefer D, et al. High-dose chemotherapy with autologous stem cell transplantation in the first line treatment of aggressive non-Hodgkin lymphoma (NHL) in adults. Cochrane Database Syst Rev 2008;(1):CD004024.

35. Greb A, Bohlius J, Trelle S, et al. High-dose chemotherapy with autologous stem cell support in first-line treatment of aggressive non-Hodgkin lymphoma – results of a comprehensive meta-analysis. Cancer Treat Rev 2007;33(4):338–46.

36. Glass B, Kloess M, Bentz M, et al, German High-Grade Non-Hodgkin Lymphoma Study Group. Dose-escalated CHOP plus etoposide (MegaCHOEP) followed by repeated stem cell transplantation for primary treatment of aggressive high-risk non-Hodgkin lymphoma. Blood 2006;107(8):3058–64.

37. Tarella C, Zanni M, Di Nicola M, et al, on behalf of the Gruppo Italiano Terapie Innovative nei Linfomi (GITIL). Prolonged survival in poor-risk diffuse large B-cell lymphoma following front-line treatment with rituximab-supplemented, early-intensified chemotherapy with multiple autologous hematopoietic stem cell support: a multicenter study by GITIL (Gruppo Italiano Terapie Innovative nei Linfomi). Leukemia 2007;21:1802–11.

38. Vitolo U, Chiappella A, Angelucci E, et al, on behalf of Gruppo Italiano Multiregionale Linfomi e Leucemie (GIMURELL). Dose-dense and high-dose chemotherapy plus rituximab with autologous stem cell transplantation for primary treatment of diffuse large B-cell lymphoma with a poor prognosis: a phase II multicenter study. Haematologica 2009;94(9):1250–8.

39. Fitoussi O, Belhadj K, Mounier N, et al. Survival impact of rituximab combined with ACVBP and upfront consolidation autotransplantation in high-risk diffuse large B-cell lymphoma for GELA. Haematologica 2011;96(8):1136–43.

40. Le Gouill S, Milpied NJ, Lamy T, et al. First-line rituximab (R) high-dose therapy (R-HDT) versus R-CHOP14 for young adults with diffuse large B-cell lymphoma: preliminary results of the GOELAMS 075 prospective multicenter randomized trial [abstract]. J Clin Oncol 2011;29(Suppl) [abstract: 8003].

41. Vitolo U, Chiappella A, Brusamolino E, et al. Rituximab dose-dense chemotherapy followed by intensified high-dose chemotherapy and autologous stem cell transplantation (HDC1ASCT) significantly reduces the risk of progression compared to standard rituximab dose-dense chemotherapy as first line treatment in young patients with high-risk (aa-IPI 2-3) diffuse large B-cell lymphoma (DLBCL): final results of phase III randomized trial DLCL04 of the Fondazione Italiana Linfomi (FIL) [abstract]. Blood 2012;120(21) [abstract: 688].

42. Schmitz N, Nickeloon M, Zioport M, et al, German High Grade Lymphoma Study Group (DSHNHL). Conventional chemotherapy (CHOEP-14) with rituximab or high-dose chemotherapy (MegaCHOEP) with rituximab for young, high-risk patients with aggressive B-cell lymphoma: an open-label, randomised, phase 3 trial (DSHNHL 2002-1). Lancet Oncol 2012;13(12):1250–9.

43. Stiff PJ, Unger JM, Cook JR, et al. Autologous transplantation as consolidation for aggressive non-Hodgkin's lymphoma. N Engl J Med 2013;369(18):1681–90.

44. Cortolazzo S, Tarella C, Gianni AM, et al. Chemoimmunotherapy with R-CHOP or high dose sequential therapy with autologous stem cell transplantation (R-HDS) for high risk diffuse large B-cell lymphomas patients: results of the randomized R-HDS0305 trial by Gruppo Italiano Terapie Innovative Nei Linfomi (GITIL). Blood 2012;120(21) [abstract: 764].

45. Friedberg JW. Double-hit diffuse large B-cell lymphoma. J Clin Oncol 2012; 30(28):3439–43.

46. Johnson NA, Slack GW, Savage KJ, et al. Concurrent expression of MYC and BCL2 in diffuse large B-cell lymphoma treated with rituximab plus

cyclophosphamide, doxorubicin, vincristine, and prednisone. J Clin Oncol 2012; 30(28):3452–9.

47. Petrich A, Gandhi M, Jovanovic B, et al. Impact of induction regimen and stem coll transplantation on outcomes in double-hit lymphoma: a multicenter retrospective analysis. Blood 2014;124(15):2354–61.

48. Dunleavy K, Pittaluga S, Shovlin M, et al. Concurrent expression of MYC/BCL2 protein in newly diagnosed DLBCL is not associated with an inferior survival following EPOCH-R therapy [abstract]. Blood 2013;122(21) [abstract: 3029].

49. Pfreundschuh M, Trümper L, Kloess M, et al. Two-weekly or 3-weekly CHOP chemotherapy with or with-out etoposide for the treatment of elderly patients with aggressive lymphomas: results of the NHL-B2 trial of the DSHNHL. Blood 2004;104(3):634–41.

50. Iioka F, Izumi K, Kamoda Y, et al. Outcomes of very elderly patients with aggressive B-cell non-Hodgkin lymphoma treated with reduced-dose chemotherapy. Int J Clin Oncol 2016;21:498–505.

51. Meguro A, Ozaki K, Sato K, et al. Rituximab plus 70% cyclophosphamide, doxorubicin, vincristine and prednisone for Japanese patients with diffuse large B-cell lymphoma aged 70 years and older. Leuk Lymphoma 2012;53:43–9.

52. Aoki K, Takahashi T, Tabata S, et al. Efficacy and tolerability of reduced-dose 21-day cycle rituximab and cyclophosphamide, doxorubicin, vincristine and prednisolone therapy for elderly patients with diffuse large B-cell lymphoma. Leuk Lymphoma 2013;54:2441–7.

53. Peyrade F, Jardin F, Thieblemont C, et al. Attenuated immunochemotherapy regimen (R-miniCHOP) in elderly patients older than 80 years with diffuse large B-cell lymphoma: a multicentre, single-arm, phase 2 trial. Lancet Oncol 2011; 12:460–8.

54. Ewer MS, Martin FJ, Henderson C, et al. Cardiac safety of liposomal anthracyclines. Semin Oncol 2004;31:161–81.

55. Luminari S, Montanini A, Caballero D, et al. Nonpegylated liposomal doxorubicin (Myocet) combination (R-COMP) chemotherapy in elderly patients with diffuse large B-cell lymphoma (DLBCL): results from the phase II EUR018 trial. Ann Oncol 2010;21:1492–9.

56. Corazzelli G, Frigeri F, Arcamone M, et al. Biweekly rituximab, cyclophosphamide, vincristine, non-pegylated liposome-encapsulated doxorubicin and prednisone (R-COMP-14) in elderly patients with poor-risk diffuse large B-cell lymphoma and moderate to high 'life threat' impact cardiopathy. Br J Haematol 2011;154:579–89.

57. Mian M, Wasle I, Gamerith G, et al. R-CHOP versus R-COMP: are they really equally effective? Clin Oncol (R Coll Radiol) 2014;26:648–52.

58. Fridrik MA, Jaeger U, Petzer A, et al. Cardiotoxicity with rituximab, cyclophosphamide, non-pegylated liposomal doxorubicin, vincristine and prednisolone compared to rituximab, cyclophosphamide, doxorubicin, vincristine, and prednisolone in frontline treatment of patients with diffuse large B-cell lymphoma: a randomised phase-III study from the Austrian Cancer Drug Therapy Working Group [Arbeitsgemeinschaft Medikamentöse umortherapie AGMT] (NHL-14). Eur J Cancer 2016;58:112–21.

59. Moccia AA, Schaff K, Hoskins P, et al. R-CHOP with etoposide substituted for doxorubicin (R-CEOP): excellent outcome in diffuse large B cell lymphoma for patients with a contraindication to anthracyclines. Blood 2009;114 [abstract: 408].

60. Rashidi A, Oak E, Carson KR, et al. Outcomes with R-CEOP for R-CHOP-ineligible patients with diffuse large B-cell lymphoma are highly dependent on cell of origin defined by Hans criteria. Leuk Lymphoma 2016;57:1191–3.

61. Zucca E, Conconi A, Mughal TI, et al. Patterns of outcome and prognostic factors in primary large-cell lymphoma of the testis in a survey by the International Extranodal Lymphoma Study Group. J Clin Oncol 2003;21:20–7.

62. Vitolo U, Chiappella A, Ferreri AJM, et al. First-line treatment for primary testicular diffuse large B-cell lymphoma with rituximab-CHOP, CNS prophylaxis, and contralateral testis irradiation: final results of an international phase II trial. J Clin Oncol 2011;29(20):2766–72.

63. Clinical trial.gov identifier NCT00945724.

64. Ryan G, Martinelli G, Kuper-Hommel M, et al. Primary diffuse large B-cell lymphoma of the breast: prognostic factors and outcomes of a study by the International Extranodal Lymphoma Study Group. Ann Oncol 2008;19(2):233–41.

65. Messina C, Ferreri AJ, Govi S, et al. Clinical features, management and prognosis of multifocal primary bone lymphoma: a retrospective study of the international extranodal lymphoma study group (the IELSG 14 study). Br J Haematol 2014; 164:834–40.

66. Wiernik PH, Lossos IS, Tuscano JM, et al. Lenalidomide monotherapy in relapsed or refractory aggressive non-Hodgkin's lymphoma. J Clin Oncol 2008;26(30): 4952–7.

67. Witzig TE, Vose JM, Zinzani PL, et al. An international phase II trial of single-agent lenalidomide for relapsed or refractory aggressive B-cell non-Hodgkin's lymphoma. Ann Oncol 2011;22(7):1622–7.

68. Zinzani PL, Pellegrini C, Gandolfi L, et al. Combination of lenalidomide and rituximab in elderly patients with relapsed or refractory diffuse large B-cell lymphoma: a phase 2 trial. Clin Lymphoma Myeloma Leuk 2011;11(6):462–6.

69. Hernandez-Ilizaliturri FJ, Deeb G, Zinzani PL, et al. Higher response to lenalidomide in relapsed/refractory diffuse large b-cell lymphoma in nongerminal center B-cell-like than in germinal center B-cell-like phenotype. Cancer 2011;117(22): 5058–66.

70. Chiappella A, Tucci A, Castellino A, et al. Lenalidomide plus cyclophosphamide, doxorubicin, vincristine, prednisone and rituximab is safe and effective in untreated, elderly patients with diffuse large B-cell lymphoma: phase I study by the Fondazione Italiana Linfomi. Haematologica 2013;98:1732–8.

71. Nowakowski GS, LaPlant B, Habermann TM, et al. Lenalidomide can be safely combined with R-CHOP (R2CHOP) in the initial chemotherapy for aggressive B-cell lymphomas: phase I study. Leukemia 2011;25:1877–81.

72. Tilly H, Morschhauser F, Salles G, et al. Phase 1b study of lenalidomide in combination with rituximab-CHOP (R2-CHOP) in patients with B-cell lymphoma. Leukemia 2013;27:252–5.

73. Nowakowski GS, LaPlant BR, Reeder C, et al. Combination of lenalidomide with R-CHOP (R2CHOP) is well-tolerated and effective as initial therapy for aggressive B-cell lymphomas—a phase II study. Blood 2012;120:689 [abstract].

74. Vitolo U, Chiappella A, Franceschetti S, et al. Lenalidomide plus R-CHOP21 in elderly patients with untreated diffuse large B-cell lymphoma: results of the REAL07 open-label, multicentre, phase 2 trial. Lancet Oncol 2014;15:730–7.

75. Efficacy and safety study of lenalidomide plus R-CHOP chemotherapy versus placebo plus R-CHOP chemotherapy in untreated ABC type diffuse large B-cell lymphoma (ROBUST). ClinicalTrials.gov identifier: NCT02285062.

76. Wilson WH, Gerecitano JF, Goy A, et al. The Bruton's tyrosine kinase (BTK) inhibitor, ibrutinib (PCI-32765), has preferential activity in the ABC subtype of relapsed/refractory de novo diffuse large B-cell lymphoma (DLBCL): interim results of a multicenter, open label, phase 2 study. Blood 2012;120:686.

77. Younes A, Thieblemont C, Morschhauser F, et al. Combination of ibrutinib with rituximab, cyclophosphamide, doxorubicin, vincristine, and prednisone (R-CHOP) for treatment-naive patients with CD20-positive B-cell non-Hodgkin lymphoma: a non-randomised, phase 1b study. Lancet Oncol 2014;15:1019–26.

78. A Study of the Bruton's tyrosine kinase inhibitor, PCI-32765 (ibrutinib), in combination with rituximab, cyclophosphamide, doxorubicin, vincristine, and prednisone in patients with newly diagnosed non-germinal center B-cell subtype of diffuse large B-cell lymphoma. ClinicalTrials.gov identifier: NCT01855750.

79. Ruan J, Martin P, Furman RR, et al. Bortezomib plus CHOP-rituximab for previously untreated diffuse large B-cell lymphoma and mantle cell lymphoma. J Clin Oncol 2011;29(6):690–7.

Molecular Classification of Diffuse Large B-cell Lymphoma: What Is Clinically Relevant?

Pierre Sujobert, MD, PhD[a,b,c], Gilles Salles, MD, PhD[b,c,d] *,
Emmanuel Bachy, MD, PhD[b,c,d]

KEYWORDS

- Aggressive lymphoma • Diffuse large B-cell lymphoma • Cell-of-origin
- Germinal center subtype • Activated B-cell like subtype • Targeted therapy
- Personalized medicine

KEY POINTS

- Molecular characterization of diffuse large B-cell lymphoma mainly relies on the distinction between germinal center B-cell like and activated B-cell like subtypes.
- Each subtype displays specific molecular specificities related to the cell of origin from which they are supposed to derive.
- Far from being merely theoretical, the distinction provides important insights into prognostic features, outcome on conventional therapy, and targeted therapy options.
- Much work must be performed to implement cell of origin (COO) assessment in routine practice with fast, widely available, and affordable techniques.

INTRODUCTION

Diffuse large B-cell lymphoma (DLBCL) accounts for approximately 30% to 40% of all non-Hodgkin lymphoma (NHL) cases. Although the course of the disease is usually aggressive, more than 50% of patients can be cured by currently available immunochemotherapy protocols. The molecular classification of DLBCL segregating germinal center B-cell like (GCB) from activated B-cell like (ABC) subtypes based on gene expression profile analysis remains a cornerstone for the understanding of DLBCL biology. This molecular classification has been proven to be significant for

[a] Laboratory of Hematology, Hospices Civils de Lyon, Hôpital Lyon Sud, 165 Chemin du Grand Revoyet, Pierre-Bénite 69310, France; [b] Université Claude Bernard Lyon1, Université de Lyon, Lyon, France; [c] Centre de Recherche en Cancérologie de Lyon, INSERM 1052 CNRS 5286, Lyon, France; [d] Department of Hematology, Hospices Civils de Lyon, Hôpital Lyon Sud, 165 Chemin du Grand Revoyet, Pierre-Bénite 69310, France
* Corresponding author. Department of Hematology, Hospices Civils de Lyon, 165, chemin du Grand Revoyet, Pierre-Bénite cedex 69495, France.
E-mail address: gilles.salles@chu-lyon.fr

Hematol Oncol Clin N Am 30 (2016) 1163–1177
http://dx.doi.org/10.1016/j.hoc.2016.07.001
0889-8588/16/© 2016 Elsevier Inc. All rights reserved.

clinical purposes, because it is closely related to patient prognosis. However, major pharmacological progress has only recently rendered specific subtype targeting by new drug compounds possible.

This article focuses on how findings in basic science and translational research have progressively shaped the understanding of DLBCL molecular biology, allowed for better prognostic determination, and uncovered a whole new perspective for treating the disease. It emphasizes the cell of origin (COO) classification of DLBCL, which is supported by many lines of biological evidence and has strong clinical implications. The case of double-hit lymphomas identified by the fluorescence in situ hybridization (FISH) analysis of the rearrangement of *MYC* and *BCL2* or *BCL6* oncogenes will be reviewed in another article on this issue.

MOLECULAR DIFFUSE LARGE B-CELL LYMPHOMA SUBTYPES, PROGNOSTIC AND CLINICAL IMPLICATIONS
Why the Need to Classify Diffuse Large B-cell Lymphoma?

The classification of lymphomas is a continuous process that has evolved with the knowledge of the pathophysiology and/or the development of new therapeutics. Since the early recognition of the histologic differences between Hodgkin and non-Hodgkin lymphomas, several classifications have been established. The actual World Health Organization (WHO) 2008 classification recognizes entities based on similar clinical, phenotypical, and/or genetic characteristics. The theoretic framework underlying the WHO classification is the concept of the COO, which proposes to assign every lymphoid cancer to its closest normal counterpart. However, DLBCLs were first considered a highly heterogeneous group of lymphomas that were still too insufficiently characterized to be discriminated.

The ultimate goal of such a classification is to recognize similar lymphomas with the same underlying biological abnormalities so that prognosis and tailored treatment modalities can be chosen. This personalized medicine is often described as the holy grail of modern medicine but is in fact already routinely applied to some lymphoma patients. Hence, therapeutic strategies are already highly differentiated according to the histologic subtype of the aggressive lymphoma (ie, Burkitt lymphoma vs DLBCL). However, many unmet needs remain for a better classification of DLBCL, which represents approximately 40% of adult lymphomas and showing highly heterogeneous clinical outcomes with conventional immunochemotherapy.

Classification of Diffuse Large B-cell Lymphoma Based on Gene Expression Profiles

Fifteen years ago, a transcriptomic analysis of fresh frozen samples of DLBCL was reported based on an analysis of approximately 17,000 probes covering genes involved in germinal center biology, lymphoma, cancer biology, and normal lymphocyte biology.[1] The unsupervised analysis of transcriptomic profiling was able to distinguish DLBCL from normal B cells and other lymphoid malignancies. Moreover, this approach clearly distinguished the following 2 classes of DLBCL based on the similarity of their gene expression profiles with normal B cells: The germinal center B-cell like (GCB) and the activated B-cell like (ABC) DLBCL. Importantly, 2 levels of evidence supported the relevance of this distinction. First, the authors noted that specific genetic alterations were associated with each subtype, suggesting distinct oncogenic mechanisms. Second, the GCB/ABC signature was highly correlated with the overall survival (OS) of patients treated with cyclophosphamide, doxorubicin, vincristine, predisolone (CHOP) chemotherapy, and the ABC subtype was associated with the worse outcome.

This pioneering work was further refined 2 years later with a large series of patients with gene expression profiling (GEP) based on 100 genes.[2] This analysis led to the distinction of the following 3 groups: GCB, ABC, and unclassifiable DLBCL. Importantly, this study confirmed the differences in the oncogenetic mechanisms between ABC and GCB DLBCL and the strong prognostic value of this classifier.

Further studies have validated that the worse prognosis associated with the ABC subtype was maintained in the rituximab era, both in frontline therapy[3] and in relapsed DLBCL.[4] Moreover, a predictive value of the COO classification potentially altering therapeutic choice was suggested in relapsed DLBCL patients, because GCB DLBCL was associated with a better survival rate with R-DHAP (containing cisplatin plus cytarabine) than R-ICE (containing carboplatin plus ifosfamide and etoposide).[4] In first-line therapy, young patients with non-GCB DLBCL receiving intensified immunochemotherapy were also reported to experience prolonged survival compared with patients treated with conventional R-CHOP.[5]

Germinal Center B-cell Like and Activated B-cell Like Diffuse Large B-cell Lymphoma: Two Roads to Oncogenesis

Since these 2 early studies, much research has been conducted to analyze the biology of both lymphoma subtypes. Combining whole-exome sequencing and functional unbiased screening with shRNA libraries, it was demonstrated that ABC lymphomas are addicted to the signaling pathways downstream of the B-cell receptor (BCR).[6] This activation of the BCR pathway in ABC DLBCL might be sustained either by mutations in genes encoding this pathway (eg, *CD79A, CD79B,* or *CARD11*) or BCR activation with self-antigens.[7] Moreover, ABC DLBCLs also frequently harbor an activating mutation of *MYD88*, resulting in the activation of the NF-κB pathway and also priming the cells for the detrimental production of interferon β (IFNβ). Interestingly, both pathways have been exploited therapeutically in ABC DLBCL with the use of ibrutinib (which inhibits the Bruton tyrosine kinase [BTK] that belongs to the BCR signaling pathway) and lenalidomide (which favors detrimental IFNβ overproduction in *MYD88*-mutated DLBCL by inhibiting interferon responsive factor 4 [IRF4]).[8] In contrast, GCB DLBCLs harbor oncogenetic hits typical of germinal center lymphomas, such as the t(14;18) translocation, the mutations of epigenetic modifiers (*EZH2, KMT2D*),[9] or mutations in the genes encoding the *S1PR2* receptor or its signal transduction protein *GNA13*.[10] The main differences in the mutational landscape between the 2 groups are summarized in **Fig. 1**.

From Bench to Bedside

The prognostic and predictive potential of DLBCL classification prompted the development of surrogate markers to easily determine the COO. Indeed, GEP using a microarray is not suitable for the clinical routine, because the technique relies on fresh-frozen biopsies, remains expensive when considering numerous samples, and requires time-consuming procedures.

The first attempt to translate the GEP signature of DLBCL for routine purposes was based on immunohistochemistry. One of the most popular algorithms for immuno-histochemistry (IHC)-based determination of COO has been proposed by Hans and colleagues,[11] who described GCB DLBCL as CD10-positive or BCL6-positive and MUM1-negative, while ABC DLBCLs were identified as CD10-negative and MUM1-positive. In an attempt to improve the Hans algorithm, Choi and colleagues[12] (the so-called Choi algorithm), Meyer and colleagues[13] (the Tally algorithm) and Visco and colleagues[14] (the Visco algorithm) proposed different combinations of GC markers (BCL6, CD10, GCET1, and LMO2) and ABC markers (MUM1/IRF4 and

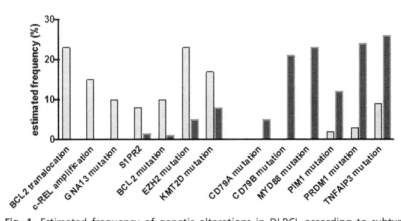

Fig. 1. Estimated frequency of genetic alterations in DLBCL according to subtype. (*Data from* Refs.[2,6,9,10])

FOXP1) to discriminate between DLBCL molecular subtypes. However, there were discrepancies in the clinical outcomes predicted by these different classifiers, and ultimately, none of them was robust enough to classify DLBCL compared with the gold standard GEP classifier.[15–17] One explanation for these disappointing results was probably the poor reproducibility of the quantitative assessment of the immunostaining.[18] Moreover, these algorithms only recognize 2 categories of lymphoma and fail to identify the unclassifiable cases described in transcriptomic analyses. Nevertheless, this approach is the only one largely available at present, and has been temporarily admitted as an alternative to molecular methods in the recent WHO revision.[19] Although the Hans algorithm is the most popular, this recent revision stipulates that others may also be used.

More recently, RNA-based techniques have been developed that evaluate the level of expression of the most significant genes of the GCB/ABC signature. cDNA-mediated annealing, selection, extension and ligation (DASL, Illumina proprietary technology, San Diego, CA) is a bead-based microarray technology able to quantify mRNA level expression of degraded mRNA from formalin-fixed-paraffin-embedded (FFPE) samples. Although no formal comparison with the GEP gold standard has been performed for ABC, GCB, or unclassified subtype assignments, the technique adequately discriminated patient outcome in a large cohort of 172 patients (of whom 140 were treated with R-CHOP).[20] The technology is currently being evaluated in a randomized clinical trial assessing the addition of bortezomib to an R-CHOP regimen backbone (NCT, ClinicalTrials.gov Identifier NCT01324596, REMoDL-B trial).

The NanoString Lymph2Cx 20 genes signature (comprising 15 genes of interest and 5 housekeeping genes) is based on oligonucleotide hybridization of a panel of probes labeled with a fluorescent barcode (digital multiplexed gene expression). For clinical use, this technique can be performed on FFPE samples with a short turnaround time (<48 h). When compared with the gold standard microarray, the Lymph2Cx signature accurately predicted the cell of origin, with less than 1% of cases being misclassified and with a high concordance level between laboratories.[21] Finally, when applied to a large cohort of DLBCL uniformly treated with R-CHOP, the Lymph2Cx signature was able to classify GC versus ABC DLBCL, and the prognosis of ABC DLBCL was poorer as expected.[22] Another study using a 20-gene set that was different from the Lymph2Cx reported the accuracy of the NanoString technology compared with the microarray gold standard.[23] No study has formally compared different gene set NanoString signatures to date. One limitation of these approaches is the need to use the proprietary NanoString platform, which remains expensive for routine use. The feasibility and accuracy of the Lympho2Cx signature in the context of a prospective trial is being assessed (NCT ClinicalTrials.gov Identifier NCT02285062, ROBUST trial).

An interesting alternative has recently been developed based on a quantitative RNA analysis called reverse transcription-multiplex ligation-dependent probe amplification (RT-MLPA).[24] Based on the expression level of 14 genes, this technique accurately assigns DLBCL subtype from fresh-frozen or FFPE biopsies, reproducing the prognostic value of the GC/ABC signature. Even if the robustness of this method has been less characterized than the Lymph2Cx signature, its low cost and flexibility support its use as an another approach to assess the COO of DLBCL.

In summary, for 15 years, no reliable technique on FFPE tissue has emerged as a satisfactory surrogate for GEP COO determination. Now that COO determination not only informs patient prognosis but might also drive therapeutic decisions (see the article on targeted therapy elsewhere in this issue), the need for an accurate, broadly accepted, and time- and cost-saving method is more warranted than ever before. Because of its poor reproducibility, there is little chance that immunohistochemistry could become the ultimate surrogate for the GEP gold standard. The NanoString technology seems the most advanced to date in terms of validation against the GEP gold standard and reproducibility between laboratories.[21] However, because of medico-economic considerations, it might be affordable for only a minority of patients. RT-MLPA is an interesting and low-cost technology that has been recognized as an acceptable surrogate in the 2016 WHO classification and warrants further assessment of its interlaboratory reproducibility. Importantly, high-throughput sequencing technologies (next-generation sequencing or NGS) are becoming increasingly available in most care centers and are able to both identify therapeutically actionable target mutations and assess degraded mRNA expression levels from FFPE samples at reasonable costs. One could imagine that a combination of gene expression level determination and targeted sequencing of mutually exclusive mutations (such as GNA13 and MYD88) would become a benchmark in the near future. The pros and cons of the different methods detailed previously are recapitulated in **Table 1**.

Beyond mutation patterns and gene expression profiles, genomic gains and losses encompassing specific oncogenes or tumor suppressors (such as MYC and CDKN1B

Table 1
Comparative analysis of the different techniques available to determine the cell of origin in diffuse large B-cell lymphoma

	Microarray	IHC	Lymp2Cx	DASL	RT-MLPA
FFPE compatible	No	Yes	Yes	Yes	Yes
Accuracy	Gold standard	Poor	Very high	Undetermined	Very high
Reproducibility	High	Low	High	Undetermined	Undetermined
Feasibility in daily use	No	Yes	Yes	Yes	Yes
Cost	High	Low	High	High	Medium

Abbreviations: DASL, cDNA-mediated Annealing, Selection, extension and Ligation; FFPE, formalin-fixed paraffin-embedded; IHC, immunohistochemistry; Lymp2Cx, Nanostring 20-gene signature; RT-MLPA, Reverse transcription multiplex ligation-dependent probe amplification.

gains or *TP53* and *CDKN2A* losses) were found to be significantly associated with outcome independently of the ABC and GCB subtypes.[25] As an alternative to genome scale comparative genomic hybridization array (CGHa), multiplex polymerase chain reaction of short fluorescent fragments or quantitative multiplex PCR of short fluorescent fragments (QMPSF) could represent alternatives for routine practice.[25] However, genomic gains and losses remain essentially prognostic and are still lacking any specific therapeutic implications.

TARGETED THERAPY FOR MOLECULAR SUBTYPES OF DIFFUSE LARGE B-CELL LYMPHOMA

Beyond prognostic issues associated with molecular subtype determination in DLBCL, biological segregation between GCB and ABC lymphomas was found to be of utmost importance for patient-tailored therapy and targeted therapy design. Although promising novel agents in aggressive lymphomas will be detailed elsewhere in this issue, the authors will briefly give an overview of how agents might be particularly attractive for treating specific molecular subtypes of DLBCL (illustrated in **Fig. 2** and summarized in **Table 2**).

Targeted Therapy for Germinal Center B-cell Like Diffuse Large B-cell Lymphoma

BCL6 inhibitor
The GCB subtype of DLBCL critically relies on *BCL6* expression and function for survival. Therefore, BCL6 has been observed as an attractive target for patients with GCB DLBCL, and *BCL6* is more highly expressed in DLBCL cells than in normal cells. In fact, preclinical data of a small-molecule BCL6 inhibitor showed encouraging in vitro and murine in vivo

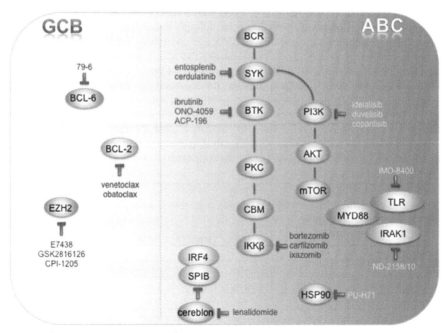

Fig. 2. Schematic representation of the targeted treatments for the GCB and ABC DLBCL subtypes. Note that the distinction is merely theoretical, as agents in 1 category might ultimately prove efficient in the other.

efficacy without major toxicity.[26–28] However, clinical data are still not available for the compound, and no active early phase clinical trial has been initiated to date.

BCL2 family member inhibitors

The overexpression of the apoptosis inhibitor BCL2 is a hallmark of GCB DLBCL, and approximately 20% of the inhibitors harbor a t(14;18) translocation, suggesting a particular interest of BCL2 inhibitors in these lymphomas. Moreover, BCL6 directly represses *BCL2* expression; therefore, an unintended effect of inhibiting BCL6 is promoting transcription of antiapoptotic family members. Interestingly, recent data have noted that BCL6 inhibitors could thus be synthetically lethal with BH3 mimetic drugs, such as ABT-737, ABT-199 (venetoclax) or GX15-070MS (obatoclax).[29] Combinations of ABT-199 and immunochemotherapy (rituximab-CHOP or obinutuzumab-CHOP) are currently being evaluated (**Table 2**). Notably, *BCL2* amplifications have been associated with the ABC subtype,[30] suggesting that this oncogene might not be an exclusive target for the GCB DLBCL subtype.

EZH2 inhibitors

Germinal center-derived lymphomas often exhibit gain-of-function mutations of the epigenetic modifier *EZH2*. GCB DLBCL roughly presents *EZH2* mutations in approximately 20% of cases.[31] Inhibitors of EZH2 displayed potent antilymphoma activity in cell lines and xenograft models.[32–34] Three different small-molecule inhibitors designed for further development in clinics are currently being evaluated in phase I and phase II trials for lymphoma patients. Interestingly, immunohistochemistry assessment of methylation profiles might further refine the choice of DLBCL patients selected for EZH2 inhibitor treatments.[35]

Targeted Therapy for Activated B-cell Like Diffuse Large B-cell Lymphoma

B-cell receptor pathway inhibitors

Certain pathways deregulating and ultimately leading to constitutive NF-κB activation is a hallmark of the ABC subtype of DLBCL. Among them, the BCR pathway is a cornerstone, and many drugs aiming at disrupting signaling have been developed. Ibrutinib is a first-in-class BTK inhibitor known for its remarkable efficacy in mantle cell lymphoma and chronic lymphoid leukemia (CLL). Better response rates have been found in ABC patients compared with GCB DLBCL patients (37% vs 5% overall response rates, respectively) using ibrutinib as a single agent,[36] and its combination with R-CHOP has also been found to be safe.[37] Results from larger phase III studies (NOT01055750) are needed to confirm the efficacy and safety of this molecule in association with chemotherapy in patients with non-GCB DLBCL. Other BTK inhibitors (GS/ONO-4059, ACP-196) are in development. Interestingly, identification of peculiar mutation patterns might predict response outcomes to BTK inhibitors (eg, resistance due to the presence of the downstream CARD11 mutation or of the MYD88 mutation associated with BCR independency).[36] Therefore, next-generation sequencing might provide the framework for therapy decisions over the next few years.[38]

Other adaptors from the BCR signaling pathway are potentially attractive targets for compound development. The SYK/PI3K cascade inhibition has yielded promising response rates and prolonged event-free survival in CLL and indolent lymphoma. Few results in aggressive lymphomas of PI3K inhibitors such as duvelisib, a dual PI3Kγ and δ inhibitor, or copanlisib, a pan-class I PI3K inhibitor, have been published,[39,40] but more data should become rapidly available. Entosplenib, a SYK inhibitor whose tolerance and potential efficacy have been studied in CLL, is also currently being evaluated in DLBCL, alone and in association with conventional chemotherapy and other targeted therapies (idelalisib or ONO-4059). PRT062070 (cerdulatinib), a dual SYK/JAK inhibitor,

Table 2
Targeted therapy for diffuse large B-cell lymphoma

	Compound	Targets	Rationale	Development Stage	Clinical Trials in DLBCL (Nonexhaustive List)
Rationally targeted toward GCB DLBCL	79-6	BCL6	• Highly expressed in DLBCL vs normal cells • Promotes genomic instability • Impedes normal differentiation	Preclinical	None
	Venetoclax	BCL2	• Overexpressed preferentially in GCB DLBCL following translocation • Overexpressed following BCL6 therapeutic inhibition	Clinical	NCT01328626 NCT01594229 NCT02265731 NCT02640833 NCT02611323 NCT01969695 NCT02055820
	Obatoclax	BCL2	Idem	Clinical	NCT00538187
	E7438	EZH2	• Gain-of-function mutations in GCB DLBCL • Represses important tumor suppressors	Clinical	NCT01897571
	CPI-1205	EZH2	Idem	Clinical	NCT02395601
	GSK2816126	EZH2	Idem	Clinical	NCT02082977
Rationally targeted toward ABC DLBCL	Entosplenib	SYK	• Constitutive activity by BCR extrinsic stimulation or upstream pathway mutation (CD79a or b) • Promotes downstream signaling and NF-κB activity	Clinical	NCT01799889 NCT01796470 NCT02457598 NCT02568683
	Cerdulatinib	SYK	Idem	Clinical	NCT01994382
	Ibrutinib	BTK	• Constitutive activity by BCR extrinsic stimulation or upstream pathway mutation • Promotes downstream signaling and NF-κB activity	Clinical	NCT01569750 NCT01479842 NCT01855750 NCT02142049 NCT02219737 NCT02055924
	ONO-4059	BTK	Idem	Clinical	NCT01659255
	ACP-196	BTK	Idem	Clinical	NCT02112526

Drug	Target	Mechanism	Status	Trials
Copanlisib	Pan class I PI3K	• Constitutive PI3K activity downstream of SYK • Promotes survival and proliferation via AKT	Clinical	NCT01660451 NCT02391116 NCT01476657 NCT01871675
Duvelisib	PI3Kγ,δ	Idem	Clinical	None
ND-2158 or ND-2110	IRAK4	• Inhibits the downstream adaptor of the MYD88 pathway • Potential efficacy in case of L265P $MYD88$ mutation	Preclinical	
Lenalidomide	Cereblon IRF4 SPIB	• Inhibition of IRF4 via cereblon • Detrimental IFNβ overproduction • Pleiotropic immunomodulatory effect on T-, NK-, and dendritic cells	Clinical	NCT01197560 NCT01122472 NCT02285062 NCT01856192 NCT02128061
IMO-8400	TLR7/8/9	• Inhibits the toll-like receptors upstream of MYD88 • Stimulation triggers activation of the MYD88/IRAK pathway	Clinical	NCT02252146
Bortezomib	26S Proteasome subunit	• Prevents degradation of IκB • Prevents translocation of NF-κB into the nucleus	Clinical	NCT02542111 NCT01965977 NCT01324596 NCT01848132
Ixazomib	20S Proteasome subunit	Idem	Clinical	NCT02481310
Carfilzomib	20S Proteasome subunit	idem	Clinical	NCT01926665 NCT02073097 NCT01959698
PU-H71	Hsp90	• Disruption of tumor-enriched Hsp90 complexes • Broad effects on BCR signaling, calcium flux and NF-κB activation	Clinical	NCT01581541 NCT01393509

Note that the distinction is merely theoretic as agents in 1 category might ultimately prove efficient in the other.

is now entering into a phase I dose escalation study. Importantly, SYK inhibitors appear to also be effective in some GCB DLBCL cell lines, underlying how a strict frontier between both subtypes might be insufficient in terms of therapy choice.[41] Safety concerns related to immune activation have emerged concerning the use of PI3K inhibitors in combination with either rituximab plus lenalidomide in relapse or with rituximab alone in frontline settings for follicular lymphoma (FL)[42] or CLL,[43] respectively.

Although currently not available for people, in vitro and in vivo data in animal models of phenothiazine-derived inhibitors of MALT1, part of the CARD11-BCL10-MALT1 (CBM) complex that is the central node for NK-κB activation, should be developed in a few years.[44,45]

MYD88 pathway inhibitors

Recently published data has paved the way for using IRAK4 adaptor inhibitors (preclinical ND-2158 and ND-2110 compounds) to treat patients with *MYD88* L265P gain-of-function mutations leading to the amplification of pathway activation.[46] Another approach with IMO-8400, a synthetic DNA-based antagonist that has demonstrated effective inhibition of TLR7/8/9[47] upstream of the MYD88/IRAK cascade, is currently under scrutiny in mutated ABC DLBCL.

Proteasome inhibitors

Given the constitutive NF-κB activation in ABC DLBCL and the known, albeit unspecific, ability of proteasome inhibitors to prevent IκB degradation, bortezomib has been evaluated in this particular subtype of lymphoma. Although results were disappointing when used as a single agent,[48] further studies reported differential and encouraging efficacy in ABC versus GCB DLBCL when combined with immunochemotherapy.[49] However, a recent randomized phase II study did not demonstrate the superiority of VR-CAP (R-CHOP where vincristine is replaced with bortezomib) over R-CHOP.[50] Other trials with bortezomib in association or as maintenance are ongoing.[51,52] Second-generation proteasome inhibitors, such as carfilzomib or ixazomib, were potent in xenograft models of DLBCL, and clinical results are eagerly awaited.[53]

Immunomodulatory agents

As previously mentioned, the development of lenalidomide and other similar compounds, used alone or in combination with chemotherapy, may also preferentially target the ABC DLBCL subtype.[54] Several ongoing randomized studies (see **Table 2**) should provide specific information regarding the spectrum of activity of these compounds in DLBCL and whether characteristic molecular subtypes benefit from this approach, as has already been suggested from single-agent studies.[55]

Heat shock protein 90 inhibitors

Disruption of tumor-enriched heat shock protein 90 (HSP90) complexes has been shown to inhibit the growth of DLBCL lines both in vitro and in vivo by attenuating BCR signaling, calcium flux, and ultimately, NF-κB activation.[56] The PU-H71 compound is now under investigation in clinical trials and could display a high level of synergy with BCR pathway inhibitors for patients with ABC DLBCL.[56]

Beyond Activated B-cell Like and Germinal Center B-cell Like Subtypes— Consideration for Targeted Therapy

Metabolic signature

The COO classification of DLBCL has yielded significant improvements in our understanding of DLBCL, as well as the prognostic stratification of patients and the design of targeted therapies. However, any classification is improvable, and alternative classifications of DLBCL could also be worthwhile. For example, another GEP-based classification of DLBCL has distinguished DLBCL with features of BCR activation, DLBCL characterized by overexpression of genes of the oxidative phosphorylation (oxphos) metabolic pathway, or DLBCL characterized by various host response transcriptomic signatures.[57] These alternative classifications also uncovered specific sensitivity of DLBCL subtypes to therapies, at least in preclinical experiments, including original treatments targeting the metabolic rewiring of oxphos DLBCL.[58]

Bromodomain and extraterminal inhibitors

Several bromodomain and extraterminal (BET) family member inhibitors have gained the interest of researchers worldwide, especially in regard to tumors overexpressing the *MYC* oncogene.[59,60] A preliminary report related the safety of the OTX-015 drug in hematological malignancies,[61] while evidence is accumulating in favor of its preclinical efficacy in DLBCL.[62] Several small-molecule inhibitors are currently in development (OTX015, CPI-0610, TEN-010 and GSK525762), with two of them being evaluated in lymphoma. The relationship between the activation of some gene pathways and the expression of MYC protein and the clinical response to these agents remains to be determined.

Stromal signature

In 2008, Lenz and colleagues[3] proposed a prognostic classification based on the 2 following different signatures. The extracellular matrix deposition and histiocytic infiltration signature were associated with a favorable outcome, whereas a high tumor blood vessel density reflected an unfavorable signature for patients treated with R-CHOP. Different microenvironments in DLBCL reflected by specific signatures might appear as appealing targets in the near future.

Immune environment

Immune checkpoint inhibitors have recently demonstrated their therapeutic efficacy in a variety of tumors, including lymphoma.[63] The characterization of the different molecules expressed by either lymphoma cells or the immune infiltrating cells may become helpful in selecting patients who could benefit from these approaches.[64,65]

SUMMARY

The evolution of DLBCL diagnosis, prognosis assessment, and treatment during the last 10 years may be observed as a prototypic paradigm shift of how molecular characterization has refined the histopathological definition of lymphoid malignancies. Although many molecular abnormalities have been found to be associated with patient outcomes, solid evidence that therapeutic decisions should be based on this information is sparse. However, the rapid development of targeted therapies may dramatically change the treatment paradigms in the near future. Besides the routine characterization of the DLBCL subtypes using IHC and other information that may be acquired through this technique (regarding specific targets or the microenvironment), the molecular characterization of DLBCL is likely to become necessary in the coming years. Whether this characterization will require only the identification of the COO using robust gene expression-derived assays or also mandate the identification of some pattern of mutations remains to be determined. More than ever, the careful and critical examination of clinical and translational data gathered in clinical trials should help in selecting the optimal approaches.

REFERENCES

1. Alizadeh AA, Eisen MB, Davis RE, et al. Distinct types of diffuse large B-cell lymphoma identified by gene expression profiling. Nature 2000;403(6769):503–11.

2. Rosenwald A, Wright G, Chan WC, et al. The use of molecular profiling to predict survival after chemotherapy for diffuse large-B-cell lymphoma. N Engl J Med 2002;346(25):1937–47.
3. Lenz G, Wright G, Dave SS, et al. Stromal gene signatures in large-B-cell lymphomas. N Engl J Med 2008;359(22):2313–23.
4. Thieblemont C, Briere J, Mounier N, et al. The germinal center/activated B-cell subclassification has a prognostic impact for response to salvage therapy in relapsed/refractory diffuse large B-cell lymphoma: a bio-CORAL study. J Clin Oncol 2011;29(31):4079–87.
5. Molina TJ, Canioni D, Copie-Bergman C, et al. Young patients with non-germinal center B-cell-like diffuse large B-cell lymphoma benefit from intensified chemotherapy with ACVBP plus rituximab compared with CHOP plus rituximab: analysis of data from the Groupe d'Etudes des Lymphomes de l'Adulte/Lymphoma Study Association Phase III Trial LNH 03-2B. J Clin Oncol 2014;32(35):3996–4003.
6. Davis RE, Ngo VN, Lenz G, et al. Chronic active B-cell-receptor signalling in diffuse large B-cell lymphoma. Nature 2010;463(7277):88–92.
7. Young RM, Wu T, Schmitz R, et al. Survival of human lymphoma cells requires B-cell receptor engagement by self-antigens. Proc Natl Acad Sci U S A 2015; 112(44):13447–54.
8. Yang Y, Shaffer AL 3rd, Emre NC, et al. Exploiting synthetic lethality for the therapy of ABC diffuse large B cell lymphoma. Cancer Cell 2012;21(6):723–37.
9. Pasqualucci L, Trifonov V, Fabbri G, et al. Analysis of the coding genome of diffuse large B-cell lymphoma. Nat Genet 2011;43(9):830–7.
10. Muppidi JR, Schmitz R, Green JA, et al. Loss of signalling via Galpha13 in germinal centre B-cell-derived lymphoma. Nature 2014;516(7530):254–8.
11. Hans CP, Weisenburger DD, Greiner TC, et al. Confirmation of the molecular classification of diffuse large B-cell lymphoma by immunohistochemistry using a tissue microarray. Blood 2004;103(1):275–82.
12. Choi WW, Weisenburger DD, Greiner TC, et al. A new immunostain algorithm classifies diffuse large B-cell lymphoma into molecular subtypes with high accuracy. Clin Cancer Res 2009;15(17):5494–502.
13. Meyer PN, Fu K, Greiner TC, et al. Immunohistochemical methods for predicting cell of origin and survival in patients with diffuse large B-cell lymphoma treated with rituximab. J Clin Oncol 2011;29(2):200–7.
14. Visco C, Li Y, Xu-Monette ZY, et al. Comprehensive gene expression profiling and immunohistochemical studies support application of immunophenotypic algorithm for molecular subtype classification in diffuse large B-cell lymphoma: a report from the International DLBCL Rituximab-CHOP Consortium Program Study. Leukemia 2012;26(9):2103–13.
15. Gutierrez-Garcia G, Cardesa-Salzmann T, Climent F, et al. Gene-expression profiling and not immunophenotypic algorithms predicts prognosis in patients with diffuse large B-cell lymphoma treated with immunochemotherapy. Blood 2011;117(18):4836–43.
16. Coutinho R, Clear AJ, Owen A, et al. Poor concordance among nine immunohistochemistry classifiers of cell-of-origin for diffuse large B-cell lymphoma: implications for therapeutic strategies. Clin Cancer Res 2013;19(24):6686–95.
17. Salles G, de Jong D, Xie W, et al. Prognostic significance of immunohistochemical biomarkers in diffuse large B-cell lymphoma: a study from the Lunenburg Lymphoma Biomarker Consortium. Blood 2011;117(26):7070–8.
18. de Jong D, Rosenwald A, Chhanabhai M, et al. Immunohistochemical prognostic markers in diffuse large B-cell lymphoma: validation of tissue microarray as a

prerequisite for broad clinical applications—a study from the Lunenburg Lymphoma Biomarker Consortium. J Clin Oncol 2007;25(7):805–12.

19. Swerdlow SH, Campo E, Pileri SA, et al. The 2016 revision of the World Health Organization classification of lymphoid neoplasms. Blood 2016;127(20):2375–90.

20. Barrans SL, Crouch S, Care MA, et al. Whole genome expression profiling based on paraffin embedded tissue can be used to classify diffuse large B-cell lymphoma and predict clinical outcome. Br J Haematol 2012;159(4):441–53.

21. Scott DW, Wright GW, Williams PM, et al. Determining cell-of-origin subtypes of diffuse large B-cell lymphoma using gene expression in formalin-fixed paraffin-embedded tissue. Blood 2014;123(8):1214–7.

22. Scott DW, Mottok A, Ennishi D, et al. Prognostic significance of diffuse large B-cell lymphoma cell of origin determined by digital gene expression in formalin-fixed paraffin-embedded tissue biopsies. J Clin Oncol 2015;33(26): 2848–56.

23. Masque-Soler N, Szczepanowski M, Kohler CW, et al. Molecular classification of mature aggressive B-cell lymphoma using digital multiplexed gene expression on formalin-fixed paraffin-embedded biopsy specimens. Blood 2013;122(11): 1985–6.

24. Mareschal S, Ruminy P, Bagacean C, et al. Accurate classification of germinal center B-cell-like/activated B-cell-like diffuse large B-cell lymphoma using a simple and rapid reverse transcriptase-multiplex ligation-dependent probe amplification assay: a CALYM study. J Mol Diagn 2015. [Epub ahead of print].

25. Jardin F, Ruminy P, Kerckaert JP, et al. Detection of somatic quantitative genetic alterations by multiplex polymerase chain reaction for the prediction of outcome in diffuse large B-cell lymphomas. Haematologica 2008;93(4):543–50.

26. Cerchietti LC, Ghetu AF, Zhu X, et al. A small-molecule inhibitor of BCL6 kills DLBCL cells in vitro and in vivo. Cancer Cell 2010;17(4):400–11.

27. Hatzi K, Jiang Y, Huang C, et al. A hybrid mechanism of action for BCL6 in B cells defined by formation of functionally distinct complexes at enhancers and promoters. Cell Rep 2013;4(3):578–88.

28. Cerchietti LC, Yang SN, Shaknovich R, et al. A peptomimetic inhibitor of BCL6 with potent antilymphoma effects in vitro and in vivo. Blood 2009;113(15): 3397–405.

29. Dupont T, Yang SN, Patel J, et al. Selective targeting of BCL6 induces oncogene addiction switching to BCL2 in B-cell lymphoma. Oncotarget 2016;7(3):3520–32.

30. Kusumoto S, Kobayashi Y, Sekiguchi N, et al. Diffuse large B-cell lymphoma with extra Bcl-2 gene signals detected by FISH analysis is associated with a "non-germinal center phenotype". Am J Surg Pathol 2005;29(8):1067–73.

31. Morin RD, Johnson NA, Severson TM, et al. Somatic mutations altering EZH2 (Tyr641) in follicular and diffuse large B-cell lymphomas of germinal-center origin. Nat Genet 2010;42(2):181–5.

32. McCabe MT, Ott HM, Ganji G, et al. EZH2 inhibition as a therapeutic strategy for lymphoma with EZH2-activating mutations. Nature 2012;492(7427):108–12.

33. Knutson SK, Wigle TJ, Warholic NM, et al. A selective inhibitor of EZH2 blocks H3K27 methylation and kills mutant lymphoma cells. Nat Chem Biol 2012;8(11): 890–6.

34. Qi W, Chan H, Teng L, et al. Selective inhibition of Ezh2 by a small molecule inhibitor blocks tumor cells proliferation. Proc Natl Acad Sci U S A 2012;109(52): 21360–5.

35. Dubois S, Mareschal S, Picquenot JM, et al. Immunohistochemical and genomic profiles of diffuse large B-cell lymphomas: implications for targeted EZH2 inhibitor therapy? Oncotarget 2015;6(18):16712–24.

36. Wilson WH, Young RM, Schmitz R, et al. Targeting B cell receptor signaling with ibrutinib in diffuse large B cell lymphoma. Nat Med 2015;21(8):922–6.

37. Younes A, Thieblemont C, Morschhauser F, et al. Combination of ibrutinib with rituximab, cyclophosphamide, doxorubicin, vincristine, and prednisone (R-CHOP) for treatment-naive patients with CD20-positive B-cell non-Hodgkin lymphoma: a non-randomised, phase 1b study. Lancet Oncol 2014;15(9):1019–26.

38. Dubois S, Viailly PJ, Mareschal S, et al. Next generation sequencing in diffuse large B cell lymphoma highlights molecular divergence and therapeutic opportunities: a LYSA study. Clin Cancer Res 2016;22(12):2919–28.

39. Morschhauser F, Bron D, Bouabdallah K, et al. Preliminary results of a phase II study of single agent Bay 80-6946, a novel PI3K inhibitor, in patients with relapsed/refractory, indolent or aggressive lymphoma. Blood 2013;122(21):87.

40. Flinn IW, Cherry M, Maris M, et al. Combination trial of Duvelisib (IPI-145) with bendamustine, rituximab, or bendamustine/rituximab in patients with lymphoma or chronic lymphocytic leukemia. Blood 2015;126(23):3928.

41. Cheng S, Coffey G, Zhang XH, et al. SYK inhibition and response prediction in diffuse large B-cell lymphoma. Blood 2011;118(24):6342–52.

42. Smith SM, Pitcher B, Jung S-H, et al. Unexpected and serious toxicity observed with combined idelalisib, lenalidomide and rituximab in relapsed/refractory B cell lymphomas: alliance A051201 and A051202. Blood 2014;124(21):3091.

43. Lampson BL, Matos T, Kim HT, et al. Idelalisib given front-line for the treatment of chronic lymphocytic leukemia results in frequent and severe immune-mediated toxicities. Blood 2015;126(23):497.

44. Nagel D, Spranger S, Vincendeau M, et al. Pharmacologic inhibition of MALT1 protease by phenothiazines as a therapeutic approach for the treatment of aggressive ABC-DLBCL. Cancer Cell 2012;22(6):825–37.

45. Ferch U, Kloo B, Gewies A, et al. Inhibition of MALT1 protease activity is selectively toxic for activated B cell-like diffuse large B cell lymphoma cells. J Exp Med 2009;206(11):2313–20.

46. Kelly PN, Romero DL, Yang Y, et al. Selective interleukin-1 receptor-associated kinase 4 inhibitors for the treatment of autoimmune disorders and lymphoid malignancy. J Exp Med 2015;212(13):2189–201.

47. Suarez-Farinas M, Arbeit R, Jiang W, et al. Suppression of molecular inflammatory pathways by Toll-like receptor 7, 8, and 9 antagonists in a model of IL-23-induced skin inflammation. PLoS One 2013;8(12):e84634.

48. Goy A, Younes A, McLaughlin P, et al. Phase II study of proteasome inhibitor bortezomib in relapsed or refractory B-cell non-Hodgkin's lymphoma. J Clin Oncol 2005;23(4):667–75.

49. Dunleavy K, Pittaluga S, Czuczman MS, et al. Differential efficacy of bortezomib plus chemotherapy within molecular subtypes of diffuse large B-cell lymphoma. Blood 2009;113(24):6069–76.

50. Offner F, Samoilova O, Osmanov E, et al. Frontline rituximab, cyclophosphamide, doxorubicin, and prednisone with bortezomib (VR-CAP) or vincristine (R-CHOP) for non-GCB DLBCL. Blood 2015;126(16):1893–901.

51. Davies AJ, Caddy J, Maishman T, et al. A prospective randomised trial of targeted therapy for diffuse large B-cell lymphoma (DLBCL) based upon real-time gene expression profiling: the RemodI-B study of the UK NCRI and SAKK lymphoma groups (ISRCTN51837425). Blood 2015;126(23):812.

52. Leonard JP, Kolibaba K, Reeves JA, et al. Randomized phase 2 open-label study of R-CHOP ± bortezomib in patients (Pts) with untreated non-germinal center B-cell-like (non-GCB) subtype diffuse large cell lymphoma (DLBCL): results from the pyramid trial (NCT00931918). Blood 2015;126(23):811.

53. Lee EC, Fitzgerald M, Bannerman B, et al. Antitumor activity of the investigational proteasome inhibitor MLN9708 in mouse models of B-cell and plasma cell malignancies. Clin Cancer Res 2011;17(23):7313–23.

54. Nowakowski GS, LaPlant B, Macon WR, et al. Lenalidomide combined with R-CHOP overcomes negative prognostic impact of non-germinal center B-cell phenotype in newly diagnosed diffuse large B-cell lymphoma: a phase II study. J Clin Oncol 2015;33(3):251–7.

55. Hernandez-Ilizaliturri FJ, Deeb G, Zinzani PL, et al. Higher response to lenalidomide in relapsed/refractory diffuse large B-cell lymphoma in nongerminal center B-cell-like than in germinal center B-cell-like phenotype. Cancer 2011;117(22): 5058–66.

56. Goldstein RL, Yang SN, Taldone T, et al. Pharmacoproteomics identifies combinatorial therapy targets for diffuse large B cell lymphoma. J Clin Invest 2015; 125(12):4559–71.

57. Monti S, Savage KJ, Kutok JL, et al. Molecular profiling of diffuse large B-cell lymphoma identifies robust subtypes including one characterized by host inflammatory response. Blood 2005;105(5):1851–61.

58. Caro P, Kishan AU, Norberg E, et al. Metabolic signatures uncover distinct targets in molecular subsets of diffuse large B cell lymphoma. Cancer Cell 2012;22(4): 547–60.

59. Ceribelli M, Kelly PN, Shaffer AL, et al. Blockade of oncogenic IkappaB kinase activity in diffuse large B-cell lymphoma by bromodomain and extraterminal domain protein inhibitors. Proc Natl Acad Sci U S A 2014;111(31):11365–70.

60. Chapuy B, McKeown MR, Lin CY, et al. Discovery and characterization of super-enhancer-associated dependencies in diffuse large B cell lymphoma. Cancer Cell 2013;24(6):777–90.

61. Odore E, Lokiec F, Cvitkovic E, et al. Phase I population pharmacokinetic assessment of the oral bromodomain inhibitor OTX015 in patients with haematologic malignancies. Clin Pharmacokinet 2015;55(3):397–405.

62. Boi M, Gaudio E, Bonetti P, et al. The BET bromodomain inhibitor OTX015 affects pathogenetic pathways in preclinical B-cell tumor models and synergizes with targeted drugs. Clin Cancer Res 2015;21(7):1628–38.

63. Cheah CY, Fowler NH, Neelapu SS. Targeting the programmed death-1/programmed death-ligand 1 axis in lymphoma. Curr Opin Oncol 2015;27(5): 384–91.

64. Chen BJ, Chapuy B, Ouyang J, et al. PD-L1 expression is characteristic of a subset of aggressive B-cell lymphomas and virus-associated malignancies. Clin Cancer Res 2013;19(13):3462–73.

65. Laurent C, Charmpi K, Gravelle P, et al. Several immune escape patterns in non-Hodgkin's lymphomas. Oncoimmunology 2015;4(8):e1026530.

Diffuse Large B-Cell Lymphoma

Should Limited-Stage Patients Be Treated Differently?

Eva Giné, MD[a], Laurie H. Sehn, MD, MPH[b],*

KEYWORDS

- Limited-stage DLBCL • Risk factors • Radiotherapy • Immunotherapy
- Late relapses

KEY POINTS

- Limited-stage diffuse large B-cell lymphoma (DLBCL) patients usually present with a favorable clinical risk profile. In the rituximab era, patients with 0 to 1 risk factors have a survival rate greater than 90% at 5 years.
- Therapeutic approaches include combined-modality (immunochemotherapy and radiotherapy) versus immunochemotherapy-alone strategies. A PET-guided approach may facilitate individualized therapy.
- Current evidence does not support the requirement for radiotherapy in all patients. Patients with poor chemotherapy tolerance or evidence of chemotherapy resistance may benefit from the inclusion of radiotherapy.
- Late relapses can occur in limited-stage DLBCL. Repeat biopsy at relapse is highly recommended to guide further management and to enable ongoing translational research.

INTRODUCTION

Diffuse large B-cell lymphoma (DLBCL) presents as localized disease in about 25% to 30% of patients, which is of clinical relevance both in terms of prognosis and treatment.[1,2] Using a practical definition of limited stage, including patients who present with Ann Arbor stages I or II nonbulky (<10 cm) disease without B-symptoms, these cases have a superior outcome compared with advanced-stage patients (**Fig. 1**). Limited-stage DLBCL patients typically present with no or few clinical risk factors, which contributes to the favorable outcome observed. For this reason, a stage-modified International Prognostic Index (IPI) was specifically proposed for these cases.[3]

[a] Hospital Clínic of Barcelona and Institut d'Investigacions Biomèdiques August Pi i Sunyer (IDIBAPS), Carrer del Rosselló, 08036 Barcelona, Spain; [b] Centre for Lymphoid Cancer, British Columbia Cancer Agency and the University of British Columbia, 600 West 10th avenue, Vancouver, BC V5Z 4E6, Canada
* Corresponding author.
E-mail address: Lsehn@bccancer.bc.ca

Hematol Oncol Clin N Am 30 (2016) 1179–1194
http://dx.doi.org/10.1016/j.hoc.2016.07.010
0889-8588/16/© 2016 Elsevier Inc. All rights reserved.

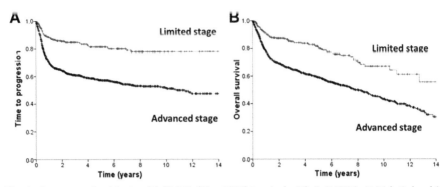

Fig. 1. Outcome of subjects with DLBCL (N = 1665) treated with R-CHOP in British Columbia between 2001 and 2015 according to stage of disease; limited (n = 361) or advanced stage (n = 1304). (A) Time to progression. (B) Overall survival (unpublished data from BC Cancer Agency).

Currently, there is no standard management approach for limited-stage DLBCL. A variety of treatment options exist, relying on either short or full-length courses of immunochemotherapy, with or without radiotherapy.[2,4,5] However, the role of radiotherapy in the rituximab era must be redefined and the use of PET-guided strategies should be explored. At present, overall outcome is excellent with expected 5-year overall survival (OS) and progression-free survival (PFS) above 90% and 80%, respectively. However, a delayed pattern of relapse has been observed and seems to persist despite the introduction of rituximab.[6,7] Whether this reflects a unique biology for limited-stage DLBCL deserves further investigation.[7,8] The aim of this article is to review the key literature in limited-stage DLBCL and how it may serve to guide current practice. Central nervous system, testicular, and primary mediastinal B-cell lymphoma are excluded because their unique biological and clinical features require specific consideration.

DEFINITION OF LIMITED-STAGE DIFFUSE LARGE B-CELL LYMPHOMA AND PROGNOSTIC FACTORS

Limited-stage DLBCL, similar to its pseudonyms, early-stage or localized DLBCL, lacks a precise definition. Limited stage is typically defined as patients who present with Ann Arbor stages I or II nonbulky disease that is confinable within a radiation field. Additional risk factors, such as lack of B-symptoms, have also been incorporated within the definition; however, these have varied among different studies, making cross-trial comparisons difficult. Similarly, the threshold used to define bulk has varied between the studies, with 10 cm most commonly used, which may further affect reported outcomes.[9]

Because most limited-stage DLBCL patients present with a favorable risk profile, the IPI is of limited utility. As such, investigators of the Southwest Oncology Group (SWOG) introduced a stage-modified IPI to better stratify patients according to risk of progression and survival (**Table 1**).[3,5,10–12] The stage-modified index retains age, lactate dehydrogenase, and performance status as risk factors but redefines stage II as a negative prognostic factor and eliminates the number of extranodal sites, which is applicable only for advanced disease. Of note, the stage-modified IPI has been validated in retrospective series both in the pre-rituximab and rituximab era.[6,13] More recently, the newly described National Comprehensive Cancer Network (NCCN)-IPI[12] has also been evaluated in a retrospective series of localized DLBCL and may be the most powerful prognostic index in patients receiving immunochemotherapy.[14]

Table 1
Prognostic indices in diffuse large B-cell lymphoma

Risk Factor	Risk Group	Pre-Rituximab Era 5-y OS (%)	Rituximab Era 3-y OS (%)
IPI[5,10,a]			
Age >60 y	Low (0–1)	73	91
LDH >Normal	Low-intermediate (2)	51	81
Stage III-IV	High-intermediate (3)	43	65
PS 2–4	High (4–5)	26	59
Extranodal >1	*R-IPI*[11,a]		
	Very good (0)	—	94
	Good (1–2)	—	79
	Poor (3–5)	—	55
aa-IPI[10,a]			
LDH >Normal	Low (0)	83	98
Stage III-IV	Low-intermediate (1)	69	92
PS 2–4	High-intermediate (2)	46	75
	High (3)	32	75
Stage-Modified IPI[3]			
Age >60 y	0–1 risk factor	82	93[b]
Stage II	2 risk factors	71	76[b]
LDH Increased	3 risk factors	48	55[b]
PS >1			
NCCN-IPI[12,a]			
Age, Years	Low 0–1	—	94
>40 to ≤60 (1)[d]	L-I 2–3	—	72
>60 to ≤75 (2)[d]	H-I 4–5	—	54
>75 (3)	High ≥6	—	35
LDH Normalized			
>1 to ≤3 (1)			
>3 (2)			
Ann Arbor III-IV (1)			
Extranodal[c] (1)			
PS ≥2 (1)			

Abbreviations: aa-IPI, age-adjusted IPI for patients ≤60 years; LDH, lactate dehydrogenase; NCCN, National Comprehensive Cancer Network; PS, performance status; R-IPI, revised-IPI.

[a] IPI, R-IPI, aa-IPI, and NCCN-IPI survival data include advanced-stage DLBCL. Survival data extracted from original prognostic index publications, Ref. 5, and unpublished results from British Columbia Cancer Agency (BCCA) series of limited-stage DLBCL treated in the rituximab era.

[b] 5-year OS in the BCCA series of limited-stage DLBCL subjects (n = 361).

[c] Extranodal disease in bone marrow, central nervous system, liver or gastrointestinal tract, or lung.

[d] Risk score applied for prognostic factor in the NCCN-IPI.

Based on the stage-modified IPI, patients with 0 or 1 adverse clinical risk factors have an excellent outcome, with an OS of more than 90% at 5 years. Consideration of less intensive strategies may be appropriate for this subgroup. In contrast, patients with 2 or more clinical risk factors have a moderately favorable outcome, with a 5-year OS of approximately 75%. Identifying the 20% to 25% of patients who will ultimately fail is an important challenge because this would allow for an individualized treatment approach. Improved insight into the biology of DLBCL and the availability of molecular markers to enable better prognostication will be paramount for this group (**Fig. 2**).

The observation that limited-stage DLBCL patients more frequently exhibit delayed relapses compared with advanced-stage patients has led to the speculation that this

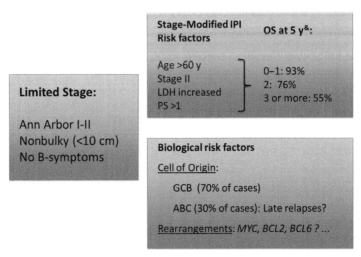

Fig. 2. Practical definition of limited-stage disease in DLBCL and outcome according to stage-modified IPI in the rituximab era. &, data from BCCA, unpublished series; ABC, activated B-cell; GCB, germinal center B-cell; LDH, lactate dehydrogenase. (*Data from* n=361 with limited-stage DLBCL treated in the rituximab era at British Columbia Cancer Agency, unpublished results.)

may represent unique biology. To date, there are few data evaluating the biological differences between limited-stage and advanced-stage patients. In a recent retrospective analysis using the Lymph2Cx assay to determine cell of origin (COO), patients with limited-stage DLBCL were found to have predominantly a germinal center B-cell (GCB) subtype, representing approximately 70% of cases. In addition, similar to what has been shown largely for advanced-stage cases, the activated B-cell (ABC) subtype is associated with worse outcomes.[15] Interestingly, it seems that delayed relapses are not observed in the GCB subgroup (**Fig. 3**).[15] A recent study using the Hans algorithm

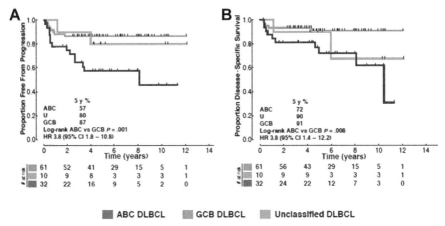

Fig. 3. Outcome of patients with limited-stage DLBCL treated with R-CHOP according to COO classification by Lymph2Cx. (*A*) Progression-free survival. (*B*) Disease-specific survival. (*From* Scott DW, Mottok A, Ennishi D, et al. Prognostic significance of diffuse large B-cell lymphoma cell of origin determined by digital gene expression in formalin-fixed paraffin-embedded tissue biopsies. J Clin Oncol 2015;33(26):2848–56; with permission.)

for COO classification has also observed a higher proportion of GCB subtype (75%) in limited-stage DLBCL, although no difference in outcome according to COO was observed, possibly due to the limitations of classification by immunohistochemistry.[13] At present, there is no information on the frequency or prognostic impact of *MYC*, *BCL2*, or *BCL6* rearrangements within limited-stage DLBCL patients and it is unknown whether this should influence treatment decisions.

CLINICAL STUDIES IN THE PRE-RITUXIMAB ERA

Most of the therapeutic evidence collected from randomized clinical trials in limited-stage DLBCL comes from studies conducted before the introduction of rituximab (**Table 2**).[3,7,16–18] Undoubtedly, among the 4 randomized trials comparing combined modality approaches with radiotherapy to chemotherapy alone, the most influential was the SWOG 8736 (S8736) study, which demonstrated the superiority at 5 years of 3 cycles of cyclophosphamide, doxorubicin, vincristine, and prednisone CHOP followed by IFRT compared with 8 cycles of CHOP alone.[3] The initial results of this study not only confirmed the lesser toxicity of a combined modality approach over full-length CHOP but also its superiority in terms of local control of disease and OS. This resulted in the broad adoption of 3 cycles of CHOP and IFRT as the standard of care for limited-stage DLBCL. However, in an updated analysis, the improvement in PFS and OS with abbreviated chemotherapy and IFRT disappeared at 7 to 9 years of follow-up due to a higher number of delayed relapses and death from lymphoma in that cohort.[19] In the final analysis of S8736 with a median follow-up time of 17.7 years, the 2 arms had almost an identical median OS of approximately 13 years and a similar pattern of delayed relapses without a plateau being observed.[7] Although this trial suggests that the use of IFRT may offer a short-term advantage, it also raises the concern that abbreviated chemotherapy may be insufficient for some patients because most relapses in the combined modality arm occurred outside of the radiation field.

A separate randomized trial performed by the Eastern Cooperative Oncology Group (ECOG) evaluated the benefit of the addition of IFRT following 8 cycles of CHOP.[16] Subjects who achieved a complete remission (CR) after CHOP were randomized to observation versus IFRT, whereas subjects who achieved only a partial remission (PR) all received IFRT. Although a borderline improvement in disease-free survival was noted with the use of IFRT in those who achieved a CR, no OS benefit was seen.[16] Subjects in PR who received IFRT had a better outcome than expected, suggesting a possible benefit in patients with an incomplete response to chemotherapy.

In a third trial, the intensive chemotherapy regimen of adriamycin, cyclophosphamide, vindesine, bleomycin, and prednisone (ACVBP) followed by consolidation with methotrexate, etoposide, ifosfamide, and cytarabine was compared with 3 cycles of CHOP and IFRT[17] in younger patients with limited-stage aggressive lymphoma. The ACVBP regimen was associated with a better event-free survival (EFS) and OS, suggesting that highly effective chemotherapy may outweigh the advantage of IFRT. However, due to concerns for both acute and delayed toxicity associated with this intensive regimen, it was not widely adopted.

In the final randomized trial, elderly subjects with no IPI risk factors were treated with 4 cycles of CHOP with or without IFRT.[18] No difference in 5-year EFS or OS was noted between the arms, suggesting that in a good-risk population the addition of IFRT did not provide benefit after abbreviated chemotherapy.[18]

A direct comparison of the 4 randomized trials is difficult, because the subject populations differed with respect to histologic subtypes included, age range, IPI risk, and inclusion of bulky disease. However, some important conclusions can be drawn. First,

Table 2
Randomized and select phase II studies in limited-stage diffuse large B-cell lymphoma

Author	Study	Subjects (N)	Treatment	5-y PFS	5-y OS	Benefit for FT P (<.05)
Studies in the Pre-Rituximab Era						
Miller et al,[3] 1998	SWOG 8736	395[a]	CHOP × 3 + IFRT CHOP × 8	77 64	82 72	Yes (PFS & OS)
Stephens et al,[7] 2016	SWOG 8736 (final subset analysis)	308[b]	CHOP × 3 + IFRT CHOP × 8	11.1 y[h] 12 y[h]	13.7 y[h] 13 y[h]	No
Horning et al,[16] 2004	ECOG 1484	172[c] (in CR)	CHOP × 8 + IFRT CHOP × 8	73[i] 56	87 73	Disease-free survival only
Reyes et al,[17] 2005	GELA LNH-93-1	647[d]	CHOP × 3 + IFRT ACVBP	74[j] 82	81 90	No[k]
Bonnet et al,[18] 2007	GELA LNH-93-4	576[e]	CHOP × 4 + IFRT CHOP × 4	64[j] 61	68 72	No
Studies in the Rituximab Era						
Persky et al,[25] 2008	SWOG 0014	60[f]	R4 + CHOP × 3 + IFRT	88% at 4 y	92% at 4 y	—
Persky et al,[26] 2015	SWOG S0313	46[f]	CHOP × 3 + IFRT + ibritumomab	82% at 5 y	87% at 5 y	—
Lamy et al,[27] 2014	Lysa/Goelams Phase III 02–03	313[g]	R-CHOP × 4 or 6 + IFRT R-CHOP × 4 or 6	91[i] 87	95 90	No

Abbreviations: ACVBP, adriamycin, cyclophosphamide, vindesine, bleomycin, and prednisone; CHOP, cyclophosphamide, doxorubicin, vincristine, and prednisone; ECOG, Eastern Cooperative Oncology Group; RT, radiotherapy.

a Aggressive lymphomas (Working Formulation), excluded bulky disease in stage II.
b Only including DLBCL-like histologies.
c Aggressive lymphomas (Working Formulation), including bulky in 30% of cases.
d Aggressive lymphomas (WHO) in young patients (<61 years) with 0 aa-IPI risk factors and bulky in 12% of cases.
e Aggressive lymphomas (WHO) in old patients (>60 years) with 0 aa-IPI risk factors and bulky in 25% of cases.
f DLBCL in 56 cases (S0014) and 44 cases (S0313), nonbulky and with at least 1 adverse stage-modified IPI risk factor.
g DLBCL only and nonbulky (<7 cm).
h Median EFS and OS.
i Six-year disease-free survival.
j Five-year EFS.
k ACVBP superior both for EFS and OS (P<.05).

even in the pre-rituximab era, limited-stage DLBCL subjects had a favorable outcome with 5-year OS exceeding 70% independent of management strategy used. Second, none of the randomized trials demonstrated a clear long-term benefit of the addition of radiotherapy.

CLINICAL STUDIES IN THE RITUXIMAB ERA

The addition of rituximab to CHOP more than a decade ago represented a major therapeutic advance, with 4 randomized studies demonstrating a significant improvement in response rate, EFS, and OS in various subpopulations of DLBCL subjects.[8,20–23] None of these trials exclusively addressed limited-stage DLBCL but the MabThera International Trial (MINT) evaluated rituximab plus CHOP (R-CHOP) for 6 cycles in young subjects with good prognosis DLBCL (age-adjusted [aa]-IPI 0–1).[21,24] Approximately 70% of subjects included in this trial had stage I or II disease, and only 3% of cases had bulky disease greater than 10 cm; therefore, most of these subjects by definition had limited-stage DLBCL. Although the results for the limited-stage subgroup were not reported separately, at 6 years of follow-up the EFS and OS for subjects with disease less than 5 cm and without risk factors were excellent: 84% and 95%, respectively. Consequently, 6 cycles of R-CHOP was established as an acceptable treatment approach for this very favorable group of patients.[5,21,24] An ongoing randomized study, the FLYER trial from the German High-Grade Non-Hodgkin's Lymphoma Study Group will evaluate reducing the number of cycles of R-CHOP in young good-risk DLBCL subjects (aa-IPI = 0 and tumor mass diameter <7.5 cm).

Very few studies have evaluated treatment strategies exclusively for patients with limited-stage DLBCL in the era of rituximab. Available data are largely limited to several phase II trials, several retrospective studies, and only 1 randomized trial that has been preliminarily reported (see **Table 2**; **Table 3**).[13,25–34]

Two phase II trials performed by SWOG explored the benefit of adding immunotherapy to a combined modality approach and retrospectively compared these results to the landmark study S8736. The S0014 study included 60 subjects with limited-stage aggressive non-Hodgkin (NHL) and at least 1 risk factor from the stage-modified IPI, and added 4 doses of rituximab to 3 cycles of CHOP followed by IFRT.[25] The addition of rituximab resulted in PFS of 88% and OS of 92% at 4 years, and seemed to be a modest improvement compared with S8736. The second phase II study S0313, explored ibritumomab tiuxetan consolidation after 3 cycles of CHOP and IFRT in subjects with the same inclusion criteria as S0014.[26] The combination was demonstrated to be feasible and obtained a similar efficacy compared with S0014.

Several retrospective analyses have explored the role of radiotherapy in patients with DLBCL in the rituximab era and have yielded conflicting results.[13,28–34] A single-center series from MD Anderson Cancer Center reported a clear advantage for the use of radiation in patients with DLBCL, including the subset of limited-stage patients, in terms of both PFS and OS, using multivariate and match pair analysis.[28] In contrast, the results from other larger single-center studies focusing on limited-stage DLBCL could not show a clear advantage for the use of radiation.[13,31] Similarly, various multicenter studies could not demonstrate significant differences in outcome with the addition of radiation.[14,30,33] Finally, 1 registry study suggested an improved tolerance without any survival advantage for combined modality therapy in a cohort of elderly subjects,[32] whereas another population-based study reported an improved survival for subjects receiving radiotherapy, despite decreasing usage of this approach in recent years.[34]

Table 3
Retrospective studies in limited-stage diffuse large B-cell lymphoma

Rituximab Era

Author	Institution or Group	Subjects (N)	Treatment	5-y PFS	5-y OS	Benefit for RT P (<.05)
Phan et al,[28] 2010	MD Anderson	190[a]	R-CHOP × 6–8 + IFRT R-CHOP × 6–8	82 68	92 73	Yes[a] (PFS & OS)
Marcheselli et al,[29] 2011	Gruppo Italiano Studio Linfomi	63	R-CHOP × 6 + IFRT R-CHOP × 6	—	—	Yes (only EFS)
Terada et al,[30] 2012	Osaka Lymphoma Study Group	137	R-CHOP × 3–4 + RT R-CHOP × 6–8	89.7[b] 74.3[b]	96.2[b] 85.5[b]	No
Kwon et al,[31] 2015	Seoul National University Hospital	198[c]	R-CHOP × 6–8 + ILRT R-CHOP × 6–8	92.7[c] 83.9[c]	95[c] 87.1[c]	Yes (PFS and OS, multivariate analysis only)
Odejide et al,[32] 2015	SEER and Dana-Farber Lymphoma CRIS	874 (≥66 y)	R-CHOP 3–4 + RT R-CHOP × 6–8	—	77 76	No
Dabaja et al,[33] 2015	US NCCN	402	R-CHOP × 6–8 + IFRT R-CHOP × 6–8	83[d] 76[d]	91[d] 83[d]	Not clear (only univariate analysis)
Vargo et al,[34] 2015	National Cancer Database	59,000 (1998–2012)	Chemotherapy + RT Chemotherapy	—	82 75	Yes (OS)
Kumar et al,[13] 2015	Memorial Sloan-Kettering Cancer Center	261	R-CHOP × 3–4 R-CHOP × 3–4 + RT R-CHOP × 6 R-CHOP × 6 + RT	94 89 80 90	100 94 85 98	No

Abbreviations: ILRT, involved lesion radiotherapy; RT, radiotherapy.
[a] 121 of 190 limited-stage DLBCL treated with 6 tc 8 cycles of R-CHOP and 103 of 190 receiving RT (of those, 49 with bulky greater than 5 cm). Matched pair analysis also significant for RT improvement in limited-stage DLBCL.
[b] PFS and OS at 3 years.
[c] DLBCL including bulky (≥7 cm) in 30% and B-symptoms in 14% of subjects.
[d] Overall results including advanced-stage DLBCL for FFS and OS.

It should be noted that results from these retrospective studies are difficult to interpret. Rather than the use of radiation was not randomized in these populations, or provided in a consistent manner, inherent selection biases in terms of which subjects received radiation may be impossible to adequately control for, even within the context of multivariate analyses. Regardless, it would seem that the benefit of radiotherapy is marginal at best, when added to highly effective immunochemotherapy regimens.

In the rituximab era, there is only 1 randomized trial, 02-03 from Lysa/Goelams Group, that evaluates the role of radiotherapy in limited-stage DLBCL.[27] Subjects with nonbulky (<7 cm) limited-stage DLBCL were treated with 4 or 6 cycles of R-CHOP according to the number of stage-modified IPI risk factors (0 vs 1 or more) and those achieving a CR were randomized either to receive radiotherapy or watchful waiting. Subjects in partial metabolic response after the fourth cycle received 2 more cycles of R-CHOP and IFRT. Although these data have not yet been published, the preliminary results confirmed the excellent outcomes of these subjects with 5-year EFS and OS of 88% and 91%, respectively, and have not shown any advantage in adding radiotherapy after 4 or 6 cycles of R-CHOP in subjects achieving a CR. Regarding the 14% of subjects who were in PR after 4 cycles of R-CHOP, the addition of 2 more cycles of R-CHOP followed by radiotherapy seemed sufficient to obtain a similar outcome to CR subjects.

IS THERE STILL A ROLE FOR RADIOTHERAPY IN THE MANAGEMENT OF LIMITED-STAGE DIFFUSE LARGE B-CELL LYMPHOMA?

Historically, radiotherapy was the first available therapy to successfully cure a significant proportion of patients with localized aggressive NHL.[35] Subsequently, chemotherapy was incorporated with the aim of treating occult systemic disease and reducing the size of the radiation field, leading to a combined-modality approach,[3,36] which coexisted with a chemotherapy-only approach for these patients.[37] Early results from the SWOG S8736 trial were influential in increasing the use of combined-modality therapy, which largely became the standard of care.[3] However, the introduction of more effective immunochemotherapy and the lack of persuasive data confirming a long-term advantage to radiotherapy has called into question the need for radiotherapy in all patients.

The primary concern related to the routine use of radiotherapy is the associated toxicity, in particular the delayed effects, such as xerostomia, coronary artery disease, and secondary malignancies occurring in the radiation field. Moreover, the risk of such toxicities is higher in younger patients and can persist for more than 30 years after initial therapy.[38–40] Although the relative contribution of radiation to the overall toxicity observed in these patients is difficult to ascertain, data suggest that the risk is augmented with combined-modality approaches.[41] The proportion of subjects reported to experience secondary malignancies in older studies is between 10% and 15%, of which only 15% occur within the radiation field.[6,17,18] In DLBCL, no clear dose-response curve for the benefit of radiation has been described, suggesting that lower doses may not compromise outcome.[42–44] As a consequence, radiotherapy techniques have evolved over time, leading to the use of smaller fields and lower doses, potentially reducing toxicity. The use of limited-field radiation seems to maintain efficacy in limited-stage DLBCL.[31,45] A population-based study of the British Columbia Cancer Agency (BCCA),[45] suggested that involved-nodal radiotherapy, which significantly reduces the radiation volume, was equivalent to IFRT in terms of time to progression (TTP), PFS, and OS in patients treated before the rituximab era.

Longer follow-up is needed to evaluate the impact of limited-field radiotherapy on the global toxicity profile.

Because 4 randomized trials in the pre-rituximab era[7,16–18] and the first randomized trial in the R-CHOP[27] era failed to demonstrate a long term benefit for radiotherapy, the routine use of radiotherapy in all limited-stage DLBCL patients is no longer justifiable. However, certain clinical situations may continue to benefit from the improved local control offered by radiotherapy. In frail patients with poor chemotherapy tolerance, the use of a combined-modality approach may offer the most favorable risk-benefit ratio. In addition, patients in PR following chemotherapy may convert to long-term disease-free survivors after irradiation of the involved region. The routine use of radiation in patients with bulkier masses continues to be controversial. The MINT study demonstrated that the adverse prognostic impact of the maximum tumor diameter was linear, and could only be partially abrogated by rituximab.[46] A cut-off of 10 cm for consideration of bulky disease seemed appropriate in the rituximab era and these patients should continue to be considered as having advanced-stage disease. The ongoing UNFOLDER study of the German High-Grade Non-Hodgkin's Lymphoma Study Group is exploring R-CHOP-21 and R-CHOP-14, as well as the benefit of radiotherapy in young subjects with tumor masses greater than 7.5 cm. However, the 2 trial arms without radiotherapy were prematurely stopped in a planned interim analysis due to excess relapse.

In summary, the routine use of radiotherapy in the management of patients with limited-stage DLBCL seems to no longer be necessary. However, it may continue to serve a role in patients with poor tolerance to chemotherapy or in patients achieving only a PR after immunochemotherapy. The benefit of radiating bulkier masses greater than 7.5 cm is still a matter of debate and more data are needed to clarify this issue.

WHAT IS THE ROLE OF PET IMAGING IN LIMITED-STAGE DIFFUSE LARGE B-CELL LYMPHOMA PATIENTS?

PET imaging increases the accuracy of staging and response assessment in DLBCL and has become instrumental in guiding treatment choice and predicting outcome. A PET-guided therapeutic approach is being actively explored in limited-stage DLBCL patients; however, few published data are available at present. The preliminary results of randomized study 02-03 of Lysa/Goelams[27] (see previous discussion) suggests that patients achieving a complete metabolic response following immunochemotherapy do not require radiotherapy, whereas those in partial metabolic response after 4 cycles of R-CHOP may benefit from 2 more cycles of R-CHOP and radiotherapy.

In 2005, the BCCA adopted a PET-based treatment algorithm for limited-stage DLBCL subjects, with the rationale of selectively administering radiation therapy to those who remained PET-positive after 3 cycles of R-CHOP, whereas subjects who were PET-negative received 1 additional cycle of R-CHOP alone.[2] Up to 80% of the 134 subjects evaluated had at least 1 negative risk factor according to the stage-modified IPI. Most subjects were PET-negative (77%) and had a 3-year TTP of 92%, whereas subjects who were PET-positive (22%) had a 3-year TTP of 60%, despite receiving radiation therapy. At the time of analysis, 4 cycles of R-CHOP seemed to be effective in most cases of limited-stage DLBCL, whereas the addition of radiation therapy alone for PET-positive cases may be insufficient and alternative approaches should be considered.

According to these preliminary results, PET-guided tailored therapy may be a useful tool to direct the treatment of limited-stage DLBCL, although more experience is required to fully assess the merit of this approach.

EXTRANODAL DISEASE

Approximately 30% of patients with DLBCL present with primary extranodal disease. Although it is well recognized that presentation within certain sites, such as the central nervous system (CNS) or testicle, represent distinct entities with unique biology and prognosis, this is less clear for other sites of origin. At present, there are few data supporting selective therapeutic approaches based on extranodal site of origin. Different outcomes according to distinct extranodal sites of involvement have been described, although with controversial results.[47,48] In the pre-rituximab era, DLBCL localized to the head and neck was reported to have a worse prognosis than nodal cases, and the addition of radiation therapy did not translate into a survival benefit.[49] Moreover, these patients also had a survival improvement with the introduction of rituximab, whereas no value for radiotherapy usage could be demonstrated.[50] DLBCL involving Waldeyer ring has been reported to have a favorable outcome, and retrospective data have suggested that radiotherapy can be omitted in patients achieving CR following chemotherapy.[47,49] Similarly, gastrointestinal lymphomas have also been reported to have a favorable prognosis.[47] Primary bone DLBCL seems to carry a favorable prognosis when treated with immunochemotherapy,[51] whereas primary breast lymphoma may be associated with poor-risk features, such as ABC subtype and a risk of involvement of the contralateral breast or CNS.[52,53] Interestingly, retrospective studies performed in the rituximab era suggest that differences in outcome according to site of primary presentation (nodal or extranodal) are no longer apparent[54,55] and that radiotherapy does not add a significant survival benefit in extranodal cases.[14] Currently, the routine use of radiation therapy in extranodal DLBCL does not seem warranted.

PRACTICAL THERAPEUTIC APPROACH FOR LIMITED-STAGE DIFFUSE LARGE B-CELL LYMPHOMA IN THE RITUXIMAB ERA

Recommendations from NCCN[4] and the European Society for Medical Oncology (ESMO)[5] guidelines include various options for the treatment of limited-stage DLBCL. Briefly, NCCN guidelines propose that patients with nonbulky (<10 cm) stage I or II disease can be treated with either 3 cycles of R-CHOP followed by involved-site radiotherapy or up to 6 cycles of R-CHOP, with optional use of radiotherapy. ESMO guidelines do not stratify treatment recommendations according to stage of disease. However, in young, low-risk patients (aa-IPI = 0) with nonbulky disease, 6 cycles of R-CHOP without radiation therapy is recommended.

From a practical viewpoint, the selection of optimum therapy should take into account several factors, including performance status of the patient, site of disease involvement, and number of clinical risk factors. Frail patients with poor chemotherapy-tolerance, or patients with very localized disease in a site that is readily amenable to radiation, may benefit from a combined-modality approach that minimizes exposure to chemotherapy. Whereas, patients with higher risk according to the stage adjusted IPI may benefit from a longer course of chemotherapy. In addition, chemotherapy responsiveness as assessed by PET scanning may help to further guide therapeutic decisions. Suggested treatment options in the management of limited-stage DLBCL are summarized in **Table 4**.

The design of future treatment strategies for limited-stage DLBCL will need to integrate both clinical and biological features to rationally select optimal therapy and to incorporate novel targeted agents. Obtaining a new biopsy at relapse is highly recommended because it will provide additional biological insight. Ultimately, long-term follow-up will be crucial to evaluate the full impact on outcome of novel approaches.

Table 4
Treatment approaches in limited-stage diffuse large B-cell lymphoma

Treatment Approach	Regimen	Limited-Field Radiotherapy	Comments
Combined-modality	R-CHOP × 3 + RT	Always	• May be preferable for patients with poor chemotherapy tolerance • The involved area must be amenable to radiotherapy
Extended immunochemotherapy	R-CHOP × 6	No	• May be preferable for patients with several risk factors or in cases in which the involved area is not safely amenable to radiotherapy
PET-guided tailored approach	R-CHOP × 3–6 ± RT	PET-guided	• Approach under evaluation • The involved area has to be amenable to radiotherapy in case of partial metabolic response

SUMMARY

Limited-stage DLBCL patients usually present with a favorable clinical risk profile. In the rituximab era, patients with 0 to 1 risk factors have a survival rate above 90% at 5 years.

Therapeutic approaches include combined-modality (immunochemotherapy and radiotherapy) versus immunochemotherapy-alone strategies. A PET-guided approach may facilitate individualized therapy.

Current evidence does not support the requirement for radiotherapy in all patients. Patients with poor chemotherapy tolerance or evidence of chemotherapy resistance may benefit from the inclusion of radiotherapy.

Late relapses can occur in limited-stage DLBCL. Repeat biopsy at relapse is highly recommended to guide further management and to enable ongoing translational research.

REFERENCES

1. Sehn LH, Gascoyne RD. Diffuse large B-cell lymphoma: optimizing outcome in the context of clinical and biologic heterogeneity. Blood 2015;125(1):22–32.
2. Sehn LH. Chemotherapy alone for localized diffuse large B-cell lymphoma. Cancer J 2012;18(5):421–6.
3. Miller TP, Dahlberg S, Cassady JR, et al. Chemotherapy alone compared with chemotherapy plus radiotherapy for localized intermediate- and high-grade non-Hodgkin's lymphoma. N Engl J Med 1998;339(1):21–6.
4. Zelenetz AD. Guidelines for NHL: updates to the management of diffuse large B-cell lymphoma and new guidelines for primary cutaneous CD30+ T-cell lymphoproliferative disorders and T-cell large granular lymphocytic leukemia. J Natl Compr Canc Netw 2014;12(5 Suppl):797–800.

5. Tilly H, Gomes da Silva M, Vitolo U, et al. Diffuse large B-cell lymphoma (DLBCL): ESMO clinical practice guidelines for diagnosis, treatment and follow-up. Ann Oncol 2015;26(Suppl 5):v116–25.
6. Shenkier TN, Voss N, Fairey R, et al. Brief chemotherapy and involved-region irradiation for limited-stage diffuse large-cell lymphoma: an 18-year experience from the British Columbia Cancer Agency. J Clin Oncol 2002;20(1):197–204.
7. Stephens DM, Li H, LeBlanc ML, et al. Continued risk of relapse independent of treatment modality in limited stage diffuse large B cell lymphoma: final and long term analysis of Southwest Oncology Group study S8736. J Clin Oncol 2016; 34(25):2997–3004.
8. Coiffier B, Thieblemont C, Van Den Neste E, et al. Long-term outcome of patients in the LNH-98.5 trial, the first randomized study comparing rituximab-CHOP to standard CHOP chemotherapy in DLBCL patients: a study by the Groupe d'Etudes des Lymphomes de l'Adulte. Blood 2010;116(12):2040–5.
9. Miller TP. The limits of limited stage lymphoma. J Clin Oncol 2004;22(15):2982–4.
10. A predictive model for aggressive non-Hodgkin's lymphoma. The International Non-Hodgkin's Lymphoma Prognostic Factors Project. N Engl J Med 1993; 329(14):987–94.
11. Sehn LH, Berry B, Chhanabhai M, et al. The revised International Prognostic Index (R-IPI) is a better predictor of outcome than the standard IPI for patients with diffuse large B-cell lymphoma treated with R-CHOP. Blood 2007;109(5):1857–61.
12. Zhou Z, Sehn LH, Rademaker AW, et al. An enhanced International Prognostic Index (NCCN-IPI) for patients with diffuse large B-cell lymphoma treated in the rituximab era. Blood 2014;123(6):837–42.
13. Kumar A, Lunning MA, Zhang Z, et al. Excellent outcomes and lack of prognostic impact of cell of origin for localized diffuse large B-cell lymphoma in the rituximab era. Br J Haematol 2015;171(5):776–83.
14. Mian M, Marcheselli L, Rossi A, et al. A diachronic-comparative analysis for the identification of the most powerful prognostic index for localized diffuse large B-cell lymphoma. Ann Oncol 2014;25(12):2398–404.
15. Scott DW, Mottok A, Ennishi D, et al. Prognostic significance of diffuse large B-cell lymphoma cell of origin determined by digital gene expression in formalin-fixed paraffin-embedded tissue biopsies. J Clin Oncol 2015;33(26): 2848–56.
16. Horning SJ, Weller E, Kim K, et al. Chemotherapy with or without radiotherapy in limited-stage diffuse aggressive non-Hodgkin's lymphoma: Eastern Cooperative Oncology Group study 1484. J Clin Oncol 2004;22(15):3032–8.
17. Reyes F, Lepage E, Ganem G, et al. ACVBP versus CHOP plus radiotherapy for localized aggressive lymphoma. N Engl J Med 2005;352(12):1197–205.
18. Bonnet C, Fillet G, Mounier N, et al. CHOP alone compared with CHOP plus radiotherapy for localized aggressive lymphoma in elderly patients: a study by the Groupe d'Etude des Lymphomes de l'Adulte. J Clin Oncol 2007;25(7): 787–92.
19. Miller T, Leblanc M, Spier C, et al. CHOP alone compared to CHOP plus radiotherapy for early stage aggressive non-Hodgkin's lymphomas: update of the Southwest Oncology Group (SWOG) Randomized Trial. Blood 2001;98:724a–5a.
20. Coiffier B, Lepage E, Briere J, et al. CHOP chemotherapy plus rituximab compared with CHOP alone in elderly patients with diffuse large-B-cell lymphoma. N Engl J Med 2002;346(4):235–42.
21. Pfreundschuh M, Trümper L, Osterborg A, et al. CHOP-like chemotherapy plus rituximab versus CHOP-like chemotherapy alone in young patients with good-

prognosis diffuse large-B-cell lymphoma: a randomised controlled trial by the MabThera International Trial (MInT) Group. Lancet Oncol 2006;7(5):379–91.

22. Pfreundschuh M, Schubert J, Ziepert M, et al. Six versus eight cycles of bi-weekly CHOP-14 with or without rituximab in elderly patients with aggressive CD20+ B-cell lymphomas: a randomised controlled trial (RICOVER-60). Lancet Oncol 2008;9(2):105–16.

23. Habermann TM, Weller EA, Morrison VA, et al. Rituximab-CHOP versus CHOP alone or with maintenance rituximab in older patients with diffuse large B-cell lymphoma. J Clin Oncol 2006;24(19):3121–7.

24. Pfreundschuh M, Kuhnt E, Trümper L, et al. CHOP-like chemotherapy with or without rituximab in young patients with good-prognosis diffuse large-B-cell lymphoma: 6-year results of an open-label randomised study of the MabThera International Trial (MInT) Group. Lancet Oncol 2011;12(11):1013–22.

25. Persky DO, Unger JM, Spier CM, et al. Phase II study of rituximab plus three cycles of CHOP and involved-field radiotherapy for patients with limited-stage aggressive B-cell lymphoma: Southwest Oncology Group study 0014. J Clin Oncol 2008;26(14):2258–63.

26. Persky DO, Miller TP, Unger JM, et al. Ibritumomab consolidation after 3 cycles of CHOP plus radiotherapy in high-risk limited-stage aggressive B-cell lymphoma: SWOG S0313. Blood 2015;125(2):236–41.

27. Lamy T, Damaj G, Gyan E, et al. R-CHOP with or without radiotherapy in non-bulky limited stage diffuse large B cell lymphoma (DLBCL): preliminary results of the prospective randomized phase III 02-03 trial from the Lysa/Goelams group. Blood 2014;124(21):393.

28. Phan J, Mazloom A, Medeiros LJ, et al. Benefit of consolidative radiation therapy in patients with diffuse large B-cell lymphoma treated with R-CHOP chemotherapy. J Clin Oncol 2010;28(27):4170–6.

29. Marcheselli L, Marcheselli R, Bari A, et al. Radiation therapy improves treatment outcome in patients with diffuse large B-cell lymphoma. Leuk Lymphoma 2011;52(10):1867–72.

30. Terada Y, Take H, Shibayama H, et al. Short cycle of immunochemotherapy followed by radiation therapy compared with prolonged cycles of immunochemotherapy for localized DLBCL: The Osaka Lymphoma Study Gropus (OLSG) retrospective analysis. Blood 2012;120(21).

31. Kwon J, Kim IH, Kim BH, et al. Additional survival benefit of involved-lesion radiation therapy after R-CHOP chemotherapy in limited stage diffuse large B-cell lymphoma. Int J Radiat Oncol Biol Phys 2015;92(1):91–8.

32. Odejide OO, Cronin AM, Davidoff AJ, et al. Limited stage diffuse large B-cell lymphoma: comparative effectiveness of treatment strategies in a large cohort of elderly patients. Leuk Lymphoma 2015;56(3):716–24.

33. Dabaja BS, Vanderplas AM, Crosby-Thompson AL, et al. Radiation for diffuse large B-cell lymphoma in the rituximab era: analysis of the National Comprehensive Cancer Network lymphoma outcomes project. Cancer 2015;121(7):1032–9.

34. Vargo JA, Gill BS, Balasubramani GK, et al. Treatment selection and survival outcomes in early-stage diffuse large B-cell lymphoma: do we still need consolidative radiotherapy? J Clin Oncol 2015;33(32):3710–7.

35. Chen MG, Prosnitz LR, Gonzalez-Serva A, et al. Results of radiotherapy in control of stage I and II non-Hodgkin's lymphoma. Cancer 1979;43(4):1245–54.

36. Connors JM, Klimo P, Fairey RN, et al. Brief chemotherapy and involved field radiation therapy for limited-stage, histologically aggressive lymphoma. Ann Intern Med 1987;107(1):25–30.

37. Cabanillas F, Bodey GP, Freireich EJ. Management with chemotherapy only of stage I and II malignant lymphoma of aggressive histologic types. Cancer 1980;46(11):2356–9.
38. Hemminki K, Lenner P, Sundquist J, et al. Risk of subsequent solid tumors after non-Hodgkin's lymphoma: effect of diagnostic age and time since diagnosis. J Clin Oncol 2008;26(11):1850–7.
39. Mudie NY, Swerdlow AJ, Higgins CD, et al. Risk of second malignancy after non-Hodgkin's lymphoma: a British Cohort Study. J Clin Oncol 2006;24(10):1568–74.
40. Tward JD, Wendland MM, Shrieve DC, et al. The risk of secondary malignancies over 30 years after the treatment of non-Hodgkin lymphoma. Cancer 2006;107(1): 108–15.
41. Pirani M, Marcheselli R, Marcheselli L, et al. Risk for second malignancies in non-Hodgkin's lymphoma survivors: a meta-analysis. Ann Oncol 2011;22(8):1845–58.
42. Lowry L, Smith P, Qian W, et al. Reduced dose radiotherapy for local control in non-Hodgkin lymphoma: a randomised phase III trial. Radiother Oncol 2011; 100(1):86–92.
43. Longo DL. Combined-modality therapy for early-stage diffuse large B-cell lymphoma: knowing when to quit. J Clin Oncol 2015;33(32):3684–5.
44. Dorth JA, Prosnitz LR, Broadwater G, et al. Radiotherapy dose-response analysis for diffuse large B-cell lymphoma with a complete response to chemotherapy. Radiat Oncol 2012;7:100.
45. Campbell BA, Connors JM, Gascoyne RD, et al. Limited-stage diffuse large B-cell lymphoma treated with abbreviated systemic therapy and consolidation radiotherapy: involved-field versus involved-node radiotherapy. Cancer 2012; 118(17):4156–65.
46. Pfreundschuh M, Ho AD, Cavallin-Stahl E, et al. Prognostic significance of maximum tumour (bulk) diameter in young patients with good-prognosis diffuse large-B-cell lymphoma treated with CHOP-like chemotherapy with or without rituximab: an exploratory analysis of the MabThera International Trial Group. Lancet Oncol 2008;9(5):435–44.
47. López-Guillermo A, Colomo L, Jiménez M, et al. Diffuse large B-cell lymphoma: clinical and biological characterization and outcome according to the nodal or extranodal primary origin. J Clin Oncol 2005;23(12):2797–804.
48. Møller MB, Pedersen NT, Christensen BE. Diffuse large B-cell lymphoma: clinical implications of extranodal versus nodal presentation–a population-based study of 1575 cases. Br J Haematol 2004;124(2):151–9.
49. Mian M, Capello D, Ventre MB, et al. Early-stage diffuse large B cell lymphoma of the head and neck: clinico-biological characterization and 18 year follow-up of 488 patients (IELSG 23 study). Ann Hematol 2013. [Epub ahead of print].
50. Murawski N, Held G, Ziepert M, et al. The role of radiotherapy and intrathecal CNS prophylaxis in extralymphatic craniofacial aggressive B-cell lymphomas. Blood 2014;124(5):720–8.
51. Pilorge S, Harel S, Ribrag V, et al. Primary bone diffuse large B-cell lymphoma: a retrospective evaluation on 76 cases from French institutional and LYSA studies. Leuk Lymphoma 2016;1–7.
52. Cheah CY, Campbell BA, Seymour JF. Primary breast lymphoma. Cancer Treat Rev 2014;40(8):900–8.
53. Ryan G, Martinelli G, Kuper-Hommel M, et al. Primary diffuse large B-cell lymphoma of the breast: prognostic factors and outcomes of a study by the International Extranodal Lymphoma Study Group. Ann Oncol 2008;19(2):233–41.

54. Hui D, Proctor B, Donaldson J, et al. Prognostic implications of extranodal involvement in patients with diffuse large B-cell lymphoma treated with rituximab and cyclophosphamide, doxorubicin, vincristine, and prednisone. Leuk Lymphoma 2010;51(9):1658–67.

55. Gutiérrez-García G, Colomo L, Villamor N, et al. Clinico-biological characterization and outcome of primary nodal and extranodal diffuse large B-cell lymphoma in the rituximab era. Leuk Lymphoma 2010;51(7):1225–32.

Management of Relapsed Diffuse Large B-cell Lymphoma

Michael Crump, MD, FRCPC

KEYWORDS

- Relapsed/refractory DLBCL • Autologous transplant • Salvage chemotherapy
- Prognosis • CD20 antibody

KEY POINTS

- Although the addition of rituximab to primary chemotherapy has reduced the incidence of primary refractory diffuse large B-cell lymphoma (DLBCL), the outcome of such patients remains very poor.
- High-dose chemotherapy and autologous stem cell transplant (ASCT) remain standard for patients with relapsed/refractory DLBCL after rituximab-containing primary chemotherapy.
- Patients older than 60 years benefit from attempts at salvage therapy; data in patients older than 70 years are more limited.
- Current evidence suggests that rituximab should be included with second-line therapy.
- For those relapsing after, or who are not eligible for, ASCT, median survival is 6 to 8 months, and eligible patients should be enrolled in clinical trials of new agents for DLBCL.

INTRODUCTION

Diffuse large B-cell lymphoma (DLBCL) is the most common subtype of B-cell lymphoma in North America, representing 30% of all lymphomas in adults.[1] The incidence of this lymphoma increases with age, and, in North America, median age at diagnosis is approximately 65 years. Although overall survival (OS) has improved with the addition of the CD20 antibody rituximab to cyclophosphamide, doxorubicin, vincristine, and prednisone (R-CHOP) chemotherapy,[2–4] treatment failure still occurs in a significant proportion of patients with limited stage disease at presentation,[3,5,6] and up to half of patients with advanced stage disease.[4,7] With a median follow-up of 10 years, results from the GELA (Groupe d'Etude des Lymphomes de l'Adulte) randomized trial showed that 40% of patients in the R-CHOP arm developed progressive disease. more than 80% of progression events occurred within the first 3 years

Division of Medical Oncology and Hematology, Princess Margaret Cancer Centre, 610 University Avenue, Room 5-209, Toronto M5G 2M9, Canada
E-mail address: michael.crump@uhn.ca

Hematol Oncol Clin N Am 30 (2016) 1195–1213
http://dx.doi.org/10.1016/j.hoc.2016.07.004
0889-8588/16/© 2016 Elsevier Inc. All rights reserved.

hemonc.theclinics.com

after treatment, 10% occurred within years 4 and 5, and 10% after 5 years.[8] Ongoing recurrence risk is much lower in patients with stage I and II disease, but late recurrences do occur.[5,6] Some late recurrences may represent reemergence of an indolent lymphoma histology,[9] emphasizing the need for biopsy of all such patients before the initiation of therapy. In a series of patients with recurrence of lymphoma more than 5 years from completion of therapy (median time to relapse 7.4 years, range 5–20 years), two-thirds had stage I/II disease at diagnosis and more than 80% had low-risk International Prognostic Factors Index (IPI). Assessment of cell of origin according to the Hans algorithm showed that such recurrences have a germinal center B-cell immunophenotype, and have other characteristics of germinal center B cells.[9,10]

What is the expected outcome of patients who progress or relapse after initial treatment? In the pre-rituximab era, despite the availability of high-dose chemotherapy and autologous stem cell transplant (ASCT), median survival after progression or relapse for patients treated with CHOP or equivalent combination regimens was only 9 months, and 2-year survival was 30%.[11] In more than 3000 patients with aggressive lymphoma treated on GELA trials over the last 20 years, OS of patients with primary refractory lymphoma was 12% at 7 years; those with late relapse more than 1 year after therapy had 7-year OS of 38%.[12] Among the patients with late relapse more than 5 years after primary therapy reported by Larouche and colleagues,[9] 5-year event-free survival from relapse was only 17% and OS 27%, suggesting that late relapse did not portend a good prognosis. Event-free survival seemed to be better for patients who underwent intensive therapy with ASCT compared with standard-dose treatments (56% vs 18%), although patient selection and inclusion of those refractory to salvage chemotherapy in the standard-dose therapy group likely account for some of this apparent difference.

HIGH-DOSE CHEMOTHERAPY AND AUTOLOGOUS STEM CELL TRANSPLANT FOR RELAPSED AND REFRACTORY DIFFUSE LARGE B-CELL LYMPHOMA

Although understanding of the diverse biology of DLBCL has evolved, and patient subsets defined by molecular profiles such as cell of origin may start to guide therapy at the time of diagnosis and at relapse, high-dose chemotherapy with ASCT support is still regarded as the standard of care for eligible patients with relapsed and refractory DLBCL. The randomized trial reported by Phillip and colleagues[13] in 1995 forms the basis of this recommendation even now. To be eligible for the Parma trial, all patients had a complete response (CR) to prior anthracycline-containing induction treatment, and patients with central nervous system (CNS) or bone marrow involvement at the time of relapse were excluded. Salvage therapy consisted of dexamethasone, cisplatin, and cytarabine (DHAP) and bone marrow was the source of stem cells, harvested following 1 course of DHAP. Patients with a CR or partial response (PR) after 2 cycles of DHAP were randomized to continuation with DHAP for 4 cycles or high-dose chemotherapy with carmustine, etoposide, cytarabine, and cyclophosphamide (BEAC). Radiotherapy was indicated in both arms for bulky disease larger than 5 cm at the time of relapse, using involved field radiation according to Ann Arbor staging. For patients in the high-dose therapy arm, the total dose of radiation was 26 Gy given twice daily before transplant, whereas in the standard arm radiation was 35 Gy in 20 fractions given following completion of DHAP.[13]

Patients undergoing ASCT for DLBCL now differ from those enrolled in this small trial reported 20 years ago: patients in the Parma trial all had a CR to first-line therapy, and were less than or equal to 60 years of age at randomization; none had transformed lymphoma, and no patient had received the CD20 antibody rituximab. Patients currently considered for salvage chemotherapy with curative intent are up to age 70 years or older, may have relapsed with CNS involvement, may have primary refractory disease, and have been treated with chemoimmunotherapy including rituximab. Although the treatment environment is currently different, other lessons from this trial remain important, including the influence of disease biology on treatment outcome: patients with higher number of IPI risk factors at relapse, and those with remission less than 1 year, derive less benefit from attempts at salvage therapy and ASCT,[14–16] and these factors have been used to stratify patients in recent randomized trials of salvage therapy. Tissue biomarkers for response to salvage therapy and ultimate outcome of stem cell transplant have been evaluated in the context of single-center reports and the randomized CORAL (collaborative trial in relapsed aggressive lymphoma) trial, suggesting that further evaluation of results according to cell of origin or presence of high-risk cytogenetic changes such as CMYC translocation are warranted.[17–20] At present, tissue biomarkers have not identified a population of patients who have an excellent prognosis, wherein omission of ASCT from second-line therapy could be considered, or a subgroup destined to receive no benefit from aggressive salvage therapy. The specific application of intensive therapy to patients with transformed lymphoma or those with dual translocation (double-hit) DLBCL are discussed elsewhere.

CHOICE OF SALVAGE THERAPY BEFORE AUTOLOGOUS STEM CELL TRANSPLANT

Recent randomized trials have explored essential questions in the application of high-dose therapy for relapsed or refractory DLBCL (**Table 1**). An important study by the HOVON (Dutch-Belgium cooperative trial group) showed that the addition of rituximab to salvage chemotherapy for relapsed DLBCL expressing CD20 resulted in significant improvement in response rate (75% vs 54%), failure-free survival at 24 months (50% vs 24%), and progression-free survival (PFS; 52% vs 31%).[21] Cox analysis adjusted for duration of first remission, performance status, and relapse IPI showed

Table 1
Randomized trials of salvage therapy before ASCT

	N	Results
CD20 Antibody		
DHAP/VIM/DHAP + rituximab[21]	239	RR: R-chemo, 74%; chemo, 54%
		PFS: R-chemo, 52%; chemo, 31%
Rituximab + DHAP vs ofatumumab + DHAP[26]	447	RR: ofatumumab, 38%; R, 42%
		2-y PFS: ofatumumab, 21%; R, 28%
		2-y OS: ofatumumab, 41%; R, 36%
Chemotherapy		
R-ICE vs R-DHAP[22]	477	CR/CRu R-ICE, 36%; R-DHAP, 40%
		RR R-ICE, 63%; R-DHAP, R-ICE, 64%
		3-y PFS, 31% vs 42%
		3-y OS, 47% vs 51%
GDP vs DHAP[23]	619	CR/CRu GDP, 13.5% vs DHAP, 14.3%
		RR GDP, 45.1% vs DHAP, 44.1%
		4-y EFS, 26% vs 28%
		4-y OS, 39% vs 39%

Abbreviations: Chemo, chemotherapy; EFS, event-free survival; GDP, gemcitabine, dexamethasone, cisplatin; ICE, ifosfamide, carboplatin, etoposide; OS, overall survival; PFS, progression-free survival; R, rituximab; RR, response rate; VIM, etoposide, ifosfamide, methotrexate.

an improvement in OS at 24 months favoring the addition of rituximab; most importantly, most patients enrolled in this trial were rituximab naive.

Two randomized trials have addressed choice of the optimum salvage chemotherapy before ASCT. The COHAL trial conducted by Gisselbrecht and colleagues[22] compared ifosfamide, carboplatin, and etoposide plus rituximab (R-ICE) with DHAP plus rituximab (R-DHAP). The primary end point of this superiority trial was mobilization-adjusted response rate after 3 cycles of chemotherapy (considering patients whose stem cell mobilization failed to achieve the target of 2×10^6 CD34 cells/kg as having experienced treatment failure, regardless of response). This trial showed a similar CR rate for R-ICE versus R-DHAP (36% vs 40%), overall response rate (63% vs 64%) and mobilization-adjusted response (52% vs 54%); ASCT with BEAM (carmustine, etoposide, cytarabine, melphalan) was performed in 51% of patients receiving R-ICE and 55% of patients receiving R-DHAP. Event-free survival and PFS were similar between the two induction regimens. The NCIC-CTG study LY.12 compared gemcitabine, dexamethasone, cisplatin (GDP) with DHAP in a noninferiority design; secondary end point was stem cell mobilization rate.[23] Rituximab was added to both chemotherapy arms for patients with CD20+ lymphoma part way through this study, through protocol amendment. This study was positive, reaching its noninferiority threshold of a difference between the study arms of less than 10%: overall response rate (CR/complete response unconfirmed (CRu), PR) following 2 cycles of GDP was 45%, compared with 44.1% for DHAP. Transplantation rates were also similar between the two study arms: GDP 51.0%, DHAP 48.9%.[19] PFS and OS at 4 years were not different between the two arms. However, DHAP chemotherapy produced significantly greater acute toxicity and need for hospitalization to manage adverse events, and GDP represents a highly cost-effective alternative to DHAP.[24]

In an effort to improve results of salvage therapy, alternative antibodies to rituximab have been tested. Matasar and colleagues[25] reported a phase II trial of the addition of the fully human monoclonal CD20 antibody ofatumumab to ICE or DHAP chemotherapy before ASCT, with an overall response in patients with refractory disease or early relapse of 55% and CR rate of 30%. However, in a randomized comparison of ofatumumab with rituximab in combination with the same salvage therapy, no differences in response rate or PFS were observed.[26]

CONDITIONING REGIMENS FOR AUTOLOGOUS STEM CELL TRANSPLANT FOR DIFFUSE LARGE B-CELL LYMPHOMA

The rationale for ASCT is to use high doses of chemotherapy to overcome drug resistance, and several regimens have historically been used based on institutional experience. There are no prospective randomized comparisons of the chemotherapy components of the high-dose therapy regimens with stem cell support for aggressive lymphomas. The impact of conditioning regimen on outcome with ASCT for lymphomas was recently reported by collaborators at the Center for International Blood and Marrow Transplant Research, including 1837 patients treated with ASCT for DLBCL.[27] The key outcomes of this large registry analysis are shown in **Table 2**. There were differences observed among the most commonly used intensive therapy regimens in recipient age, duration of follow-up, and prior rituximab exposure; age-adjusted IPI was similar across the cohorts. The choice of regimen had no independent influence on treatment-related mortality (TRM), which was higher patients who were older, had worse performance status, had chemotherapy-resistant disease, and had a larger number of prior therapy regimens.[28] The incidence of idiopathic pneumonia syndrome (IPS), an important cause of transplant-related morbidity and

Table 2
Outcomes post-ASCT for DLBCL according to intensive therapy regimen

Outcome at 3 y	BEAM N = 731	CBV^{LOW} N = 465	CBV^{HIGH} N = 187	BU-CY N = 273
Relapse/Progression (%)	44 (40–47)	40 (36–45)	46 (40–54)	41 (35–47)
PFS (%)	47 (44–51)	47 (43–52)	39 (32–44)	45 (39–52)
OS (%)	58 (55–62)	55 (50–59)	43 (35–51)	52 (46–58)
1-y Treatment-related Mortality (%)	4 (3–5)	7 (5–8)	8 (6–11)	7 (6–9)

Abbreviations: BEAM, carmustine (BCNU), etoposide, cytarabine, melphalan; BU-CY, busulfan + cyclophosphamide; CBV^{high}, cyclophosphamide, carmustine greater than 300 mg/m^2, etoposide; CBV^{low}, cyclophosphamide, carmustine less than 300 mg/m^2, etoposide.
Adapted from Chen YB, Lane AA, Logan BR, et al. Impact of conditioning regimen on outcomes for patients with lymphoma undergoing high-dose therapy with autologous hematopoietic cell transplantation. Biol Blood Marrow Transplant 2015;21:1046–53; with permission.

mortality, at 1 year ranged from 3% to 6% and was related to carmustine (BCNU) doses more than 300 mg/m^2, age, and chemotherapy-resistant disease; patients who experienced IPS had higher TRM. In this analysis, for patients with DLBCL undergoing ASCT with high-dose cyclophosphamide carmustine etoposide (CBV), relapse rate was similar to other high-dose regimens but overall mortality was higher, and the use of this regimen is not recommended.

In order to improve the efficacy of the BEAM regimen, trials of the addition of a radioimmunoconjugate to high-dose chemotherapy have been performed, with encouraging results.[29,30] The Bone Marrow Transplant Clinical Trials Network performed a randomized phase III trial comparing BEAM combined with rituximab or with ^{131}I tositumomab in patients with chemotherapy-sensitive DLBCL. Patients with persistent (PR to initial therapy) or relapsed DLBCL were included: after a median follow-up of 25 months, PFS was 48.6% for patients receiving rituximab-BEAM and 47.9% for patients receiving ^{131}I tositumomab-BEAM, with no difference in OS.[27] Time to neutrophil recovery and platelet transfusion independence were similar between the 2 high-dose treatments; grade 3 or greater mucositis was the only significant toxicity that was more frequent in the tositumomab arm. Day 100 transplant-related mortality was also similar in both arms (4.1% vs 4.9%).

THE PROBLEM OF PRIMARY REFRACTORY DIFFUSE LARGE B-CELL LYMPHOMA

Failure to achieve at least a PR following initial chemotherapy, or progression within 3 months of treatment completion, have been used to define primary refractory DLBCL.[31] Although the addition of rituximab has reduced the incidence of this from between 10% and 20% to between 5% and 10% in trials of up-front therapy,[2,3,32] the outcome of this patient population remains poor. Several studies suggest that this population may be enriched with lymphoma bearing molecular features such as dual expression of BCL2 and CMYC protein and presence of cmyc translocation, alone or with bcl2 or bcl6 translocation (double-hit lymphoma). The response rate to salvage therapy in patients with primary refractory DLBCL who are potentially eligible for ASCT is significantly lower than for those who experience relapse after achieving complete remission.[23,33,34] Although patients with primary refractory DLBCL may still be considered for ASCT, the limitations of current salvage therapy regimens in this patient population need to be acknowledged in discussions of treatment options and outcomes, and enrollment of such patients in clinical trials of novel salvage therapy approaches is encouraged.

Patients with relapsed or primary refractory DLBCL whose lymphoma does not respond to initial salvage treatment (refractory relapse) represent an additional therapeutic challenge. Although many centers routinely offer second-line salvage (third-line chemotherapy) to this patient population, the proportion of patients who are able to proceed to ASCT is small. Seshadri and colleagues[35] evaluated 120 patients with DLBCL who had no response to or progression after cisplatin-containing salvage treatment before intended ASCT; the response rate to a second salvage regimen was 14% (10 out of 71; 1 CR, 9 partial PRs) and only 1 of 43 patients who were primary refractory to CHOP responded to third-line therapy. In this series, only 8 of 71 patients receiving second-line salvage therapy were able to proceed to ASCT, with PFS at 2 years of 31%. In an analysis of patients in the CORAL trial who did not proceed to ASCT because of treatment failure after initial salvage with R-ICE or R-DHAP, the response rate to second salvage for those with stable or progressive disease was 32% (43 out of 135), and 44 patients ultimately underwent autologous (n = 37) or allogeneic (n = 7) transplant.[36] Median survival for those undergoing transplant was 10.6 months, and 2-year OS was 34%; PFS for this group of patients was not reported. Patients with low-risk IPI scores and who are not refractory to primary therapy may benefit from a second salvage attempt, but the probability of undergoing ASCT and long-term PFS are very low in this population.

There are currently no data to support the notion that patients with primary refractory DLBCL derive greater benefit from matched related or unrelated allogeneic stem cell transplant compared with ASCT. A recent report from the European Society for Blood and Marrow Transplantation (EBMT) Lymphoma Working Party[37] showed that 4-year non-relapse mortality is significantly higher for patients receiving allogeneic transplant (either myeloablative or reduced-intensity conditioning), and 4-year PFS and OS were superior for patients undergoing ASCT for relapsed or refractory DLBCL. After adjusting for baseline factors (including chemotherapy-resistant lymphoma, which was more common in patients receiving an allotransplant), relapse incidence was not different between patients undergoing ASCT or allogeneic transplant, although mortality was significantly worse for patients receiving an allogeneic transplant (**Fig. 1**). PFS at 4 years for patients with chemorefractory disease was 23% for ASCT, 20% for myeloablative allotransplant, and 4% for reduced-intensity allotransplant.

CENTRAL NERVOUS SYSTEM RECURRENCE OF DIFFUSE LARGE B-CELL LYMPHOMA

Relapse or progression in the CNS is an uncommon but generally fatal event in patients with DLBCL. There is considerable controversy over the population of patients who are at increased risk of CNS relapse, and the benefit of prophylactic therapies such as intrathecal (IT) chemotherapy or high-dose methotrexate (HD-MTX) in reducing the rate of relapse in the CNS.[38–40] In the pre-rituximab era, most CNS progression occurred during or within 3 months of completion of systemic therapy.[11] Data from trials evaluating the addition of rituximab to CHOP suggest that CNS progression may be an early event in younger patients with high-intermediate or high IPI score at presentation, and the addition of rituximab has done little to reduce this risk.[38] In older patients, addition of rituximab has reduced the risk of CNS progression, although IPI at the time of diagnosis remains the most relevant risk factor for relapse in the CNS.[41] Risk of treatment failure in the CNS is very low in patients with low IPI regardless of age: the 2-year rate of CNS failure in the recent Cancer Research UK comparison of R-CHOP-21 with R-CHOP-14 was less than 1%.[32] Although specific sites of extranodal involvement have generally not been reliable predictors of CNS relapse, it has been

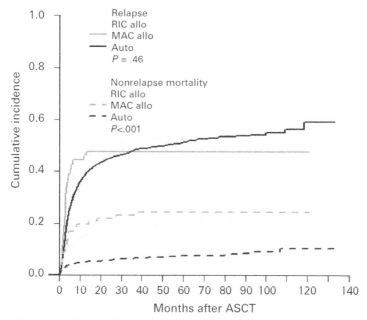

Fig. 1. Incidence of relapse and nonrelapse mortality for patients with DLBCL undergoing autologous transplant (Auto), myeloablative allotransplant (MAC allo), or reduced-intensity allotransplant (RIC allo). (*From* Robinson SP, Boumendil A, Finel H, et al. Autologous stem cell transplantation for relapsed/refractory diffuse large B-cell lymphoma: efficacy in the rituximab era and comparison to first allogeneic transplants. A report from the EBMT Lymphoma Working Party. Bone Marrow Transplant 2016;51(3):365–71; with permission.)

reported that CNS involvement at diagnosis and as a site of relapse is more common in patients with dual translocation or dual protein expression DLBCL, as discussed elsewhere.[42–44]

CNS recurrence of DLBCL portends a poor prognosis, with median survival ranging from 2 to 7 months.[11,45,46] Patients with isolated parenchymal brain recurrence after induction therapy may represent a unique patient subgroup with regard to treatment options and outcomes.[47] In one retrospective analysis of 110 patients (80% DLBCL), the median time to recurrence was 1.8 years, and following CNS-directed therapy with HD-MTX, whole-brain radiotherapy or both, median PFS was 1.0 years, with 23% of patients alive at 3 years. PFS and OS seemed to be better with the use of HD-MTX compared with whole-brain irradiation, although most second progression events still occurred in the CNS. These results must be interpreted cautiously, because considerable selection bias may underlie the choice of treatments received in this patient cohort collected from a large number of centers; specifically, the ability to administered HD-MTX versus whole-brain irradiation. HD-MTX is a reasonable treatment option for fit patients with good performance status and normal renal function. For most patients, whole-brain irradiation represents an important palliative treatment option, with an overall response rate of 67% and median survival of 8.6 months reported by Khimawi and colleagues[48] with 40-Gy whole-brain radiotherapy.

Earlier reports highlighted the poor outcome of patients with CNS involvement undergoing ASCT with CNS involvement, compared with patients with systemic relapse alone.[49] However, recent case series have suggested that long-term survival may be achieved in selected patients undergoing intensive therapy and ASCT.[50,51] A recent international retrospective collaboration reported that patients treated with ASCT (most commonly using thiotepa and carmustine) had improved 3-year survival compared with those not receiving intensive therapy (42% vs 14%).[46] It is likely that patient selection is partly responsible for these improved results, because the cohort reported was younger overall (median age 58 years) than expected for patients with DLBCL, and those undergoing ASCT had better performance status and chemotherapy-sensitive disease, compared with those not transplanted.[46]

However, prospective trials of ASCT have recently been reported, supporting the observation from retrospective series that some patients with secondary CNS lymphoma may benefit from this approach. Korfel and colleagues[52] evaluated induction treatment in 30 patients (6 with systemic involvement at study entry) with 2 cycles of HD-MTX and ifosfamide and IT liposomal ara-C, followed by high-dose cytarabine and thiotepa for stem cell mobilization. Twenty patients had a CR or PR to induction treatment and 24 proceeded to high-dose therapy with carmustine, thiotepa, and etoposide. Two-year time to treatment failure (TTF) was 49% for the whole cohort and 58% for those undergoing ASCT; OS at 2 years was 63%. Thirteen of 16 patients with treatment failure had CNS progression.

Ferrari and colleagues[53] reported a phase II multicenter study of high-dose sequential therapy in 38 patients with secondary CNS involvement with (n = 23) or without (n = 15) concomitant systemic lymphoma. Induction therapy consisted of rituximab with HD-MTX, cytarabine, and IT liposomal ara-C; responding patients had stem cell mobilization with ara-C or MTX, followed by additional therapy for those with systemic DLBCL. Twenty patients underwent intensive therapy with carmustine and thiotepa followed by ASCT. The CR rate to all therapy was 20 out of 38; event-free survival at 5 years was 40%, with events including progressive disease (PD) in 10 patients, relapse from CR in 7, and toxic death in 4 patients. Thirteen patients experienced relapse or progression in the CNS.

Intensive therapy and ASCT are appropriate therapy for patients with CNS relapse, with or without systemic recurrence, following response to CNS-directed therapy; high-dose therapy regimens containing agents that cross the blood-brain barrier, such as thiotepa and carmustine (with or without etoposide), seem to produce the best results. Regimen-related toxicity is significant but manageable with these approaches, and long-term follow-up of neurocognitive function in survivors is needed.[54]

SHOULD CD20 ANTIBODY TREATMENT BE ADDED TO SALVAGE CHEMOTHERAPY?

Despite the widespread use of rituximab in combination with second-line chemotherapy, prospective data supporting its role in this setting are sparse. The study by Vellenga and colleagues,[17] described previously, showed a clear benefit from the addition of rituximab to second-line therapy before ASCT for patients who were rituximab naive, and inclusion of rituximab in salvage therapy for such patients should be considered standard. However, most patients who currently experience treatment failure do so following R-CHOP or an equivalent rituximab-containing regimen. Several retrospective studies suggest that chemoimmunotherapy may be beneficial in the second-line setting, although these reports frequently include a mixture of patients with and without prior rituximab exposure.[55–57] Recently, Baetz and colleagues[58] reported on the results of salvage therapy with or without rituximab in the context of the NCIC-CTG LY.12 trial. Among patients with aggressive B-cell lymphoma and prior treatment with R-CHOP, overall response rates to GDP or DHAP were higher when rituximab was added to salvage therapy (51.9% vs 31.3%) and more patients were able to proceed to ASCT (45.6% vs 25.0%) compared with chemotherapy alone. Despite this, there was no improvement in event-free survival or OS for patients who underwent ASCT. However, when patients with primary refractory lymphoma (defined as progressive disease or less than a PR to induction therapy) were excluded, PFS and OS were statistically significantly better with the addition of rituximab to salvage therapy.[58] Although this is a retrospective analysis, it was undertaken within the context of a prospective randomized trial in which the addition of rituximab to salvage chemotherapy was instituted by a protocol amendment. It seems appropriate, based on current reports, to include rituximab as part of second-line therapy for patients who have achieved a response to primary chemoimmunotherapy, either before stem cell transplant or in the nontransplant setting. The retrospective analysis by Baetz and colleagues[58] was underpowered to assess the benefit of rituximab in R-CHOP-refractory patients, and the benefit of adding rituximab in this population is uncertain.

MANAGEMENT OF RELAPSED AND REFRACTORY DIFFUSE LARGE B-CELL LYMPHOMA IN OLDER PATIENTS
The Role of Autologous Stem Cell Transplant

Prospective trials evaluating high-dose therapy with ASCT support have generally restricted eligibility of patients to those aged less than 65 years. There is increasing awareness that with careful patient assessment, using comorbidity risk scoring and assessment of instrumental activities of daily living, intensive therapy and ASCT can be successfully used in fit patients more than 60 years of age.[59–61] There are numerous single-institution and transplant registry reports of outcomes in elderly patients with DLBCL undergoing ASCT. Some of these reports indicate higher rates of TRM compared with younger patients, especially for patients more than age 70 years, as well as worse outcomes with regard to relapse of lymphoma. However, because of the issues of patient selection, comparisons of treatment efficacy between patients more than 60 years of age and those younger has been difficult. Some investigators have reported outcomes in elderly patients according to the Hematopoietic Stem Cell Transplant Comorbidity Index (HCT-CI), developed for allogeneic transplantation.[62] In the study reported by Hosing and colleagues,[63] higher HCT-CI scores were predictive of increased grade 3 or greater toxicity but not TRM or OS. Elstrom and colleagues[64] reported 21 patients aged more than 70 years undergoing ASCT for DLBCL; in that small study, high-risk HCT-CI was predictive of significantly higher TRM and worse transplant outcomes. Additional data from prospective evaluation of older patients assessed with the HCT-CI are needed to understand the role of such indices in appropriate patient selection for ASCT.

A subanalysis of the NCIC-CTG LY.12 trial provides prospective data addressing the effectiveness of an aggressive approach using salvage therapy and ASCT in patients more than 60 years of age with relapsed DLBCL. This intention-to-transplant analysis showed that response rates to salvage chemotherapy (GDP or DHAP, with or without rituximab) was very similar between patients aged less than 60 years and those more than 60 years. Successful stem cell mobilization and ability to proceed to transplant were also comparable between the two age groups. Furthermore, TRM for those undergoing stem cell transplant was low in both age groups, and 2-year event-free survival after transplant seemed to be similar.[65] The number of patients enrolled in this trial more than 70 years of age was very small, and this study was undertaken without specific use of comorbidity indices to evaluate patient selection. Overall, it seems that patients between 60 and 70 years of age derive similar benefit from salvage therapy attempts with platinum-containing chemotherapy, and have similar long-term outcomes to younger patients following ASCT. Uncertainly remains as to the benefit of ASCT for relapsed and refractory DLBCL in patients more than 70 years of age, especially those with high risk HCT-CI assessments.[64,66]

Nontransplant Approaches to Older Patients with Relapsed and Refractory Diffuse Large B-cell Lymphoma

Age remains a significant risk factor for treatment failure with current chemoimmuno-therapy for DLBCL. This finding may reflect higher incidence of activated B cell sub-type and a greater incidence of CMYC translocation and protein overexpression in patients more than 60 years of age. Median survival of patients in the GELA trial following progression was 6 to 8 months, and long-term survival was achieved in only a minority of older patients not undergoing ASCT.[8] Intensive platinum-based salvage regimens such as R-ICE or R-DHAP are not appropriate for an older patient population in which the focus is on disease control and maintaining quality of life. Several gemcitabine-containing second-line regimens have been reported in this patient population, usually including oxaliplatin or cisplatin, and, where combination chemotherapy is deemed appropriate, these regimens have good disease control and acceptable toxicity (**Table 3**). Phase II trials suggest that PFS is on the order of 6 months, and response rate and PFS may be improved by the inclusion of rituximab, although this likely again applies to patients who were previously rituximab naive.

Retrospective studies of bendamustine in DLBCL with or without rituximab have also shown response rates of approximately 60% with relatively little toxicity. Ohmachi and colleagues[67] studied rituximab day 1 and bendamustine 120 mg/m^2 days 2 and 3 along with high-dose dexamethasone as antiemetic in 59 patients with relapsed DLBCL. Two-thirds of patients were aged 65 years or older and two-thirds had 1 prior regimen; only 8 of 59 were refractory to their last regimen. The overall response rate was 63%, and median PFS was 6.7 months. Cytomegalovirus (CMV) infection occurred in 6 patients (10%), which may have resulted from the significant lymphopenia and decrease in CD4+ lymphocytes seen with this bendamustine dose and anti-emetic schedule; antiviral prophylaxis and monitoring for CMV reactivation is recommended. This combination represents another effective and relatively nontoxic regimen, and forms the basis of novel combinations in DLBCL with the Bruton tyrosine kinase inhibitor ibrutinib.[68]

LOCAL RADIOTHERAPY FOR REFRACTORY DIFFUSE LARGE B-CELL LYMPHOMA

Radiation therapy is an important treatment consideration for patients with symptoms or impending organ compromise arising from large tumor masses. In a study by Haas and colleagues,[69] low-dose involved field radiotherapy (1 × 4 Gy or 2 × 2 Gy) was delivered to 71 patients with relapsed or refractory indolent and aggressive lymphoma (median 2 prior chemotherapy regimens), including elderly patients with localized symptomatic disease for whom systemic therapy was judged to be too toxic. In the subset of 30 patients with aggressive lymphoma, the overall response rate was 80%, with 37% of patients achieving CR, 43% achieving a PR, and 20% achieving disease stabilization. The median time to progression in this subgroup was 9 months, the median time to local progression was 20 months, and the median OS was 8 months.[69] Martens and colleagues[70] retrospectively reviewed local control and toxicity in 34 patients with chemotherapy-resistant lymphoma, including 14 with DLBCL, treated with hyperfractionated accelerated radiotherapy. The radiation dose was 39.9 to 40.5 Gy in 30 fractions, given twice daily. Seventeen patients had a CR/CRu, and 16 had a PR.

Table 3
Selected regimens for transplant-ineligible patients

Regimen	# of Patients with Recurrent NHL	ORR		PFS and OS	Toxicity
		CR (%)	PR (%)		
GDP[a,80]	17	23	29	Median PFS, 3 mo; Median OS, 9 mo	Neutropenia Gr 3/4, 33%/31%; Thrombocytopenia Gr 3/4, 26%/4%; Gr 2 ototoxicity, 25%; Gr 2 creat, 6%
Gem-Ox[b,81]	17	47	12	Median FFS, 9 mo	Neutropenia Gr 3, 35%; Gr 4, 16%; Thrombocytopenia Gr 3/4, 26%; Vomiting Gr 2–3, 34%; Infection Gr 2–3, 14%
Gem-Ox + rituximab[b,8?]	16	56	19	Median FFS, 18.5 mo	Neutropenia Gr 3, 29%; Gr 4, 18%; Thrombocytopenia Gr 3, 17%; Vomiting Gr 2–3, 34%; Infection Gr 2–3, 25%
Gemcitabine-vinorelbine[c,82]	22	14	35	Median TTP, 8 mo; Median OS, 13 mo	Neutropenia Gr 3–4, 41%; Thrombocytopenia Gr 3–4, 18%
Rituximab-gem-ox[d,83]	49	44[e]	17	Median PFS, 5 mo; 5-y PFS, 12%	Neutropenia Gr 3 31%, Gr 4 42%; Thrombocytopenia Gr 3 32%, Gr 4 21%; Gr 3/4 infection, 22% of cycles
Bendamustine-rituximab[f,67]	59	37	25	Median PFS, 6.7 mo	Neutropenia Gr3, 30%; Gr4, 46%; Thrombocytopenia Gr 3, 15%; Gr4, 7%; CD 4 lymphopenia Gr 3, 22%; Gr4, 44%; Infection Gr3, 12%

Abbreviations: FFS, failure-free survival; Gem-Ox, gemcitabine and oxaliplatin; Gr, grade; ORR, overall response rate; TTP, time to progression.

[a] GDP: gemcitabine 1000 mg/m² days 1 and 8, dexamethasone 40 mg days 1 to 4, cisplatin 75 mg/m² every 21 days.
[b] Gem-ox ± rituximab: gemcitabine 1200 mg/m² days 1 and 8, oxaliplatin 120 mg/m² day 2, rituximab 375 mg/m² day 1, every 3 weeks (gem-ox) or 2 weeks (gem-ox + R).
[c] Gemcitabine 1000 mg/m², vinorelbine 30 mg/m² days 1 and 8 every 21 days.
[d] Rituximab 375 mg/m² day 1, gemcitabine 1000 mg/m² + oxaliplatin 100 mg/m² day 2 every 14 days.
[e] Response assessed after 4 cycles.
[f] Rituximab 375 mg/m² day 1, bendamustine 20 mg/m² days 2 and 3 every 21 days.

Table 4
Potential new agents for the management of relapsed DLBCL

Agent (Ref)	DLBCL (N)	Response Rate (%)	Median PFS (mo)	Median Response Duration (mo)	Potential Biomarker for Response?
Lenalidomide[84,85]	26	CR, 3; PR, 2 (18)	ns	—	ABC subtype
	108	CR, 8; PR, 22 (28)	2.7	4.6	
Everolimus[86]	47	CR, 0; PR, 14 (30)	3.0	5.7	
Ibrutinib[87]	58	ABC, 14/38 (37)	2.0	4.8	ABC subtype
		GCB, 1/20 (5)	1.3	NS	
Obinutuzumab[88]	25	CR, 1; PR, 7 (28)	2.7	6.3	CD20+
Brentuximab vedotin[89]	48	CR, 8; PR, 13 (44)	4.0	5.8	CD30+

Abbreviations: GCB, germinal center B cell; NS, not stated.

The local control rate was 73% at 1, 2, and 3 years. The most commonly reported side effect was grade 1 dermatitis. This study suggests that hyperfractionated radiotherapy can provide durable local control without significant side effects.

NEW THERAPEUTIC AGENTS IN RELAPSED AND REFRACTORY DIFFUSE LARGE B-CELL LYMPHOMA

A complete review of developmental DLBCL therapy and the underlying biology is beyond the scope of this article. A large number of new drugs are currently undergoing testing, some based on rational targeting of pathways critical to the pathophysiology of DLBCL, and others further expanding the role of monoclonal antibodies and chemoimmunoconjugates (**Table 4**). Recent reports of exome sequencing studies of biopsy samples from patients with relapsed and refractory DLBCL describe numerous mutations in important signaling pathway genes that may influence sensitivity to emerging novel agents, such as CD79a, MYD88, JAK-STAT, NFκB, and XPO-1.[71,72]

For patients relapsing after ASCT or for whom ASCT is not indicated, a retrospective review by Nagle and colleagues[73] suggested that patients treated with novel approaches (alternative CD20 antibodies, lenalidomide, kinase inhibitors, or radioimmunotherapy) had superior survival compared with those treated with standard agents or supportive care alone. Although these favorable results may reflect obvious selection bias in patients treated with newer therapies, they do emphasize the need to consider clinical trials as the best option for fit patients who are refractory to their most recent systemic therapy. Early results of studies incorporating lenalidomide, ibrutinib, and other targeted agents into salvage chemotherapy,[74–77] and the use of new immunologic approaches such as chimeric antigen receptor T cells (CAR-T) and bispecific T cell–engaging antibodies,[78,79] are promising, and provide the next generation of treatment approaches to improve the outcome for patients with relapsed and refractory DLBCL.

SUMMARY

For patients with relapsed and refractory DLBCL, including patients up to age 70 years, those with transformed indolent lymphoma, and selected patients with CNS recurrence, the use of salvage chemotherapy with ASCT for those with chemotherapy-sensitive disease is the preferred initial approach. Among salvage chemotherapy regimens, the optimum treatment choice should consider toxicity, cost, and ability to collect peripheral blood stem cells; based on the randomized LY.12 trial, GDP represents an evidence-based treatment choice. For those who are not candidates for ASCT because of age or comorbidities, combination therapy may be considered, with myelosuppression usually the limiting toxicity. For this patient population, and those experiencing disease recurrence following ASCT, enrollment in a clinical trial of new, targeted agents is strongly recommended.

REFERENCES

1. Morton LM, Wang SS, Devesa SS, et al. Lymphoma incidence patterns by WHO subtype in the United States, 1992-2001. Blood 2006;107:265–76.
2. Coiffier B, Lepage E, Briere J, et al. CHOP chemotherapy plus rituximab compared with CHOP alone in elderly patients with diffuse large B-cell lymphoma. N Engl J Med 2002;346:235–42.
3. Pfreundschuh M, Trümpe L, Österborg A, et al. CHOP-like chemotherapy plus rituximab versus CHOP-like chemotherapy alone in young patients with

good-prognosis diffuse large-B-cell lymphoma: a randomized controlled trial by the MabThera International Trial (MInT) Group. Lancet Oncol 2006;7(5):379–91.

4. Feugier P, Van Hoof A, Sebban C, et al. Long term results of the R-CHOP study in the treatment of elderly patients with diffuse large B-cell lymphoma: A study by the Group D'Etude des Lymphomes de L'Adulte. J Clin Oncol 2005;23:4117–26.

5. Persky DO, Unger JM, Spier CM, et al. Phase II Study of rituximab plus three cycles of CHOP and involved-field radiotherapy for patients with limited-stage aggressive B-cell lymphoma: Southwest Oncology Group Study 0014. J Clin Oncol 2008;26(14):2258–63.

6. Lee AY, Connors JM, Klimo P, et al. Late relapse in patients with diffuse large-cell lymphoma treated with MACOP-B. J Clin Oncol 1997;15:1745–53.

7. Zhou Z, Sehn LH, Rademaker AW, et al. An enhanced International Prognostic Index (NCCN-IPI) for patients with diffuse large B-cell lymphoma treated in the rituximab era. Blood 2014;123(6):837–42.

8. Coiffier B, Thieblemont C, Van Den Neste E, et al. Long-term outcome of patients in the LNH-98.5 trial, the first randomized study comparing rituximab-CHOP to standard CHOP chemotherapy in DLBCL patients: a study by the Groupe d'Etudes des Lymphomes de l'Adulte. Blood 2010;116(12):2040–5.

9. Larouche JF, Berger F, Chassagne-Clément C, et al. Lymphoma recurrence 5 years or later following diffuse large b-cell lymphoma: clinical characteristics and outcome. J Clin Oncol 2010;28(12):2094–100.

10. de Jong D, Glas AM, Boerrigter L, et al. Very late relapse in diffuse large B-cell lymphoma represents clonally related disease and is marked by germinal center cell features. Blood 2003;102:324–7.

11. Bernstein SH, Unger JM, Leblanc M. Natural history of CNS relapse in patients with aggressive non-Hodgkin's lymphoma: a 20-year follow-up analysis of SWOG 8516 – the Southwest Oncology Group. J Clin Oncol 2009;27(1): 114–9.

12. Coiffier B, Salles G, Bosly A, et al. Characteristics of refractory and relapsing patients with diffuse large B-cell lymphoma. Blood 2008;112(11) [abstract 2589].

13. Philip T, Guglielmi C, Hagenbeek A, et al. Autologous bone marrow transplantation as compared with salvage chemotherapy in relapses of chemotherapy-sensitive non-Hodgkin's lymphoma. N Engl J Med 1995;333:1540–5.

14. Blay JY, Gomez F, Sebban C, et al. The International Prognostic Index correlates to survival in patients with aggressive lymphoma in relapse: analysis of the PARMA trial. Blood 1998;92(10):3562–8.

15. Hamlin PA, Zelenetz AD, Kewalramani T, et al. Age-adjusted International Prognostic Index predicts autologous stem cell transplantation outcome for patients with relapsed or primary refractory diffuse large B-cell lymphoma. Blood 2003; 102:1989–96.

16. Guglielmi C, Gomez F, Philip T, et al. Time to relapse has prognostic value in patients with aggressive lymphoma enrolled onto the Parma trial. J Clin Oncol 1998; 16(10):3264–9.

17. Miura K, Takahashi H, Nakagawa M, et al. Clinical significance of co-expression of MYC and BCL2 protein in aggressive B-cell lymphomas treated with a second line immunochemotherapy. Leuk Lymphoma 2015;22:1–7.

18. Thieblemont C, Briere J, Mounier N, et al. The germinal center/activated B-cell subclassification has a prognostic impact for response to salvage therapy in relapsed/refractory diffuse large B-cell lymphoma: a bio-CORAL study. J Clin Oncol 2011;29(31):4079–87.

19. Cuccuini W, Briere J, Mounier N, et al. MYC+ diffuse large B-cell lymphoma is not salvaged by classical R-ICE or R-DHAP followed by BEAM plus autologous stem cell transplantation. Blood 2012;119(20):4619–24.

20. Moskowitz CH, Zelenetz AD, Kewalramani T, et al. Cell of origin, germinal center versus non-germinal center, determined by immunohistochemistry on tissue microarray, does not correlate with outcome in patients with relapsed and refractory DLBCL. Blood 2005;106(10):3383–5.

21. Vellenga E, van Putten WL, van't Veer MB, et al. Rituximab improves the treatment results of DHAP-VIM-DHAP and ASCT in relapsed/progressive aggressive CD20+ NHL: a prospective randomized HOVON trial. Blood 2008;111(2): 537–43.

22. Gisselbrecht C, Glass B, Mournier N, et al. Salvage regimens with autologous transplantation for relapsed large B-cell lymphoma in the rituximab era. J Clin Oncol 2010;28(27):4184–90.

23. Crump M, Kuruvilla J, Couban S, et al. Randomized comparison of gemcitabine, dexamethasone and cisplatin versus dexamethasone, cytarabine, and cisplatin chemotherapy before autologous stem-cell transplantation for relapsed and refractory aggressive lymphomas: NCIC-CTG LY.12. J Clin Oncol 2014;32(31): 3490–6.

24. Cheung MC, Hay AE, Crump M, et al. Gemcitabine/dexamethasone/cisplatin vs cytarabine/dexamethasone/cisplatin for relapsed or refractory aggressive-histology lymphoma: cost-utility analysis of NCIC CTG LY.12. J Natl Cancer Inst 2015;107(7) [pii: djv106].

25. Matasar MJ, Czuczman MS, Rodriguez MA, et al. Ofatumumab in combination with ICE or DHAP chemotherapy in relapsed or refractory intermediate grade B-cell lymphoma. Blood 2013;122(4):499–506.

26. van Imhoff GW, McMillan A, Matasar MJ, et al. Ofatumumab Versus Rituximab Salvage Chemoimmunotherapy in Relapsed or Refractory Diffuse Large B-Cell Lymphoma: The Orcharrd Study (OMB110928). Blood 2014;124(21):630 [abstract].

27. Vose JM, Carter S, Burns LJ, et al. Phase III randomized study of rituximab/carmustine, etoposide, cytarabine, and melphalan (BEAM) compared with iodine-131 tositumomab/BEAM with autologous hematopoietic cell transplantation for relapsed diffuse large B-cell lymphoma: results from the BMT CTN 0401 trial. J Clin Oncol 2013;31(13):1662–8.

28. Chen YB, Lane AA, Logan BR, et al. Impact of conditioning regimen on outcomes for patients with lymphoma undergoing high-dose therapy with autologous hematopoietic cell transplantation. Biol Blood Marrow Transplant 2015;21:1046–53.

29. Decaudin D, Mounier N, Tilly H, et al. (90)Y Ibritumomab tiuxetan (Zevalin) combined with BEAM (Z-BEAM) conditioning regimen plus autologous stem cell transplantation in relapsed or refractory low-grade CD20-positive B-cell lymphoma: A GELA phase II prospective study. Clin Lymphoma Myeloma Leuk 2011;11:212–8.

30. Vose JM, Bierman PJ, Enke C, et al. Phase I trial of iodine-131 tositumomab with high-dose chemotherapy and autologous stem-cell transplantation for relapsed non-Hodgkin's lymphoma. J Clin Oncol 2005;23:461–7.

31. Josting A, Reiser M, Rueffer U, et al. Treatment of primary progressive Hodgkin's and aggressive non-Hodgkin's lymphoma: is there a chance for cure? J Clin Oncol 2000;18(2):332–9.

32. Cunningham D, Hawkes EA, Jack A, et al. Rituximab plus cyclophosphamide, doxorubicin, vincristine, and prednisolone in patients with newly diagnosed

diffuse large B-cell non-Hodgkin lymphoma: a phase 3 comparison of dose inten-sification with 14-day versus 21-day cycles. Lancet 2013;381(9880):1817–26.

33. Hitz F, Connors JM, Gascoyne RD, et al. Outcome of patients with primary refrac-tory diffuse large B cell lymphoma after R-CHOP treatment. Ann Hematol 2015; 94(11):1839–43.

34. Telio D, Fernandes K, Ma C, et al. Salvage chemotherapy and autologous he-matopoietic cell transplantation in primary refractory DLBCL: outcomes and prognostic factors. Leuk Lymphoma 2012;53(5):836–41.

35. Seshadri T, Stakiw J, Pintilie M, et al. Utility of subsequent conventional dose chemotherapy in relapsed/refractory transplant eligible patients with diffuse large B cell lymphoma failing platinum-based salvage chemotherapy. Hematology 2008;13(5):261–6.

36. Van Den Neste E, Schmitz N, Mounier N, et al. Outcome of patients with relapsed diffuse large B-cell lymphoma who fail second-line salvage regimens in the Inter-national CORAL study. Bone Marrow Transplant 2016;51(1):51–7.

37. Robinson SP, Boumendil A, Finel H, et al. Autologous stem cell transplantation for relapsed/refractory diffuse large B-cell lymphoma: efficacy in the rituximab era and comparison to first allogeneic transplants. A report from the EBMT Lym-phoma Working Party. Bone Marrow Transplant 2016;51(3):365–71.

38. Schmitz N, Zeynalova N, Glass B, et al. CNS disease in younger patients with aggressive B-cell lymphoma: an analysis of patients treated on the MabThera In-ternational Trial and trials of the German High-Grade Non-Hodgkin Lymphoma Study Group. Ann Oncol 2012;23:1267–73.

39. Guirguis HR, Cheung MC, Mahrous M, et al. Impact of central nervous system (CNS) prophylaxis on the incidence and risk factors for CNS relapse in patients with diffuse large B-cell lymphoma treated in the rituximab era: a single centre experience and review of the literature. Br J Haematol 2012;159(1):39–49.

40. Kumar A, Vanderplas A, LaCasce AS, et al. Lack of benefit of central nervous sys-tem prophylaxis for diffuse large B-cell lymphoma in the rituximab era: findings from a large national database. Cancer 2012;118(11):2944–51.

41. Boehme V, Schmitz N, Zeynalova S, et al. CNS events in elderly patients with aggressive lymphoma treated with modern chemotherapy (CHOP-14) with or without rituximab: an analysis of patients treated in the RICOVER-60 trial of the German High-Grade Non-Hodgkin Lymphoma Study Group (DSHNHL). Blood 2009;113(17):3896–902.

42. MØ Pedersen, Gang AO, Poulsen TS, et al. Double-hit BCL2/MYC translocations in a consecutive cohort of patients with large B-cell lymphoma - a single centre's experience. Eur J Haematol 2012;89(1):63–71.

43. Petrich AM, Gandhi M, Jovanovic B. Impact of induction regimen and stem cell transplantation on outcomes in double-hit lymphoma: a multicenter retrospective analysis. Blood 2014;124(15):2354–61.

44. Savage KJ, Slack GW, Mottok A, et al. The impact of dual expression of MYC and BCL2 by immunohistochemistry on the risk of CNS relapse in DLBCL. Blood 2016;127(18):2182–8.

45. Jahnke K, Thiel E, Martus P, et al. Retrospective study of prognostic factors in non-Hodgkin lymphoma secondarily involving the central nervous system. Ann Hematol 2006;85(1):45–50.

46. Bromberg JE, Doorduijn JK, Illerhaus G, et al. Central nervous system recurrence of systemic lymphoma in the era of stem cell transplantation – an International Pri-mary Central Nervous System Lymphoma Study Group project. Haematologica 2013;98(5):808–13.

47. Doolittle ND, Abrey LE, Shenkier TN, et al. Brain parenchyma involvement as isolated central nervous system relapse of systemic non-Hodgkin lymphoma: an International Primary CNS Lymphoma Collaborative Group report. Blood 2008; 111(3):1085–93.

48. Khimani NB, Ng AK, Chen HY, et al. Salvage radiotherapy in patients with recurrent or refractory primary or secondary central nervous system lymphoma after methotrexate-based chemotherapy. Ann Oncol 2011;22:979–84.

49. Williams CD, Pearce R, Taghipour G, et al. Autologous bone marrow transplantation for patients with non-Hodgkin's lymphoma and CNS involvement: those transplanted with active CNS disease have a poor outcome–a report by the European Bone Marrow Transplant Lymphoma Registry. J Clin Oncol 1994; 12(11):2415–22.

50. Cote GM, Hochberg EP, Muzikansky A, et al. Autologous stem cell transplantation with thiotepa, busulfan, and cyclophosphamide (TBC) conditioning in patients with CNS involvement by non-Hodgkin lymphoma. Biol Blood Marrow Transplant 2012;18(1):76–83.

51. Welch MR, Sauter CS, Matasar MJ, et al. Autologous stem cell transplant in recurrent or refractory primary or secondary central nervous system lymphoma using thiotepa, busulfan and cyclophosphamide. Leuk Lymphoma 2015;56(2): 361–7.

52. Korfel A, Elter T, Thiel E, et al. Phase II study of central nervous system (CNS)-directed chemotherapy including high-dose chemotherapy with autologous stem cell transplantation for CNS relapse of aggressive lymphomas. Haematologica 2013;98(3):364–70.

53. Ferreri AJM, Donadoni G, Cabras MG, et al. High doses of antimetabolites followed by high-dose sequential chemoimmunotherapy and autologous stem cell transplantation in patients with systemic B-cell lymphoma and secondary CNS involvement: final results of a multicentre phase II trial. J Clin Oncol 2015; 33(33):3903–10.

54. Doolittle ND, Korfel A, Lubow MA, et al. Long-term cognitive function, neuroimaging, and quality of life in primary CNS lymphoma. Neurology 2013;81(1):84–92.

55. Kewarlarmani T, Zelenetz AD, Nimer SD, et al. Rituximab and ICE as second-line therapy before autologous stem cell transplantation for relapsed or primary refractory diffuse large B-cell lymphoma. Blood 2004;103:3684–8.

56. Mey UJM, Olivieri A, Orlopp KS, et al. DHAP in combination with rituximab vs DHAP alone as salvage treatment for patients with relapsed or refractory diffuse large B-cell lymphoma: a matched-pair analysis. Leuk Lymphoma 2006;47(12): 2558–66.

57. Redondo AM, Pomares H, Vidal MJ, et al. Impact of prior rituximab on outcomes of autologous stem-cell transplantation in patients with relapsed or refractory aggressive B-cell lymphoma: a multicentre retrospective Spanish group of lymphoma/autologous bone marrow transplant study. Br J Haematol 2014;164(5): 668–74.

58. Baetz T, Chen BE, Couban S, et al. Addition of rituximab to salvage chemotherapy in aggressive CD20+ lymphoma prior to autologous stem cell transplant (ASCT): a cohort comparison from the NCIC CTG Study LY.12. Blood 2014;124: 1712 [abstract].

59. McCarthy PL Jr, Hahn T, Hassebroek A, et al. Trends in use of and survival after autologous hematopoietic cell transplantation in North America, 1995-2005: significant improvement in survival for lymphoma and myeloma during a period of increasing recipient age. Biol Blood Marrow Transplant 2013;19:1116–23.

60. Dahi PB, Tamari R, Devlin SM, et al. Favorable outcomes in elderly patients undergoing high-dose therapy and autologous stem cell transplantation for non-Hodgkin lymphoma. Biol Blood Marrow Transplant 2014;20(12):2004–9.

61. Gohil SH, Ardeshna KM, Lambert JM, et al. Autologous stem cell transplantation outcomes in elderly patients with B cell non-Hodgkin lymphoma. Br J Haematol 2015;171:197–204.

62. Sorror ML, Maris MB, Storb R, et al. Hematopoietic cell transplantation (HCT)-specific comorbidity index: a new tool for risk assessment before allogeneic HCT. Blood 2005;106:2912–9.

63. Hosing C, Saliba RM, Okoroji G-J, et al. High-dose chemotherapy and autologous hematopoietic progenitor cell transplantation for non-Hodgkin's lymphoma in patients >65 years of age. Ann Oncol 2008;19:1166–71.

64. Elstrom RL, Martin P, Hurtado Rua S, et al. Autologous stem cell transplant is feasible in very elderly patients with lymphoma and limited comorbidity. Am J Hematol 2012;87(4):433–5.

65. Davison K, Chen B, Kukreti V, et al. Treatment outcomes for older patients with relapsed/refractory aggressive lymphoma receiving salvage chemotherapy and autologous stem cell transplantation (ASCT) are similar to younger patients: a subgroup analysis from the phase III NCIC CTG LY12 trial. Hematol Oncol 2013;31(Supplement S1) [Abstract 022].

66. Hermet E, Cabrespine A, Guièze A, et al. Autologous hematopoietic stem cell transplantation in elderly patients (≥70 years) with non-Hodgkin's lymphoma: A French Society of Bone Marrow Transplantation and Cellular Therapy retrospective study. J Geriatr Oncol 2015;6(5):346–52.

67. Ohmachi K, Niitsu N, Uchida T, et al. Multicenter phase II study of bendamustine plus rituximab in patients with relapsed or refractory diffuse large B-cell lymphoma. J Clin Oncol 2013;31(17):2103–9.

68. Maddocks K, Christian B, Jaglowski S, et al. A phase 1/1b study of rituximab, bendamustine, and ibrutinib in patients with untreated and relapsed/refractory non-Hodgkin lymphoma. Blood 2015;125(2):242–8.

69. Haas RL, Poortmans P, de Jong D, et al. Effective palliation by low dose local radiotherapy for recurrent and/or chemotherapy refractory non-follicular lymphoma patients. Eur J Cancer 2005;41(12):1724–30.

70. Martens C, Hodgson DC, Wells WA, et al. Outcome of hyperfractionated radiotherapy in chemotherapy-resistant non-Hodgkin's lymphoma. Int J Radiat Oncol Biol Phys 2006;64(4):1183–7.

71. Morin RD, Assouline S, Alcaide M, et al. Genetic landscapes of relapsed and refractory diffuse large B-Cell lymphomas. Clin Cancer Res 2015;22(9):2290–300.

72. Dubois S, Viailly PJ, Mareschal S, et al. Next generation sequencing in diffuse large B cell lymphoma highlights molecular divergence and therapeutic opportunities: a LYSA study. Clin Cancer Res 2016;22(12):2919–28.

73. Nagle S, Woo K, Schuster S, et al. Outcomes of patients with relapsed/refractory diffuse large B-cell lymphoma with progression of lymphoma after autologous stem cell transplantation in the rituximab era. Am J Hematol 2013;88:890–4.

74. Wang M, Fowler N, Wagner-Bartak N, et al. Oral lenalidomide with rituximab in relapsed or refractory diffuse large cell, follicular and transformed lymphoma: a phase II clinical trial. Leukemia 2013;27(9):1902–9.

75. Feldman T, Mato AR, Chow KF, et al. Addition of lenalidomide to rituximab, ifosfamide, carboplatin, etoposide (RICER) in first-relapse/primary refractory diffuse large B-cell lymphoma. Br J Haematol 2014;166(1):77–83.

76. Martín A, Redondo AM, Dlouhy I, et al. Lenalidomide in combination with R-ESHAP in patients with relapsed or refractory diffuse large B-cell lymphoma: a phase 1b study from GELTAMO group. Br J Haematol 2016;173(2):245–52.

77. Straus DJ, Hamlin PA, Matasar MJ, et al. Phase I/II trial of vorinostat with rituximab, cyclophosphamide, etoposide and prednisone as palliative treatment for elderly patients with relapsed or refractory diffuse large B-cell lymphoma not eligible for autologous stem cell transplantation. Br J Haematol 2015;168(5): 663–70.

78. Kochenderfer JN, Dudley ME, Kassim SH, et al. Chemotherapy-refractory diffuse large B-cell lymphoma and indolent B-cell malignancies can be effectively treated with autologous T cells expressing an anti-CD19 chimeric antigen receptor. J Clin Oncol 2015;33(6):540–9.

79. Goebeler ME, Knop S, Viardot A, et al. Bispecific T-cell engager (BiTE) antibody construct blinatumomab for the treatment of patients with relapsed/refractory non-Hodgkin lymphoma: final results from a phase I study. J Clin Oncol 2016; 34(10):1104–11.

80. Crump M, Baetz T, Belch A, et al. Gemcitabine, dexamethasone and cisplatin in patients with relapsed or refractory aggressive histology B-cell non-Hodgkin's lymphoma: a phase II study by the National Cancer Institute of Canada Clinical Trials Group. Cancer 2004;101(8):1835–42.

81. Corazzelli C, Capobianco G, Arcamone M, et al. Long-term results of gemcitabine plus oxaliplatin with and without rituximab as salvage treatment for transplant-ineligible patients with refractory/relapsing B-cell lymphoma. Cancer Chemother Pharmacol 2009;64:907–16.

82. Papageorgiou ES, Tsirigotis P, Dimopoulos M, et al. Combination chemotherapy with gemcitabine and vinorelbine in the treatment of relapsed or refractory diffuse large B-cell lymphoma: a phase-II trial by the Hellenic Cooperative Oncology Group. Eur J Haematol 2005;75:124–9.

83. Mounier N, El Gnaoui T, Tilly H, et al. Rituximab plus gemcitabine and oxaliplatin in patients with refractory/relapsed diffuse large B-cell lymphoma who are not candidates for high-dose therapy. A phase II Lymphoma Study Association trial. Haematologica 2013;98(11):1726–31.

84. Wiernik PH, Lossos IS, Tuscano JM, et al. Lenalidomide monotherapy in relapsed or refractory aggressive non-Hodgkin's lymphoma. J Clin Oncol 2008;26(30): 4952–7.

85. Witzig TE, Vose JM, Zinzani PL, et al. An international phase II trial of single agent lenalidomide for relapsed or refractory aggressive B-cell non-Hodgkin's lymphoma. Ann Oncol 2011;22(7):1622–7.

86. Witzig TE, Reeder CB, LaPlant BR, et al. A phase II trial of the oral mTOR inhibitor everolimus in relapsed aggressive lymphoma. Leukemia 2011;25:341–7.

87. Wilson WH, Young RM, Schmitz R, et al. Targeting B cell receptor signaling with ibrutinib in diffuse large B cell lymphoma. Nat Med 2015;21(8):922–6.

88. Morschhauser FA, Cartron G, Thieblemont C, et al. Obinutuzumab (GA101) monotherapy in relapsed/refractory diffuse large b-cell lymphoma or mantle-cell lymphoma: results from the phase II GAUGUIN study. J Clin Oncol 2013; 31(23):2912–9.

89. Jacobsen ED, Sharman JP, Oki Y, et al. Brentuximab vedotin demonstrates objective responses in a phase 2 study of relapsed/refractory DLBCL with variable CD30 expression. Blood 2015;125(9):1394–402.

Role of Positron Emission Tomography in Diffuse Large B-cell Lymphoma

Gunjan L. Shah, Craig H. Moskowitz*

KEYWORDS

- Positron emission tomography • Diffuse large B-cell lymphoma • Transplant

KEY POINTS

- Positron emission tomography (PET) is standard of care at diagnosis and for determining remission status at the end of treatment, but remains investigational when performed in the middle of therapy.
- Surveillance PET is not beneficial in the majority of patients.
- PET pre-auto hematopoietic stem cell transplant is prognostic of outcome.
- Improvements in interpretation and standardization of PET across institutions, and the use of new tracers, can improve this modality.

INTRODUCTION

Positron emission tomography-low dose computed tomography with 18F-fluorodeoxy-glucose (PET) has become a valuable imaging modality studied at all stages of diffuse large B-cell lymphoma (DLBCL) management. In 2007, the first guidelines for the use of PET in lymphoma were presented by the International Harmonization Project and incorporated into response criteria.[1,2] In an effort to standardize the results of PET scans, a 5-point scale, known as the Deauville criteria, was accepted in 2009.[3] Consensus guidelines were then most recently updated in 2013 and known as the Lugano Classification.[4,5] This article discusses the literature at each phase of treatment including the role of PET scans periautologous and allogeneic hematopoietic stem cell transplant (HSCT) and newer semiquantitative measurements such as metabolic tumor volume.

DEAUVILLE CRITERIA

The 5-point scale is depicted in **Table 1**.[3] One of the major values of this system is that it is reproducible between centers. In addition, it allows for altering the positive and

Department of Medicine, Memorial Sloan Kettering Cancer Center, Lymphoma and Adult BMT Services, 1275 York Avenue, New York, NY 10065, USA
* Corresponding author.
E-mail address: moskowic@mskcc.org

Hematol Oncol Clin N Am 30 (2016) 1215–1228
http://dx.doi.org/10.1016/j.hoc.2016.07.003
0889-8588/16/© 2016 Elsevier Inc. All rights reserved.

Table 1 Deauville criteria 5-point scale	
Score	Definition
1	No uptake
2	Uptake ≤ mediastinum
3	Uptake > mediastinum but ≤ liver
4	Uptake moderately higher than liver
5	Uptake markedly higher than liver and/or new lesions
X	New areas of uptake unlikely to be related to lymphoma

negative thresholds in the context of a clinical trial. For example, to avoid undertreatment, a lower score would be considered negative. Similarly, a higher score can be used to define a positive scan to avoid overtreatment. More recently, definitions for the distinction between standardized uptake value (SUV) (ie, moderately or markedly [scores 4 and 5] greater than the liver) have been suggested, with scores of 5 applied when the uptake is 2 to 3 times greater than the maximum SUV (SUVmax) of the liver.[6]

INITIAL STAGING

PET scanning with the accompanying low-dose computed tomography (CT) is uniformly agreed upon as more accurate than contrast enhanced CECT alone for initial staging of DLCBL due to increased sensitivity for both nodal and extranodal disease.[7,8] One of the remaining questions is the use of CECT in addition to PET. There are no studies comparing PET with low-dose CT to PET with CECT. The main limitations include the availability of performing the dedicated CT at the same time and the cost of the additional study if it cannot be done simultaneously. When possible, the optimal recommendation is to have both studies at diagnosis for better anatomic staging, as the inclusion of CECT has been shown to upstage 10% to 25% of patients.[9–12] However, as studies have not shown improved survival in those upstaged patients treated more aggressively, in patients who cannot have a CECT performed with the PET, a diagnostic CT is likely only needed in patients with localized disease for which precise anatomy needs to be defined for the consideration of radiotherapy.

Another remaining question is the ability to eliminate a bone marrow biopsy (BMBx) from routine staging work-up based on the results of the PET. Patients eligible for curative treatment are recommended to have a BMBx under the current guidelines.[4] However, other authors suggest that not all patients require this procedure at diagnosis. The 2 main considerations include the pattern of involvement on the PET scan and the prognostic significance of the presence of concordant DLBCL versus discordant small cleaved cells histologically.

On PET scan, the marrow may have no, focal, or diffuse uptake, with each having a different association with a positive BMBx.[13–17] Adams and colleagues[13] conducted a meta-analysis of 7 studies, from which they concluded that a negative PET did not rule out the presence of lymphoma, but a focally or diffusely positive scan obviated the need for a biopsy given a pooled sensitivity and specificity of 88.7% (95% confidence interval, CI, 82.5%–93.3%) and 99.8% (95% CI 98.8%–100%), respectively. A subsequent retrospective study showed that 31% of patients with a negative PET had a positive BMBx, exemplifying the benefit of a biopsy in staging those with a negative marrow on PET.[17] On the other hand, Khan and colleagues[16] demonstrated that PET can identify all clinically important marrow DLBCL and that patients with a positive bone marrow (BM) identified by PET-CT but not BMBx had a progression-free survival (PFS) and overall survival (OS) similar to stage IV disease without marrow involvement.

Sehn and colleagues[18] suggest that discordant marrow positivity does not impact OS as long as there is no change in the International Prognostic Index (IPI), while concordant BM involvement negatively affects both OS and PFS independently. As such, although marrow involved with discordant lymphoma may be missed by a false-negative PET scan, a patient's overall course may be unchanged by omitting the BMBx.

Therefore, it would be reasonable for patients with negative or diffusely positive marrow by PET to undergo BM evaluation with aspirate, biopsy, and flow cytometry, while those with focal or focal and diffuse PET uptake would likely have marrow involvement and should be treated as such if a biopsy is omitted.

INTERIM

Interim PET scans (iPET) remain among the most controversial and least standardized uses of this modality in lymphoma management (**Table 2**). Although the purpose would be to exclude progression and possibly individualize therapy based on response, several issues exist including timing of the scan, interobserver reproducibility without a standard definition of positive and negative, and false positivity due to inflammatory responses from immunotherapy.[19–21]

Two large meta-analyses have been recently published with conflicting results. Zhu and colleagues[22] included 11 studies of DLBCL patients treated with rituximab-based immunochemotherapy who underwent scans after 2 to 4 cycles of therapy. They found that PFS was significantly shorter for those with a positive interim scan with a pooled hazard ratio (HR) of 2.96 (95% CI, 2.25–3.89). On the other hand, Sun and colleagues[23] limited their analysis to patients receiving rituximab, cyclophosphamide, adriamycin, vincristine, and prednisone (R-CHOP). In 6 studies including 605 patients, the pooled sensitivity and specificity in predicting outcomes were 52.4% and 67.8%, respectively.

One explanation for the difference across studies is the variable time at which the scan is done, with PET scans after 2 cycles evaluating chemosensitivity and after 4 cycles possibly portraying regrowth of disease.[24]

Studies have been done as early as after 1 cycle of chemotherapy, again with contradictory results. In a cohort of DLBCL and Hodgkin lymphoma patients, Kostakoglu and colleagues[25] found that all patients with a negative PET after 1 cycle had a sustained remission with a median follow-up of 28 months. More recently, however, Mylam and colleagues[26] report that in 112 DLBCL patients, there was no difference in PFS for PET-negative versus -positive patients when using a Deauville score of greater than 3.

Several suggestions have been evaluated to improve on the reproducibility of the interpretation beyond visual scales including semiquantitative measurements, such as ΔCUVmax and metabolic tumor volumes, or biopsy of the area with increased uptake.

The percent change in maximum SUV (ΔSUVmax) from baseline to the subsequent scan can be quantified and has been shown to improve interobserver agreement when compared with visual assessment.[6] Thresholds predicting response vary between studies based on the time point of the scans and range from 66% to 92%.[6,27–31] Lin and colleagues[32] reported the first large quantitative study and found an optimal cutoff of 66% for PET done after 2 cycles of chemotherapy (PET2) using receiver operating characteristic (ROC) analysis. Patients with a ΔSUVmax greater than the cutoff had a

Table 2
Selected interim PET scan studies

Reference	DLBCL Patients (n)	Type of Study	Treatment	# Cycles Before iPET	Median Follow-Up (mo)	iPET Negative	PPV	NPV	PFS w/Neg iPET	PFS w/Pos iPET	OS w/Neg iPET	OS w/Pos iPET
Cashen et al,[79] 2011	52	SC, R	R-CHOP-21 x6	2	33.9	52%	42%	77%	2 yr: 85%	2 yr: 63%	2 yr: 85%	2 yr: 65%
Cassanovas et al,[27] 2011	113	MC, P	R-CHOP or R-AVCBP	2 & 4	19	deltaSUV: after 2: 78%, after 4: 88%	NR	NR	2 yr: after 2: 77%, after 4: 83%	2 yr: after 2: 57%, after 4: 40%	2 yr: after 2: 93%, after 4: 94%	2 yr: after 2: 60%, after 4: 5C%
Itti et al,[80] 2010	80	MC, P	CHOP or AVCBP ± Rituximab	4	41	deltaSUV: 78.7%	70.6%	79.4%	2 yr: 79%	2 yr: 32%	NR	NR
Kostakoglu et al,[25] 2006	24/47	SC, R	CHOP ± Rituximab x 6-8	1	21	45%	75%	100%	2 yr: 100%	2 yr: 12.5%	NR	NR
Lin et al,[32] 2007	92	MC, P	CHOP or AVCBP ± Rituximab	2	42	deltaSUV: 82.6%	81.3%	75%	2 yr: 79%	2 yr: 21%	NR	NR

Moskowitz et al,[42] 2010	98	SC, R	R-CHOP-14x4 then a. If iPET neg or iPET pos w/neg bx: ICEx3 b. If iPET pos w/pos bx: ICEx2/ R-CE/Auto HSCT	4	44	61% (33/38 w/pos iPET had neg bx)	NR	NR	2 yr: >90%	2 yr: Neg bx 80%–85%, Pos bx 60%	NR	NR
Nols et al,[30] 2014	73	MC, R	R-CHOP or R-AVCBP	3–4	28	deltaSUV: 82%	46%	75%	2 yr: 78%	2 yr: 50%	2 yr: 88%	2 yr: 56%
Pregno et al,[20] 2012	88	MC, R	R-CHOP	2–4	26.2	72%	36%	82.5%	85%	72%	NR	NR
Safar et al,[81] 2012	112	MC, P	R-CHOP or R-AVCBP	2	38	62.5%	NR	NR	3 yr: 84%	3 yr: 47%	3 yr: 88%	3 yr: 62%
Yang et al,[82] 2011	161	SC, P	R-CHOP-21 x6-8	3–4	30	72%	NR	NR	3 yr: 88.3%	3 yr: 52.5%	3 yr: 91.4%	3 yr: 53.3%
Yoo et al,[83] 2011	155	MC, R	R-CHOP	2–4	20	64.5%	62%	93%	3 yr: 84%	3 yr: 66%	3 yr: 84%	3 yr: 77%

Abbreviations: Auto HSCT autologous hematopoietic stem cell transplant; Bx, biopsy; DLBCL, diffuse large B-cell lymphoma; iPET, interim PET; MC, multicenter; NPV, negative predictive value; NR, not reported OS, overall survival; P, prospective; PFS, progression-free survival; PPV, positive predictive value; R, retrospective; SC, single center.

2-year event-free survival (EFS) of 79% compared with 21% in those with a lesser reduction ($P = .001$). The same group found that for PET after 4 cycles of chemotherapy (PET4), the threshold increased to 73% with a 2-year EFS of 79 versus 32%, and concluded that while semiquantification after 2 cycles of chemotherapy reduced false-positive scans, it was equivalent to visual analysis after 4 cycles.[28]

Other groups have also shown that ΔSUVmax is able to predict outcomes. Casasnovas and colleagues[27] showed an OS benefit of 93% versus 60% ($P<.0001$) with a PET2 ΔSUVmax cutoff of 66% and 94% versus 50% ($P<.0001$) with a PET4 ΔSUVmax cutoff of 70%. On the other hand, using the same 66% threshold, Pregno and colleagues[20] were unable to show a difference in outcome based on iPET after 2 to 4 cycles of therapy.

To evaluate changing treatment based on an unfavorable iPET, the PETAL (Positron Emission Tomography guided therapy of Aggressive non-Hodgkin Lymphomas) trial prospectively applied a ΔSUVmax threshold of 66% on PET2 with patients not meeting the cutoff escalated to a Burkitt-like regimen. With 926 patients, iPET was unfavorable in 13% and highly predictive of outcome with a 2-year time to treatment failure of 79% versus 47% ($P<.0001$), but they were unable to show a benefit to switching therapy.[33] The GAINED (GA in Newly Diagnosed Diffuse Large B-cell Lymphomas) trial and the UK Clinical Research Network iPET study are ongoing.

Other semiquantitative approaches under investigation include the use of metabolic tumor volume (MTV) and total lesion glycolysis (TLG), with prognostic significance both at diagnosis[34–39] and at interim restaging.[31,40] MTV is defined as the volume of hypermetabolic tissue with an SUV greater than a threshold value of 2.5 (MTV2.5) and is thought to better represent tumor burden by measuring the viable tumor fraction. TLG goes 1 step further and quantifies the metabolic disease burden by multiplying the glucose utilization rate (SUVmean) and the MTV.[39] Yang and colleagues compared the ΔMTV2.5 with the Deauville 5-point scale and ΔSUVmax in 186 patients after 3 to 4 cycles of R-CHOP and found that patients with a worse scan by each method had a shorter PFS. In addition, when given a point for each method patients scored positively in, any score greater than zero predicted for worse outcomes. Interestingly, the mean MTV2.5 reduction rate on the iPET was not significantly different between patients who relapsed and those who did not (98.2 vs 93%). Using ROC analysis, they determined that the ΔMTV2.5 cutoff for interim scanning was 99.3% and found a 2-year PFS of 84.2 versus 64.9% for those above and below the threshold, respectively.[31] Similarly, Malek and colleagues[40] retrospectively evaluated iPET after 2 to 4 cycles of R-CHOP or dose-adjusted R-EPOCH in 140 patients. In their ROC analysis, the ΔMTV was 52% with an HR of 1.37 ($P = .02$) for PFS when comparing achieving a ΔMTV greater than 52% versus less than 52%. Given the wide variation in ΔMTV thresholds, further research is clearly necessary to determine the optimal cutoff for this methodology.

Histologic confirmation of areas of increased SUV on interim scans can help increase the accuracy of interpretation if therapy changes are being considered based on the results. However, Moskowitz and colleagues[41,42] found that 33 of 38 patients with positive iPET had a negative biopsy, and their outcome was similar to the PET-negative patients. The use of an induction/consolidation strategy with all patients receiving escalated immunochemotherapy and the timing of the scan may have contributed to the high false-positive rate. Therefore, this strategy is limited by the possibility of subjecting many patients to unnecessary biopsies when their scan positivity was based visual scales.

Finally, the use of an alternative tracer, 18F-fluorodeoxythymidine (FLT), may allow for better early discrimination of inflammation versus tumor proliferation.[43–46]

Minamimoto and colleagues[45] conducted a prospective multicenter study evaluating which of FDG or FLT PET after 2 cycles of chemotherapy was better able to predict response after 6 cycles. They found FLT iPET had a significantly higher positive predictive value (PPV), but similar negative predictive value. On the other hand, Schoder and colleagues[43] prospectively used FLT PET in the induction/consolidation DLBCL patients and showed that while FLT PET predicts PFS and OS, the PPV too low to justify changes in therapy. Additional investigations remain ongoing to improve this methodology.

Overall, even If these issues are solved, the number of scans a patient will have in a few months' span and the cost of these scans without significant benefit remain problems. In addition, there are little data supporting improved outcomes with a risk-adapted treatment strategy. Therefore, interim PET for DLBCL is not recommended outside the context of a clinical trial.

END OF TREATMENT

According to the guidelines, PET at the completion of therapy should be performed at least 3 weeks after chemotherapy or 8 to 12 weeks after radiotherapy to allow for inflammatory reactions to abate.[2] In this setting, PET has been shown to be more accurate than CECT alone, especially in evaluating residual masses, which are often just fibrosis.[47–50]

Two large systematic reviews have been conducted including patients with both non-Hodgkin (NHL) and HL. Zijlstra and colleagues[50] included 15 studies with 350 NHL patients published through 2004. For these patients, the pooled sensitivity and specificity for detection of residual disease were 72% (95% CI: 61%–82%) and 100% (95% CI: 97%–100%), respectively. Terasawa and colleagues[49] then presented an updated analysis refining the inclusion criteria evaluating 19 studies with 254 aggressive NHL patients published through 2006. The reported ranges for sensitivity and specificity of predicting relapse were 33% to 77% and 82% to 100%, respectively. In addition, using the end point of time to next treatment (TNT), Brespoels and colleagues[51] showed that while patients with PET partial response (PR) have similar outcomes to the patients defined as having a complete response (CR) or unconfirmed complete response (CRu) by the older CT criteria, they have a shorter TNT than the patients achieving PET CR. Finally, a third meta-analysis by Adams and colleagues[52] incorporated 737 R-CHOP treated DLBCL patients in 7 studies published through 2014 and found a relapse rate of 7% to 20% in patients in CR by the end-of-treatment PET.

Hence, PET remains the standard of care for determination of remission status at the completion of therapy for DLBCL patients.

SURVEILLANCE

On the other hand, PET scan is not recommended for scheduled post treatment monitoring in all patients. Ideally, surveillance imaging would detect relapse early allowing for intervention prior to symptomatic disease. However, several studies have shown that most relapses in patients with DLBCL are identified clinically between scans.[53–59] Thompson and colleagues[59] note that in a cohort of 552 DLBCL patients, 112 relapsed with only 9 of these (1.6%) identified first by surveillance imaging. Furthermore, they were unable to show a survival difference between those patients whose relapse was identified at scheduled follow-up versus outside of those times, likely due to lead time bias.

In addition, there is a high false-positive rate, prompting unnecessary biopsies with meaningful mental and financial cost to the patient and society.[54–61] El-Galaly and colleagues[54] report the sensitivity and specificity of surveillance PET were 100% and 89%, respectively, with the positive and negative predictive values 21% and 100%, respectively. Furthermore, the cost of PET imaging every 6 months during the first 2 years in CR was $8552 per patient and accounted for 81% of the total follow-up costs. Similarly in patients with aggressive NHL, Liedtke and colleagues[55] report that the cost of detecting 1 asymptomatic relapse with surveillance imaging over 5 years was between $42,750 and $85,500.

Some authors have suggested a role for surveillance PET imaging in DLBCL patients at high risk for relapse.[62] For example, Cheah and colleagues[61] found that the PPV in patients who had achieved a complete metabolic response at the completion of therapy was 56% if the IPI was less than 3 compared with 80% in patients with IPI of at least 3. In further support of this, Hiniker and colleagues[63] reported on stage I to II DLBCL patients and found that although the median duration of time to starting treatment was 14.3 versus 59.8 months depending on radiographically or clinically detected relapse respectively, there was no difference in OS from the initiation of initial therapy or relapse.

Therefore, for the majority of patients, CECT every 6 months for 5 years, as in the current National Comprehensive Cancer Network guidelines, is more than adequate follow-up.[64] Although some would not recommend surveillance CT scans at all, the use of PET scans in this phase of care should be individualized and is likely most useful in patients with high-risk disease and in those whose original tumors were only seen on PET.

BEFORE/AFTER TRANSPLANT

High-dose therapy (HDT) with autologous HSCT (auto-HSCT) is standard of care for chemosensitive relapsed DLBCL, while allogeneic HSCT (allo-HSCT) can be undertaken after a subsequent relapse or instead of auto-HSCT in certain cases. PET scanning has been studied before and after both auto- and allo-HSCT.

Several studies report on the prognostic significance of a negative PET scan prior to auto-HSCT.[65–73] As with all of the studies already discussed, comparisons between studies are difficult, as the criteria for positive and negative have varied over time. Using the modern Deauville criteria, Sauter and colleagues[69] establish the importance of PET negativity prior to auto-HSCT. For patients achieving a Deauville score of 1 to 3 after salvage therapy, the PFS and OS at 3 years were significantly longer than those with a Deauville 4 (77% vs 49% and 86% vs 54%, respectively).

PET prior to reduced-intensity allo-HSCT has also been evaluated, with some studies reporting prognostic significance,[71,74,75] while others do not.[76,77] Dodero and colleagues[75] report significantly better OS and PFS in a combined NHL and HL cohort who were PET negative prior to HSCT with 3-year OS of 76% versus 33% ($P = .001$) and PFS of 73% versus 31% ($P = .001$). Similarly, Ulaner and colleagues[71] found a 2-year PFS of 68% versus 35% ($P = .014$) for those without FDG-avid lesions compared to those with them. On the other hand, in an observational prospective study including 78 patients, Lambert and colleagues[76] were unable to show a prognostic impact on relapse rate or OS, although this trial also included a mixture of histologies. The larger Center for International Blood and Marrow Transplant Registry (CIBMTR) study showed mixed results on multivariate analysis with a positive pre-allo HSCT PET associated with an increased risk of relapse or progression (risk ratio [RR]1.86, $P = .001$), but no association with increased mortality (RR 1.29, $P = .08$),

PFS (RR 1.32, P = .1), or nonrelapse mortality (RR 0.75, P = .22).[74] However, the authors point out that all patients included had chemosensitive disease by CT criteria and regardless of status before transplant, had a 3-year survival close to 60%.

Post-allo HSCT surveillance PET imaging also remains controversial. Lambert and colleagues[76] report that surveillance PET detected relapse before CECT in half of the cases, which allowed for earlier donor lymphocyte infusion (DLI) when given to patients with abnormal PET. They noted that DLIs were not given in patients with stable CT abnormalities who had a normal PET scan and full-donor chimerism. Similarly, Hart and colleagues[78] also concluded that surveillance PET after allo-HSCT allowed for guidance in DLI administration in HL and NHL patients. On the other hand, Ulaner and colleagues[72] cautioned that benign FDG-avid lymph nodes no more than 1.5 cm can mimic malignancy, with 21 of 22 patients biopsied having benign disease. In addition, disease-free survival of patients with the smaller FDG-avid nodes was similar to those with FDG-avid masses.

Overall, PET prior to auto-HSCT is standard of care and has well documented prognostic significance. PET scans in the allo-HSCT setting have less established benefit, but are likely useful prior to transplant. Surveillance imaging requires further study to assess the impact of early DLI on outcomes.

SUMMARY

In summary, PET is standard of care at diagnosis and for determining remission status at the end of treatment, but remains investigational when performed in the middle of therapy. Surveillance PET is not beneficial in the majority of patients, while PET pre-auto HSCT is prognostic of outcome. The impact of peri-allo HSCT remains unclear. Improvements in interpretation and standardization of PET across institutions will allow for further comparative research. In addition, the use of non-FDG tracers remains under investigation and may provide future benefit. Overall, PET remains an integral component in the management of patients with DLBCL.

REFERENCES

1. Juweid ME, Stroobants S, Hoekstra OS, et al. Use of positron emission tomography for response assessment of lymphoma: consensus of the Imaging Subcommittee of International Harmonization Project in Lymphoma. J Clin Oncol 2007; 25(5):571–8.

2. Cheson BD, Pfistner B, Juweid ME, et al. Revised response criteria for malignant lymphoma. J Clin Oncol 2007;25(5):579–86.

3. Meignan M, Gallamini A, Haioun C. Report on the First International Workshop on Interim-PET-Scan in Lymphoma. Leuk Lymphoma 2009;50(8):1257–60.

4. Barrington SF, Mikhaeel NG, Kostakoglu L, et al. Role of imaging in the staging and response assessment of lymphoma: consensus of the International Conference on Malignant Lymphomas Imaging Working Group. J Clin Oncol 2014; 32(27):3048–58.

5. Cheson BD, Fisher RI, Barrington SF, et al. Recommendations for initial evaluation, staging, and response assessment of Hodgkin and Non-Hodgkin Lymphoma: the Lugano Classification. J Clin Oncol 2014;32(27):3059–68.

6. Itti E, Meignan M, Berriolo-Riedinger A, et al. An international confirmatory study of the prognostic value of early PET/CT in diffuse large B-cell lymphoma: comparison between Deauville criteria and ΔSUVmax. Eur J Nucl Med Mol Imaging 2013; 40(9):1312–20.

7. Buchmann I, Reinhardt M, Elsner K, et al. 2-(fluorine-18)fluoro-2-deoxy-D-glucose positron emission tomography in the detection and staging of malignant lymphoma. A bicenter trial. Cancer 2001;91(5):889–99.

8. Isasi CR, Lu P, Blaufox MD. A meta-analysis of 18F-2-deoxy-2-fluoro-D-glucose positron emission tomography in the staging and restaging of patients with lymphoma. Cancer 2005;104(5):1066–74.

9. Raanani P, Shasha Y, Perry C, et al. Is CT scan still necessary for staging in Hodgkin and non-Hodgkin lymphoma patients in the PET/CT era? Ann Oncol 2006; 17(1):117–22.

10. Schaefer NG, Hany TF, Taverna C, et al. Non-Hodgkin lymphoma and Hodgkin disease: coregistered FDG PET and CT at staging and restaging–do we need contrast-enhanced CT? Radiology 2004;232(3):823–9.

11. Elstrom RL, Leonard JP, Coleman M, et al. Combined PET and low-dose, noncontrast CT scanning obviates the need for additional diagnostic contrast-enhanced CT scans in patients undergoing staging or restaging for lymphoma. Ann Oncol 2008;19(10):1770–3.

12. Pelosi E, Pregno P, Penna D, et al. Role of whole-body [18F] fluorodeoxyglucose positron emission tomography/computed tomography (FDG-PET/CT) and conventional techniques in the staging of patients with Hodgkin and aggressive non Hodgkin lymphoma. Radiol Med 2008;113(4):578–90.

13. Adams HJ, Kwee TC, de Keizer B, et al. FDG PET/CT for the detection of bone marrow involvement in diffuse large B-cell lymphoma: systematic review and meta-analysis. Eur J Nucl Med Mol Imaging 2014;41(3):565–74.

14. Cerci JJ, Györke T, Fanti S, et al. Combined PET and biopsy evidence of marrow involvement improves prognostic prediction in diffuse large B-cell lymphoma. J Nucl Med 2014;55(10):1591–7.

15. Hong J, Lee Y, Park Y, et al. Role of FDG-PET/CT in detecting lymphomatous bone marrow involvement in patients with newly diagnosed diffuse large B-cell lymphoma. Ann Hematol 2012;91(5):687–95.

16. Khan AB, Barrington SF, Mikhaeel NG, et al. PET-CT staging of DLBCL accurately identifies and provides new insight into the clinical significance of bone marrow involvement. Blood 2013;122(1):61–7.

17. Adams HJ, Kwee TC, Fijnheer R, et al. Bone marrow 18F-fluoro-2-deoxy-D-glucose positron emission tomography/computed tomography cannot replace bone marrow biopsy in diffuse large B-cell lymphoma. Am J Hematol 2014; 89(7):726–31.

18. Sehn LH, Scott DW, Chhanabhai M, et al. Impact of concordant and discordant bone marrow involvement on outcome in diffuse large B-cell lymphoma treated with R-CHOP. J Clin Oncol 2011;29(11):1452–7.

19. Gallamini A, Borra A. Role of PET in lymphoma. Curr Treat Options Oncol 2014; 15(2):248–61.

20. Pregno P, Chiappella A, Bellò M, et al. Interim 18-FDG-PET/CT failed to predict the outcome in diffuse large B-cell lymphoma patients treated at the diagnosis with rituximab-CHOP. Blood 2012;119(9):2066–73.

21. Moskowitz CH. Interim PET-CT in the management of diffuse large B-cell lymphoma. Hematology Am Soc Hematol Educ Program 2012;2012:397–401.

22. Zhu D, Xu XL, Fang C, et al. Prognostic value of interim (18)F-FDG-PET in diffuse large B cell lymphoma treated with rituximab-based immune-chemotherapy: a systematic review and meta-analysis. Int J Clin Exp Med 2015;8(9):15340–50.

23. Sun N, Zhao J, Qiao W, et al. Predictive value of interim PET/CT in DLBCL treated with R-CHOP: meta-analysis. Biomed Res Int 2015;2015:648572.

24. Mylam KJ, Nielsen AL, Pedersen LM, et al. Fluorine-18-fluorodeoxyglucose positron emission tomography in diffuse large B-cell Lymphoma. PET Clin 2014;9(4): 443–55, vi.

25. Kostakoglu L, Goldsmith SJ, Leonard JP, et al. FDG-PET after 1 cycle of therapy predicts outcome in diffuse large cell lymphoma and classic Hodgkin disease. Cancer 2006;107(11):2678–87.

26. Mylam KJ, Kostakoglu L, Hutchings M, et al. (18)F-fluorodeoxyglucose-positron emission tomography/computed tomography after one cycle of chemotherapy in patients with diffuse large B-cell lymphoma: results of a Nordic/US intergroup study. Leuk Lymphoma 2015;56(7):2005–12.

27. Casasnovas RO, Meignan M, Berriolo-Riedinger A, et al. SUVmax reduction improves early prognosis value of interim positron emission tomography scans in diffuse large B-cell lymphoma. Blood 2011;118(1):37–43.

28. Itti E, Lin C, Dupuis J, et al. Prognostic value of interim 18F-FDG PET in patients with diffuse large B-Cell lymphoma: SUV-based assessment at 4 cycles of chemotherapy. J Nucl Med 2009;50(4):527–33.

29. Fuertes S, Setoain X, Lopez-Guillermo A, et al. Interim FDG PET/CT as a prognostic factor in diffuse large B-cell lymphoma. Eur J Nucl Med Mol Imaging 2013;40(4):496–504.

30. Nols N, Mounier N, Bouazza S, et al. Quantitative and qualitative analysis of metabolic response at interim positron emission tomography scan combined with International Prognostic Index is highly predictive of outcome in diffuse large B-cell lymphoma. Leuk Lymphoma 2014;55(4):773–80.

31. Yang DH, Ahn JS, Byun BH, et al. Interim PET/CT-based prognostic model for the treatment of diffuse large B cell lymphoma in the post-rituximab era. Ann Hematol 2013;92(4):471–9.

32. Lin C, Itti E, Haioun C, et al. Early 18F-FDG PET for prediction of prognosis in patients with diffuse large B-cell lymphoma: SUV-based assessment versus visual analysis. J Nucl Med 2007;48(10):1626–32.

33. Duehrsen U, Hüttmann A, Müller S, et al. Positron emission tomography (PET) guided therapy of aggressive lymphomas – a randomized controlled trial comparing different treatment approaches based on interim PET results (PETAL Trial). Blood 2014;124(21):391.

34. Song MK, Chung JS, Shin HJ, et al. Clinical significance of metabolic tumor volume by PET/CT in stages II and III of diffuse large B cell lymphoma without extranodal site involvement. Ann Hematol 2012;91(5):697–703.

35. Kim J, Hong J, Kim SG, et al. Prognostic value of metabolic tumor volume estimated by (18)F-FDG positron emission tomography/computed tomography in patients with diffuse large B-cell lymphoma of stage II or III disease. Nucl Med Mol Imaging 2014;48(3):187–95.

36. Song MK, Yang DH, Lee GW, et al. High total metabolic tumor volume in PET/CT predicts worse prognosis in diffuse large B cell lymphoma patients with bone marrow involvement in rituximab era. Leuk Res 2016;42:1–6.

37. Kim TM, Paeng JC, Chun IK, et al. Total lesion glycolysis in positron emission tomography is a better predictor of outcome than the international prognostic index for patients with diffuse large B cell lymphoma. Cancer 2013;119(6):1195–202.

38. Kostakoglu L, Chauvie S. PET-derived metabolic volume metrics in lymphoma. Clin Transl Imaging 2015;3(4):331–41.

39. Xie M, Wu K, Liu Y, et al. Predictive value of F-18 FDG PET/CT quantization parameters in diffuse large B cell lymphoma: a meta-analysis with 702 participants. Med Oncol 2015;32(1):446.

40. Malek E, Sendilnathan A, Yellu M, et al. Metabolic tumor volume on interim PET is a better predictor of outcome in diffuse large B-cell lymphoma than semiquantitative methods. Blood Cancer J 2015;5:e326.

41. Moskowitz CI I, Schöder H. Current status of the role of PET imaging in diffuse large B-cell lymphoma. Semin Hematol 2015;52(2):138–42.

42. Moskowitz CH, Schöder H, Teruya-Feldstein J, et al. Risk-adapted dose-dense immunochemotherapy determined by interim FDG-PET in advanced-stage diffuse large B-Cell lymphoma. J Clin Oncol 2010;28(11):1896–903.

43. Schoder H, Zelenetz A, Hamlin P, et al. Prospective Study of FLT PET for early interim response assessment in advanced stage B-cell lymphoma. J Nucl Med 2016;57(5):728–34.

44. Herrmann K, Buck AK, Schuster T, et al. Week one FLT-PET response predicts complete remission to R-CHOP and survival in DLBCL. Oncotarget 2014;5(12): 4050–9.

45. Minamimoto R, Fayad L, Advani R, et al. Diffuse large B-cell lymphoma: prospective multicenter comparison of early interim FLT PET/CT versus FDG PET/CT with IHP, EORTC, Deauville, and PERCIST criteria for early therapeutic monitoring. Radiology 2016;280(1):220–9.

46. Wang R, Zhu H, Chen Y, et al. Standardized uptake value based evaluation of lymphoma by FDG and FLT PET/CT. Hematol Oncol 2014;32(3):126–32.

47. Mikhaeel NG, Timothy AR, Hain SF, et al. 18-FDG-PET for the assessment of residual masses on CT following treatment of lymphomas. Ann Oncol 2000; 11(Suppl 1):147–50.

48. Spaepen K, Stroobants S, Dupont P, et al. Prognostic value of positron emission tomography (PET) with fluorine-18 fluorodeoxyglucose ([18F]FDG) after first-line chemotherapy in non-Hodgkin's lymphoma: is [18F]FDG-PET a valid alternative to conventional diagnostic methods? J Clin Oncol 2001;19(2):414–9.

49. Terasawa T, Nihashi T, Hotta T, et al. 18F-FDG PET for posttherapy assessment of Hodgkin's disease and aggressive Non-Hodgkin's lymphoma: a systematic review. J Nucl Med 2008;49(1):13–21.

50. Zijlstra JM, Lindauer-van der Werf G, Hoekstra OS, et al. 18F-fluoro-deoxyglucose positron emission tomography for post-treatment evaluation of malignant lymphoma: a systematic review. Haematologica 2006;91(4):522–9.

51. Brepoels L, Stroobants S, De Wever W, et al. Aggressive and indolent non-Hodgkin's lymphoma: response assessment by integrated international workshop criteria. Leuk Lymphoma 2007;48(8):1522–30.

52. Adams HJ, Nievelstein RA, Kwee TC. Prognostic value of complete remission status at end-of-treatment FDG-PET in R-CHOP-treated diffuse large B-cell lymphoma: systematic review and meta-analysis. Br J Haematol 2015;170(2): 185–91.

53. El-Galaly TC, Mylam KJ, Bøgsted M, et al. Role of routine imaging in detecting recurrent lymphoma: a review of 258 patients with relapsed aggressive non-Hodgkin and Hodgkin lymphoma. Am J Hematol 2014;89(6):575–80.

54. El-Galaly T, Prakash V, Christiansen I, et al. Efficacy of routine surveillance with positron emission tomography/computed tomography in aggressive non-Hodgkin lymphoma in complete remission: status in a single center. Leuk Lymphoma 2011;52(4):597–603.

55. Liedtke M, Hamlin PA, Moskowitz CH, et al. Surveillance imaging during remission identifies a group of patients with more favorable aggressive NHL at time of relapse: a retrospective analysis of a uniformly-treated patient population. Ann Oncol 2006;17(6):909–13.

56. Petrausch U, Samaras P, Haile SR, et al. Risk-adapted FDG-PET/CT-based follow-up in patients with diffuse large B-cell lymphoma after first-line therapy. Ann Oncol 2010;21(8):1694–8.

57. Zinzani PL, Stefoni V, Tani M, et al. Role of [18F]fluorodeoxyglucose positron emission tomography scan in the follow-up of lymphoma. J Clin Oncol 2009; 27(11):1781–7.

58. Hong J, Kim JH, Lee KH, et al. Symptom-oriented clinical detection versus routine imaging as a monitoring policy of relapse in patients with diffuse large B-cell lymphoma. Leuk Lymphoma 2014;55(10):2312–8.

59. Thompson CA, Ghesquieres H, Maurer MJ, et al. Utility of routine post-therapy surveillance imaging in diffuse large B-cell lymphoma. J Clin Oncol 2014; 32(31):3506–12.

60. Avivi I, Zilberlicht A, Dann EJ, et al. Strikingly high false positivity of surveillance FDG-PET/CT scanning among patients with diffuse large cell lymphoma in the rituximab era. Am J Hematol 2013;88(5):400–5.

61. Cheah CY, Hofman MS, Dickinson M, et al. Limited role for surveillance PET-CT scanning in patients with diffuse large B-cell lymphoma in complete metabolic remission following primary therapy. Br J Cancer 2013;109(2):312–7.

62. Tirumani SH, LaCasce AS, Jacene HA. Role of 2-Deoxy-2-[18F]-fluoro-d-glucose-PET/computed tomography in lymphoma. PET Clin 2015;10(2):207–25.

63. Hiniker SM, Pollom EL, Khodadoust MS, et al. Value of surveillance studies for patients with stage I to II diffuse large B-cell lymphoma in the rituximab era. Int J Radiat Oncol Biol Phys 2015;92(1):99–106.

64. Zelenetz AD, Wierda WG, Abramson JS, et al. Non-Hodgkin's lymphomas, version 3.2012. J Natl Compr Canc Netw 2012;10(12):1487–98.

65. Armand P, Welch S, Kim HT, et al. Prognostic factors for patients with diffuse large B cell lymphoma and transformed indolent lymphoma undergoing autologous stem cell transplantation in the positron emission tomography era. Br J Haematol 2013;160(5):608–17.

66. Derenzini E, Musuraca G, Fanti S, et al. Pretransplantation positron emission tomography scan is the main predictor of autologous stem cell transplantation outcome in aggressive B-cell non-Hodgkin lymphoma. Cancer 2008;113(9): 2496–503.

67. Dickinson M, Hoyt R, Roberts AW, et al. Improved survival for relapsed diffuse large B cell lymphoma is predicted by a negative pre-transplant FDG-PET scan following salvage chemotherapy. Br J Haematol 2010;150(1):39–45.

68. Roland V, Bodet-Milin C, Moreau A, et al. Impact of high-dose chemotherapy followed by auto-SCT for positive interim [18F] FDG-PET diffuse large B-cell lymphoma patients. Bone Marrow Transplant 2011;46(3):393–9.

69. Sauter CS, Matasar MJ, Meikle J, et al. Prognostic value of FDG-PET prior to autologous stem cell transplantation for relapsed and refractory diffuse large B-cell lymphoma. Blood 2015;125(16):2579–81.

70. Svoboda J, Andreadis C, Elstrom R, et al. Prognostic value of FDG-PET scan imaging in lymphoma patients undergoing autologous stem cell transplantation. Bone Marrow Transplant 2006;38(3):211–6.

71. Ulaner GA, Goldman DA, Sauter CS, et al. Prognostic value of FDG PET/CT before allogeneic and autologous stem cell transplantation for aggressive lymphoma. Radiology 2015;277(2):518–26.

72. Ulaner GA, Lilienstein J, Gönen M, et al. False-positive [18F]fluorodeoxyglucose-avid lymph nodes on positron emission tomography-computed tomography after

allogeneic but not autologous stem-cell transplantation in patients with lymphoma. J Clin Oncol 2014;32(1):51–6.

73. Akhtar S, Al-Sugair AS, Abouzied M, et al. Pre-transplant (18)F-fluorodeoxyglucose positron emission tomography-based survival model in patients with aggressive lymphoma undergoing high-dose chemotherapy and autologous SCT. Bone Marrow Transplant 2013;48(4):551–6.

74. Bachanova V, Burns LJ, Ahn KW, et al. Impact of pretransplantation (18)F-fluorodeoxy glucose-positron emission tomography status on outcomes after allogeneic hematopoietic cell transplantation for Non-Hodgkin lymphoma. Biol Blood Marrow Transplant 2015;21(9):1605–11.

75. Dodero A, Crocchiolo R, Patriarca F, et al. Pretransplantation [18-F] fluorodeoxyglucose positron emission tomography scan predicts outcome in patients with recurrent Hodgkin lymphoma or aggressive non-Hodgkin lymphoma undergoing reduced-intensity conditioning followed by allogeneic stem cell transp. Cancer 2010;116(21):5001–11.

76. Lambert JR, Bomanji JB, Peggs KS, et al. Prognostic role of PET scanning before and after reduced-intensity allogeneic stem cell transplantation for lymphoma. Blood 2010;115(14):2763–8.

77. Kletter K, Kalhs P. (18)F-deoxyglucose PET: useful in the management of patients with stem cell transplantation for lymphoma? Expert Rev Hematol 2010;3(4): 405–10.

78. Hart DP, Avivi I, Thomson KJ, et al. Use of 18F-FDG positron emission tomography following allogeneic transplantation to guide adoptive immunotherapy with donor lymphocyte infusions. Br J Haematol 2005;128(6):824–9.

79. Cashen AF, Dehdashti F, Luo J, et al. 18F-FDG PET/CT for early response assessment in diffuse large B-cell lymphoma: poor predictive value of international harmonization project interpretation. J Nucl Med 2011;52(3):386–92.

80. Itti E, Juweid ME, Haioun C, et al. Improvement of early 18F-FDG PET interpretation in diffuse large B-cell lymphoma: importance of the reference background. J Nucl Med 2010;51(12):1857–62.

81. Safar V, Dupuis J, Itti E, et al. Interim [18F]fluorodeoxyglucose positron emission tomography scan in diffuse large B-cell lymphoma treated with anthracycline-based chemotherapy plus rituximab. J Clin Oncol 2012;30(2):184–90.

82. Yang DH, Min JJ, Song HC, et al. Prognostic significance of interim 18F-FDG PET/CT after three or four cycles of R-CHOP chemotherapy in the treatment of diffuse large B-cell lymphoma. Eur J Cancer 2011;47(9):1312–8.

83. Yoo C, Lee DH, Kim JE, et al. Limited role of interim PET/CT in patients with diffuse large B-cell lymphoma treated with R-CHOP. Ann Hematol 2011;90(7): 797–802.

Promising Novel Agents for Aggressive B-Cell Lymphoma

Anas Younes, MD

KEYWORDS

- Diffuse large B-cell lymphoma • B-cell receptor • BCL2 inhibitor • EZH2 inhibitor

KEY POINTS

- DLBCL is the most common type of lymphoma in the western world.
- No single agent has been approved for the treatment of DLBCL in more than a decade.
- Agents targeting B-cell receptor signaling, Bcl2 protein, and PD1 immune checkpoint, have modest single-agent activity in relapsed DLBCL.

INTRODUCTION

Diffuse large B-cell lymphoma (DLBCL) is the most common subtype of adult lymphomas, accounting for approximately 25,000 new cases per year in the United States. Today, the most widely used regimen for the treatment of DLBCL is RCHOP (rituximab, cyclophosphamide, doxorubicin, vincristine, and prednisone). Historically, the CHOP regimen was introduced in the early 1970s. More than 40 years later, the only major therapeutic advancement has been incorporation of the monoclonal antibody rituximab with CHOP, creating the RCHOP regimen. Despite this progress, approximately 50% of patients have disease progression or relapse after RCHOP, and most die of their disease. Accordingly, new treatment modalities are necessary to improve the cure rate of patients with DLBCL.

At the molecular level, DLBCL is a heterogeneous disease. Hence, it is not surprising that many patients do not respond to standard RCHOP therapy. Gene expression profiling studies demonstrated that DLBCL is broadly classified into germinal center B-cell (GCB)-like and activated B-cell (ABC)-like subtypes. Using this "cell of origin" classification, it has been shown that treatment with standard RCHOP regime results in a better cure and overall survival in patients with the GCB subtype when compared with those with the ABC subtype. However, relapses are observed in both subsets after RCHOP therapy, suggesting the existence of additional oncogenic events that

Lymphoma Service, Memorial Sloan Kettering Cancer Center, 1275 York Avenue, New York, NY 10021, USA
E-mail address: younesa@mskcc.org

Hematol Oncol Clin N Am 30 (2016) 1229–1237
http://dx.doi.org/10.1016/j.hoc.2016.07.007
0889-8588/16/© 2016 Elsevier Inc. All rights reserved.

mediate resistance to RCHOP, irrespective of the cell of origin. More recent genome sequencing studies revealed a more complex molecular heterogeneity of DLBCL, with genetic alterations frequently observed in GCB and ABC subtypes. Other, less common genetic alterations can preferentially be detected in either GCB or ABC subsets. Novel treatment strategies that are based on lymphoma-associated oncogenic alterations are needed to improve the cure rate of patients with DLBCL.

One of the biggest challenges in drug development for patients with cancer, including DLBCL, is the high failure rate caused by excessive toxicity, low response rates, or both (**Fig. 1**). The success of future drug development in DLBCL depends on using biomarkers to identify patients who are likely to benefit from a specific therapy. The following is a focused review on the most promising agents for the treatment of DLBCL, with a discussion on how to select patients for these novel drugs based on genetic and molecular biomarkers. This article also provides a brief update on recent advances in immune therapy of DLBCL.

B-CELL RECEPTOR SIGNALING INHIBITORS

The B-cell receptor (BCR) complex is composed of membrane IgM that is linked with transmembrane heterodimer protein (CD79a/CD79b). Both CD79 proteins contain an immunoreceptor tyrosine-based activation motif in their intracellular tails. On BCR crosslinking by an antigen, the CD79a immunoreceptor tyrosine-based activation motif tyrosines (Tyr188 and Tyr199) are phosphorylated, creating a docking site for Src-homology 2 domain-containing kinases, such Lyn, Blk, and Fyn, with subsequent activation of downstream kinases, such as spleen tyrosine kinase (Syk) and bruton tyrosine kinase (Btk). Aberrant and sustained activation of BCR signaling pathway is implicated in the pathogenesis of a variety of B-cell malignancies, including DLBCL.

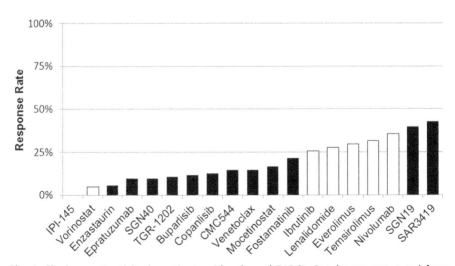

Fig. 1. Single-agent activity in patients with relapsed DLBCL. Results are generated from published data from phase I or phase II studies. Some of these trials are either ongoing and/or enrolled a small number of patients, and therefore these response rates may change with time. *Black bars* indicate investigational agents with no Food and Drug Administration–approved indication. *White bars* identify agents with Food and Drug Administration approval for different types of lymphoma, but none are approved for DLBCL.

Novel drugs targeting various components of BCR signaling pathway have been developed, initially targeting SYK, and subsequently targeting BTK.

Spleen Tyrosine Kinase Inhibitors

SYK is a nonreceptor tyrosine kinase important for the development of the lymphatic system. SYK is expressed in cells of the hematopoietic lineage, such as B cells, mast cells, basophils, neutrophils, macrophages, and osteoclasts, but is also present in cells of nonhematopoietic origin, such as epithelial cells, hepatocytes, fibroblasts, neuronal cells, and vascular endothelial cells. Thus, SYK seems to play a general physiologic function in a wide variety of cells. $Syk^{-/-}$ knockout mice die during embryonic development of hemorrhage and show severe defects in the development of the lymphatic system. Fostamatinib disodium (R788), a competitive inhibitor for ATP binding to the Syk catalytic domain, demonstrated a 55% response rate in patients with relapsed chronic lymphocytic leukemia (CLL).[1] Patients with other B-cell malignancies had a lower response rate to fostamatinib. In a recent study, 68 patients with relapsed or refractory DLBCL, fostamatinib treatment resulted in a 3% response rate. None of the patients with clinical benefit had ABC genotype.

Bruton Tyrosine Kinase Inhibitors

BTK inactivating mutations impair B-cell development and are associated with the absence of mature B cells and agammaglobulinemia. Ibrutinib is a selective and irreversible inhibitor of BTK. Although ibrutinib demonstrated a significant clinical activity in patients with CLL, mantle cell lymphoma, and Waldenström macroglobulinemia, it has a modest clinical activity in DLBCL and follicular lymphoma. In relapsed DLBCL, ibrutinib treatment resulted in an overall response rate of 23%. In contrast to the results that were observed with the SYK inhibitor fostamatinib, most responses to ibrutinib were observed in patients with the ABC DLBCL subtype.[2] This observation generated interest in further investigating ibrutinib in combination with standard chemotherapy regimens for the treatment of patients with newly diagnosed ABC DLBCL.[3] A phase 3 randomized trial comparing RCHOP with RCHOP with ibrutinib combination (the Phoenix study) has already completed enrollment of patients with newly diagnosed non-GCB DLBCL, and the results should become available in the near future.

Ibrutinib is generally more tolerated than SYK inhibitors. The most common toxicities are diarrhea and skin rash. Grade 3 to 4 neutropenia and thrombocytopenia are seen in less than 10% of patients. Other toxicities include atrial fibrillation and bleeding. Ibrutinib covalently binds to a cysteine 481 (C-481) residue in the BTK kinase domain (**Fig. 2**). Several other kinases that contain C-481, including members of the TEC family, EGFR, and JAK3, are also inhibited by ibrutinib, which may contribute to its toxicity. To reduce toxicity, several pharmaceutical companies are developing more selective BTK inhibitors. These second-generation, selective, BTK inhibitors, including acalabrutinib and BGB-3111,[4,5] also bind to C481. Accordingly, these newer inhibitors are not expected to be more effective than ibrutinib, nor they are expected to work in ibrutinib failures. However, because these selective inhibitors may be more tolerable than ibrutinib, they may be administered without dose interruption or reduction. Whether an uninterrupted treatment schedule will be associated with a more favorable treatment outcome is currently unknown.

B-CELL CHRONIC LYMPHOCYTIC LEUKEMIA/LYMPHOMA 2 INHIBITORS

The B-cell CLL/lymphoma 2 (BCL2) family of proteins is divided into three functional subgroups: (1) the BCL2-like prosurvival proteins (Bcl2, Bcl-xL, and Mcl1),

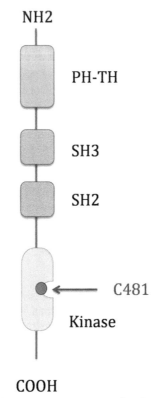

Fig. 2. Schematic structure of bruton tyrosine kinase (BTK). Most small molecule inhibitors, including ibrutinib, bind to the cysteine 481 residue in the kinase domain. PH-TH, pleckstrin homology (PH), TEC homology (TH) domain; SH, SRC homology domain (SH3 followed by SH2).

(2) the proapoptotic BCL2-associated X (BAX)/BCL2-antagonist/killer (BAK) effector proteins, and (3) the proapoptotic BCL2 homology domain 3 (BH3)-only proteins (**Fig. 3**). The BH3-only proteins are further divided into activating proteins (Bim, Puma, and Bid) and sensitizing proteins (Noxa and Bad). To date, most therapeutic strategies are focused on inhibiting the antiapoptotic Bcl-2 family members.

Navitoclax

Navitoclax (ABT-263) is the first-generation, oral, BH3 mimetic that inhibits Bcl-2, Bcl-XL, and Bcl-w, but not Mcl-1. In a phase I study of 55 patients with relapsed lymphoid malignancies, navitoclax demonstrated no clinical activity in relapsed DLBC. Treatment was associated with dose-dependent thrombocytopenia, which is related to inhibition of Bcl-XL.[6–8] Because thrombocytopenia created challenges for future combination strategies, especially with chemotherapy, the development of navitoclax was stopped.

Venetoclax

Venetoclax (ABT-199) is a Bcl-2 selective inhibitor with 100-fold affinity for Bcl2 over Bcl-XL. Consequently, it has a minimal or no effect on platelet counts.[9] Similar to

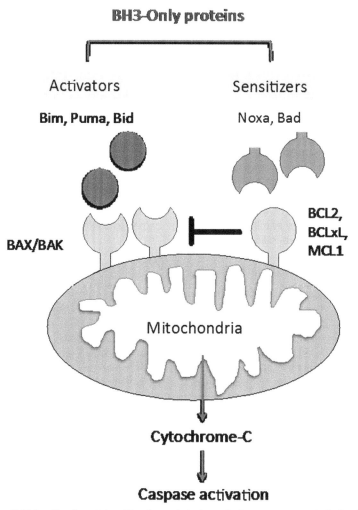

Fig. 3. The Bcl2 family of proteins. The dynamic balance between proapoptotic Bax/Bak and prosurvival Bcl2, Bcl-xL, and Mcl1 is further regulated by activating (Bim, Puma, and Bid) and sensitizing (Noxa and Bad) proteins.

navitoclax, venetoclax has no effect on Mcl1. Venetoclax demonstrated remarkable activity in patients with relapsed CLL and mantle cell lymphoma, with response rates exceeding 70%, leading to its initial Food and Drug Administration approval for the treatment of patients with relapsed CLL carrying p53 genetic alterations.[10] However, the response rate in patients with relapsed DLBCL was only 18%.[11] Because initial studies were associated with fatal tumor lysis, subsequent studies implemented strict monitoring and treatment of tumor lysis, in addition to a ramped dose schedule over several weeks. Despite the low response rate in relapsed DLBCL, venetoclax-based combination strategies remains of a high interest. Ongoing clinical trials are investigating the efficacy and safety of venetoclax in combination with standard chemotherapy regimens (rituximab plus bendamustine, and RCHOP), and with other small molecule inhibitors.

ENHANCER OF ZESTE HOMOLOG 2 INHIBITORS

Enhancer of zeste homolog 2 (EZH2) is a histone-lysine N-methyltransferase enzyme, responsible for methylation of lysine 27 of histone H3 (H3K27). This histone modification is associated with repressed gene transcription when trimethylated (H3K27me3). EZH2 is critical for normal development and EZH2 knockout results in lethality at early stages of mouse development. EZH2-activating mutations or overexpression has been observed in a variety of cancers, including lymphoma.[12–14] Wild-type and mutant EZH2 functions are essential for GCB-type DLBCLs but not for ABC DLBCLs, suggesting that EZH2 inhibitors should primarily be effective in GCB-type DLBCLs. Preclinical experiments demonstrated the potential therapeutic value of EZH2 inhibitors in lymphoma.[15,16] In a phase I study, the oral EZH2 inhibitor, tazemetostat, was evaluated in 45 patients, including 19 with relapsed lymphoma. Responses were observed in 9 of 15 evaluable patients, including those with wild-type EZH2.[17] A phase II study is currently enrolling patients to further confirm the clinical activity in patients with DLBCL. The study will enroll ABC and GCB subtypes to confirm whether there is preferential activity in a specific DLBCL subtype.

IMMUNE CHECKPOINT INHIBITORS

The immune system is physiologically regulated by a set of cell surface proteins to downregulate T-cell activation to maintain self-tolerance and prevent autoimmunity.[18] This process is frequently hijacked by tumor cells to enable them to evade T-cell mediated antitumor immunity. Cytotoxic T-lymphocyte-associated protein 4/CD152 (CTLA-4), is an immune checkpoint protein that is expressed on the surface of T cells. The ligands for CTLA-4 are CD80 or CD86, which are typically expressed by antigen-presenting cells. Engagement of CTAL-4 with its ligands results in T-cell inactivation. Another checkpoint system involves the engagement between programmed death-1 (PD-1), which is expressed by T cells, and its ligands (PDL-1 and PDL-2). CTLA-4 knockout mice succumb to a lethal multiorgan lymphoproliferative disease, whereas inactivating PD-1, and its ligands PD-L1 and PD-L2, result in a milder phenotype that is associated with late-onset organ-specific inflammation.[19,20]

CTLA-4 and PD-1 are currently being targeted for the treatment of cancer, including lymphoma. Earlier studies with the anti-CTLA-4 antibody, ipilimumab, produced modest clinical activity in patients with relapsed B-cell non-Hodgkin lymphoma and Hodgkin lymphoma.[21] More recently, trials using blocking antibodies to PD-1 showed a more promising clinical activity in patients with relapsed Hodgkin lymphoma.[22–24] The experience in patients with relapsed DLBCL remains limited to a small number of patients treated in a phase I study, demonstrating a 40% response rate. Other studies are currently evaluating the efficacy of various antibodies targeting PD-L1, such as MPDL3280A, but the results are still pending.

CHIMERIC ANTIGEN RECEPTOR T CELLS

Chimeric antigen receptors (CARs) are composed of a single-chain variable fragment (scFv) derived from a murine or humanized antibody that redirects T cells to a specific antigen that is expressed by tumor cells. In B-cell lymphoma, CARs have been typically directed to CD19.[25] CAR T cells can recognize and kill tumor cells in an HLA-independent manner. Several CAR T-cell platforms are currently in clinical trials, with no clear superiority of one platform over the other.[26] Although clinical results were achieved in patients with B-cell acute lymphoblastic leukemia,[27] results in patients with B-cell lymphoma were more modest. Future directions will focus on further enhancing T-cell activation, including combination strategies with immune checkpoint inhibitors.

Adverse events associated with CAR T-cell therapy include cytokine release syndrome, encephalopathy, and B-cell aplasia. Cytokine release syndrome includes fever, tachycardia, hypotension, capillary leak syndrome, and respiratory distress.[28,29] Encephalopathy may manifest as mild confusion to obtundation, aphasia, and seizures.[30] B-cell aplasia has been noted in CAR T-cell therapy caused by depletion of nonmalignant CD19 B lymphocytes.[27,30,31]

SUMMARY

Patients with relapsed DLBCL who are not candidates for stem cell transplant, or whose disease relapses after stem cell transplant, have clear unmet medical needs and are candidates for drug development. Although, there are currently no agents approved by the Food and Drug Administration for the treatment of relapsed DLBCL, the landscape of new agents is promising. Future direction should focus on the development of mechanism-based combination regimens, and biomarker-driven patients' selection.

REFERENCES

1. Friedberg JW, Sharman J, Sweetenham J, et al. Inhibition of Syk with fostamatinib disodium has significant clinical activity in non-Hodgkin lymphoma and chronic lymphocytic leukemia. Blood 2010;115:2578–85.

2. Wilson WH, Young RM, Schmitz R, et al. Targeting B cell receptor signaling with ibrutinib in diffuse large B cell lymphoma. Nat Med 2015;21:922–6.

3. Younes A, Thieblemont C, Morschhauser F, et al. Combination of ibrutinib with rituximab, cyclophosphamide, doxorubicin, vincristine, and prednisone (R-CHOP) for treatment-naive patients with CD20-positive B-cell non-Hodgkin lymphoma: a non-randomised, phase 1b study. Lancet Oncol 2014;15:1019–26.

4. Byrd JC, Harrington B, O'Brien S, et al. Acalabrutinib (ACP-196) in relapsed chronic lymphocytic leukemia. N Engl J Med 2016;374(4):323–32.

5. Tam C, Grigg AP, Opat S, et al. The BTK inhibitor, Bgb-3111, is safe, tolerable, and highly active in patients with relapsed/refractory B-cell malignancies: initial report of a phase 1 first-in-human trial. Blood 2015;126:832.

6. Davids MS, Letai A. ABT-199: taking dead aim at BCL-2. Cancer Cell 2013;23: 139–41.

7. Roberts AW, Advani RH, Kahl BS, et al. Phase 1 study of the safety, pharmacokinetics, and antitumour activity of the BCL2 inhibitor navitoclax in combination with rituximab in patients with relapsed or refractory CD20+ lymphoid malignancies. Br J Haematol 2015;170:669–78.

8. Wilson WH, O'Connor OA, Czuczman MS, et al. Navitoclax, a targeted high-affinity inhibitor of BCL-2, in lymphoid malignancies: a phase 1 dose-escalation study of safety, pharmacokinetics, pharmacodynamics, and antitumour activity. Lancet Oncol 2010;11:1149–59.

9. Souers AJ, Leverson JD, Boghaert ER, et al. ABT-199, a potent and selective BCL-2 inhibitor, achieves antitumor activity while sparing platelets. Nat Med 2013;19:202–8.

10. Roberts AW, Davids MS, Pagel JM, et al. Targeting BCL2 with venetoclax in relapsed chronic lymphocytic leukemia. N Engl J Med 2016;374(4):311–22.

11. Gerecitano JF, Roberts AW, Seymour JF, et al. A phase 1 study of venetoclax (ABT-199/GDC-0199) monotherapy in patients with relapsed/refractory non-Hodgkin lymphoma. Blood 2015;126:254.

12. Morin RD, Johnson NA, Severson TM, et al. Somatic mutations altering EZH2 (Tyr641) in follicular and diffuse large B-cell lymphomas of germinal-center origin. Nat Genet 2010;42:181–5.

13. Beguelin W, Popovic R, Teater M, et al. EZH2 is required for germinal center formation and somatic EZH2 mutations promote lymphoid transformation. Cancer Cell 2013;23:677–92.

14. Velichutina I, Shaknovich R, Geng H, et al. EZH2-mediated epigenetic silencing in germinal center B cells contributes to proliferation and lymphomagenesis. Blood 2010;116:5247–55.

15. Qi W, Chan H, Teng L, et al. Selective inhibition of Ezh2 by a small molecule inhibitor blocks tumor cells proliferation. Proc Natl Acad Sci U S A 2012;109: 21360–5.

16. McCabe MT, Ott HM, Ganji G, et al. EZH2 inhibition as a therapeutic strategy for lymphoma with EZH2-activating mutations. Nature 2012;492:108–12.

17. Ribrag V, Soria J-C, Michot J-M, et al. Phase 1 study of tazemetostat (EPZ-6438), an inhibitor of enhancer of zeste-homolog 2 (EZH2): preliminary safety and activity in relapsed or refractory non-Hodgkin lymphoma (NHL) patients. Blood 2015; 126:473.

18. Pardoll DM. The blockade of immune checkpoints in cancer immunotherapy. Nat Rev Cancer 2012;12:252–64.

19. Waterhouse P, Penninger JM, Timms E, et al. Lymphoproliferative disorders with early lethality in mice deficient in CTLA-4. Science 1995;270:985–8.

20. Tivol EA, Borriello F, Schweitzer AN, et al. Loss of CTLA-4 leads to massive lymphoproliferation and fatal multiorgan tissue destruction, revealing a critical negative regulatory role of CTLA-4. Immunity 1995;3:541–7.

21. Ansell SM, Hurvitz SA, Koenig PA, et al. Phase I study of ipilimumab, an anti-CTLA-4 monoclonal antibody, in patients with relapsed and refractory B-cell non-Hodgkin lymphoma. Clin Cancer Res 2009;15:6446–53.

22. Ansell SM, Lesokhin AM, Borrello I, et al. PD-1 blockade with nivolumab in relapsed or refractory Hodgkin's lymphoma. N Engl J Med 2015;372:311–9.

23. Armand P, Shipp MA, Ribrag V, et al. PD-1 blockade with pembrolizumab in patients with classical Hodgkin lymphoma after brentuximab vedotin failure: safety, efficacy, and biomarker assessment. Blood 2015;126:584.

24. Zinzani PL, Ribrag V, Moskowitz CH, et al. Phase 1b study of PD-1 blockade with pembrolizumab in patients with relapsed/refractory primary mediastinal large B-cell lymphoma (PMBCL). Blood 2015;126:3986.

25. Sadelain M. CAR therapy: the CD19 paradigm. J Clin Invest 2015;125: 3392–400.

26. Ramos CA, Heslop HE, Brenner MK. CAR-T cell therapy for lymphoma. Annu Rev Med 2016;67:165–83.

27. Brentjens RJ, Davila ML, Riviere I, et al. CD19-targeted T cells rapidly induce molecular remissions in adults with chemotherapy-refractory acute lymphoblastic leukemia. Sci Transl Med 2013;5:177ra38.

28. Maude SL, Barrett D, Teachey DT, et al. Managing cytokine release syndrome associated with novel T cell-engaging therapies. Cancer J 2014;20:119–22.

29. Lee DW, Gardner R, Porter DL, et al. Current concepts in the diagnosis and management of cytokine release syndrome. Blood 2014;124:188–95.

30. Lee DW, Kochenderfer JN, Stetler-Stevenson M, et al. T cells expressing CD19 chimeric antigen receptors for acute lymphoblastic leukaemia in children and young adults: a phase 1 dose-escalation trial. Lancet 2015; 385(9967):517–28.
31. Grupp SA, Kalos M, Barrett D, et al. Chimeric antigen receptor-modified T cells for acute lymphoid leukemia. N Engl J Med 2013;368:1509–18.

The Spectrum of Double Hit Lymphomas

Jeremy S. Abramson, MD

KEYWORDS

- Double-hit lymphomas • Double-expressing lymphomas
- High grade B-cell lymphoma • MYC • BCL2

KEY POINTS

- Double-hit lymphomas (DHLs) constitute a unique high-risk biologic and clinical subset of aggressive B-cell non-Hodgkin lymphomas characterized by translocations of MYC in addition to BCL2, BCL6, or both.
- DHLs typically present in older adults with high-risk clinical features including advanced stage, extranodal involvement, elevated lactate dehydrogenase (LDH), and often with involvement of bone marrow, peripheral blood, and the central nervous system.
- Prognosis of DHL is overall far inferior to typical diffuse large B-cell lymphoma (DLBCL), but selected low-risk patients can be identified with a favorable prognosis including limited stage, LDH less than 3 times upper limit of normal, and absence of central nervous system (CNS), bone marrow, and leukemic disease.
- Intensive treatment strategies such as DA-EPOCH-R (dose-adjusted etoposide, prednisone, vincristine, cyclophosphamide, doxorubicin, rituximab) appear associated with an improved outcome compared with R-CHOP (rituximab, cyclophophamide, doxorubicin, vincristine, prednisone).
- Double-expressing lymphomas are a subset of DLBCL with dual immunohistochemical expression of BCL-2 and MYC, but without chromosomal translocations, and also constitute a high-risk subset of DLBCL, though more favorable than DHL.

INTRODUCTION

Diffuse large B-cell lymphoma (DLBCL) is the most common non-Hodgkin lymphoma (NHL) in United States and worldwide, and approximately two-thirds of newly diagnosed patients can be expected to be cured using modern therapies. Over the last decade, a particularly high-risk entity within DLBCL has been identified, characterized molecularly by carrying translocations of the MYC proto-oncogene along with BCL2, or less commonly BCL6, or both. Presence of a MYC translocation in concert with either BCL2 or BCL6 is now known as a double-hit lymphoma (DHL), or as a triple-hit lymphoma (THL) if all 3 rearrangements are present. More recently, an

Disclosure: Dr J.S. Abramson consults for Amgen, Gilead, Incyte, Infinity, Juno, and Pharmacyclics.
Center for Lymphoma, Massachusetts General Hospital Cancer Center, Harvard Medical School, 55 Fruit Street, Yawkey 9A, Boston, MA 02114, USA
E-mail address: jabramson@mgh.harvard.edu

Hematol Oncol Clin N Am 30 (2016) 1239–1249
http://dx.doi.org/10.1016/j.hoc.2016.07.005
0889-8588/16/© 2016 Elsevier Inc. All rights reserved.

adverse prognosis in DLBCL has also been attributed to dual immunohistochemical expression of both MYC and BCL2. Such cases of dual expression of MYC/BCL2 in the absence of dual genomic translocations should not be considered cases of DHL, but rather double-expressing lymphomas (DELs), which constitute a distinct phenotypic entity and have unique considerations in terms of prognosis and therapy. DHL and THL follow a highly aggressive natural history with disappointing responses to standard chemoimmunotherapy platforms, and a poor overall prognosis. The literature guiding understanding of these high-grade lymphomas is almost entirely retrospective in nature, and therefore limited by the biases inherent in such analyses. That said, recent large retrospective series have contributed to the current prognostication and therapeutic selection.

DIAGNOSIS OF DOUBLE-HIT LYMPHOMA

DHLs constitute an uncommon but high-risk subset within DLBCL. It is estimated that approximately 5% to 10% of DLBCLs will be characterized by double-hit cytogenetics.[1,2] In addition to MYC, the most common additional translocation is BCL2 in approximately 85% of DHL cases, with a minority having a BCL6 translocation, or both (THL). It is important to recognize that karyotyping shows that these discrete chromosomal rearrangements occur in the broader context of a complex karyotype in virtually all cases, speaking to overall genomic instability.[1,3,4] The majority of DHLs presents as a de novo DLBCL, while others will have their disease transform out of a low-grade follicular lymphoma.[5–9] In 2008, the World Health Organization (WHO) created a provisional diagnostic category known as B-cell lymphoma unclassifiable with features intermediate between DLBCL and Burkitt lymphoma (BCLu).[10] Cases in this category may have more aggressive morphologic features than a typical case of DLBCL, such as a high proliferation index and starry sky appearance, but are lacking in strict features diagnostic of Burkitt lymphoma such as having more pleomorphic morphology, immunohistochemical expression of BCL2, or presence of a complex karyotype. Though DHLs represent a distinct minority of DLBCLs as a whole, both retrospective and prospective cohorts suggest that DHL constitutes 50% to 75% of cases classified within the BCLu category.[6,11,12] Increasingly, the identification of double-hit cytogenetics within a case of DLBCL has prompted hematopathologists to sign out these cases as BCLu rather than grouping them in with traditional DLBCLs, leading to a migration of DHLs out of the traditional DLBCL diagnostic category and into the provisional diagnosis of BCLu. Most recently, however, the WHO has issued a revision of the classification of lymphoid tumors and has eliminated the BCLu category.[13] In recognition of the unique characteristics of DHL, these cases now have a distinct classification known as high-grade B-cell lymphoma (HGBCL), with MYC and BCL2 and/or BCL6 translocations. DEL will still largely be included in the traditional DLBCL, not otherwise specified (NOS) category, although cases with blastoid morphology or other highly aggressive histologic features will be included in a new category of HGBCL, NOS.

DLBCL is commonly subclassified based on cell of origin (COO) as either germinal center B-cell like (GCB) or activated B-cell like (ABC). Though this classification is defined by gene expression profiling (GEP), immunohistochemical correlates are commonly employed as imperfect surrogates for GEP, which can classify cases as either GCB or non-GCB.[14] Nearly all true DHLs will be classified as GCB DLBCL,[3,7,9,15–18] making them a particularly high-risk subset within the DLBCL COO category typically associated with the more favorable prognosis. Similarly, nearly all cases of DHL will also have immunohistochemical expression of MYC and BCL-2 at the protein level, most commonly defined as MYC expression of at least 40% of cells, and BCL-2 expression in at least 70% of cells. As noted previously, however, most cases with dual MYC/BCL2 immunohistochemical expression will not have true double-hit cytogenetics. In fact, these DEL cases are usually classified as ABC or non-GCB DLBCL.[5,19] An additional pathologic feature identified in nearly all retrospective analyses in DHL is a high Ki-67 proliferation index with a median typically reported in the 80% to 90% range, and often approaching 100%.[1,3,5,16,20] A controversial diagnostic question is whether all newly diagnosed cases of aggressive B-cell lymphoma should be evaluated with fluorescence in situ hybridization (FISH) for MYC, BCL2, and BCL6. Among all newly diagnosed lymphomas characterized morphologically and immunohistochemically as BCLu (or HGBCL using the revised 2016 classification), it would be prudent to perform FISH given the high prevalence of double-hit cytogenetics within this cohort. Among DLBCLs, however, the extensive testing of all patients may not be justified given that only a minority will be DHL, and it adds significant cost. Although no single pathologic correlate exists that perfectly predicts for double-hit cytogenetics, it is clear that there is an overall pathologic pattern that tracks with a diagnosis of DHL. As noted, DHL in DLBCL is enriched for GCB cell of origin, MYC and BCL-2 immunohistochemical expression, and proliferation index greater than 80%, although none of these features alone constitutes a definitive rule-in or rule-out test. It is a safe assertion, however, that a newly diagnosed DLBCL with none of these aforementioned features would have an extremely low risk of being a true DHL, and therefore may not justify the additional expense of FISH analysis in this subset of patients.

CLINICAL FEATURES AND PROGNOSIS IN DOUBLE-HIT LYMPHOMA

Clinical features of DHL are summarized in **Table 1**. DHL is predominantly a disease of older adults, with a median age in the 60s, although it can occur in both young adults and in the very elderly.[1,3–6,20–22] The majority of patients will present with advanced stage disease, involvement of extranodal locations, significantly elevated lactate dehydrogenase (LDH), and high-intermediate or high-risk international prognostic index (IPI) score. Among extranodal locations, a high proportion of patients will have involvement of the bone marrow at the time of diagnosis, and this may involve a circulating leukemic phase in the peripheral blood, a finding that is rarely seen in typical DLBCL.[3,21] Central nervous system (CNS) involvement at diagnosis, or subsequently at relapse, is also increased in DHL relative to other DLBCLs.[1,3,4,6]

Initially published retrospective series in DHL reported a dismal prognosis with median survivals well less than 1 year, and long-term survivorship in less than 10% of patients.[5–8,17,18] These initial series, however, suffer from selection bias based on which patients at their institutions were tested for MYC and BCL-2 translocations in the first place, and therefore available for analysis. The result is databases that are enriched for patients with highly aggressive disease and either clinical or pathologic features suggestive of a Burkitt or Burkitt–like disease, which prompted FISH for MYC evaluation, a test not typically performed until recently in most cases of DLBCL. Broadly testing all cases of DLBCL, on the other hand, would include subjects who were missed in early analyses, and capture patients with lower-risk clinical and pathologic features that might correlate with an improved overall outcome. Further, older series included patients predominantly treated with CHOP-like therapy, and would not fully reflect any impact of modern therapeutic advances. Indeed, the largest and most contemporary analyses in DHL reflect a significantly improved prognosis relative to initial reports (**Table 2**). Modern data suggest that the long-term survival in DHL can be estimated at approximately 40% to 50%,[4,20–23] demonstrating that a significant minority of

Table 1
Clinical and pathologic features of double-hit lymphoma in contemporary series

Series	n	Prior iNHL	GCB (IHC)	DLBCL Morphology	Median Age	Stage III-IV	IPI >1	t-BCL2	t-BCL6	THL	Elevated LDH	>1 EN Site	CNS Involved	Marrow Involved	Leukemic Disease
Abramson et al,[21] 2012	37	27%	NR	38%	63	86%	86%	87%	11%	3%	89%	54%	16%	43%	24%
Copie-Bergman et al,[22] 2015	32	NR	81%	90%	63	84%	84%	NR	NR	NR	75%	56%	NR	30%	NR
Oki et al,[3] 2014	129	11%	93%	65%	62	84%	87%	84%	12%	11%	69%	49%	10%	42%	12%
Petrich et al,[4] 2014	311	22%	87%	50%	60	81%	NR	87%	5%	8%	76%	28%	11%	44%	NR (22% elevated WBC)

Abbreviations: CNS, central nervous system; DLBCL, diffuse large B-cell lymphoma; GCB, germinal center-B-cell; IHC, immunohistochemistry; iNHL, indolent non-Hodgkin lymphoma; IPI, international prognostic index; NR, not reported; t-BCL2, translocation BCL2; t-BCL6, translocation BCL6; THL, triple hit lymphoma; WBC, white blood cell count.

Table 2
Outcome for double-hit lymphoma in contemporary series

Series	n	Treatments (n)	PFS	OS	Treatment Differences
Abramson et al,[21] 2012	37	R-CHOP (15) DA-EPOCH-R (15) R-CODOX-M/R-IVAC (6) Upfront SCT (3)	Median 19 m	Median 34 m	DA-EPOCH-R superior to other regimens for PFS and OS
Copie-Bergman et al,[22] 2015	32	R-CHOP (19) R-ACVBP (13)	27% at 5 y	32% at 5 y	NR
Oki et al,[3] 2014	129	R-CHOP (57) R-hyperCVAD/MA (34) DA-EPOCH-R (28) R-CODOX-M/R-IVAC (28) Other (10) Upfront SCT (23)	33% at 2 y	44% at 2 y	DA-EPOCH-R superior to other regimens for CRR, PFS and OS. No statistically significant benefit for SCT in first CR
Petrich et al,[4] 2014	311	R-CHOP (100) R-hyperCVAD/MA (65) DA-EPOCH-R (64) R-CODOX-M/R-IVAC (42) Other (40) Upfront SCT (53)	Median 11 m 40% at 2 y	Median 22 m 49% at 2 y	DA-EPOCH-R superior to other regimens for CRR Intensive regimens (DA-EPOCH-R, R-CODOX-M/R-IVAC, R-hyperCVAD/MA) superior to R-CHOP for PFS. No statistically significant benefit for SCT in first CR CNS prophylaxis with MTX associated with improved OS

Abbreviations: CNS, central nervous system; CR, complete response; DA-EPOCH-R, dose adjusted etoposide, prednisone, vincristine, cyclophosphamide, doxorubicin, rituximab; NR, not reported; OS, overall survival; PFS, progression-free survival; R-CODOX-M/R-IVAC, rituximab, cyclophosphamide, vincristine, doxorubicin, methotrexate/rituximab, ifosfamide, etoposide, cytarabine; R-hyperCVAD/MA, rituximab, hyperfractionated cyclophosphamide, vincristine, doxorubicin, dexamethasone/methotrexate, cytarabine; SCT, stem cell transplant.

patients with DHL may indeed fare well, and that DHL does not predict the uniform death sentence that was initially suggested.

Given the heterogeneity in outcome among patients with DHL, prognostic variables have been extensively evaluated. In the 2 largest analyses to date, the IPI is predictive in this population, with patients with 0 to 1 risk factors having a very favorable overall prognosis of approximately 90%, compared with approximately 25% within IPI scores of 3 to 5.[3,4] In both series, the majority of subjects did present with high-risk disease, so the low-risk prognostic subgroup included only a minority of patients; it does, however, validate that a small subgroup of DHL will have low risk disease and a favorable prognosis. In the largest multicenter analysis in DHL, predictors of inferior survival on multivariable analysis included advanced Ann Arbor stage, CNS involvement, LDH greater than 3 times the upper limit of normal, and leukocytosis. Subjects with no risk factors had a long-term survival of approximately 90%, compared with approximately 55% with 1 or 2 risk factors, and 25% in the highest risk patients. As with the IPI, the largest group was indeed the high-risk patients, accounting for 58%, compared with only 4% in the lowest risk subgroup. The significance of the adverse impact of leukocytosis on multivariable analysis is not entirely clear, since further differentiation of the WBC subsets is not provided; however, it may reflect high risk associated with circulating leukemic phase disease, which has been associated with an inferior prognosis in other DHL studies.[3,21] Pathologic features have also been evaluated for prognostic impact, including prior follicular lymphoma histology, DLBCL morphology, BCL2 versus BCL6 translocation, and MYC translocation partner, none of which have been consistently identified as an independent prognostic variable.[3,5,6,9,16,22] It should also be noted that most DHL cases included in the literature to date have been with BCL2 as opposed to BCL6, so further study is required in the latter subset to determine if observations in MCY/BCL2 DHL cases are truly applicable to those harboring dual translocations of MYC and BCL6.

TREATMENT OF DOUBLE-HIT LYMPHOMA

No standard of care exists for the management of DHL, and the literature that informs choice of therapy is retrospective in nature (see **Table 2**). There is clear evidence that R-CHOP (rituximab, cyclophosphamide, doxorubicin, vincristine and prednisone) does not produce a sustained remission in the majority of patients. The largest datasets suggest that approximately 20% of R-CHOP treated patients will be free from progression 2 years from diagnosis.[3,21] More intensive induction strategies have been employed including R-CODOX-M/R-IVAC (rituximab, cyclophosphamide, vincristine, doxorubicin, methotrexate/rituximab, ifosfamide, etoposide, cytarabine), R-hyperCVAD/MA (rituximab, hyperfractionated cyclophosphamide, vincristine, doxorubicin, dexamethasone/methotrexate, cytarabine), and DA-EPOCH-R (dose-adjusted etoposide, prednisone, vincristine, cyclophosphamide, doxorubicin, rituximab). In a 311-subject multicenter analysis, there was no clear difference identified among these 3 intensive strategies, but all were associated with an improved progression-free survival (PFS) relative to R-CHOP, with a 2-year PFS of approximately 50%. Despite the improvement in PFS, no clear difference emerged in terms of overall survival (OS). A single-center analysis of 129 patients from the MD Anderson Cancer Center (MDACC) suggested improved outcome in patients treated with DA-EPOCH-R, with a 2-year event free survival of 67%, which was superior to other regimens, but median follow-up in this series is still brief at 18 months. Both studies also evaluated the role of stem cell transplant consolidation in first complete remission, and neither identified a statistically significant improved survival favoring transplant consolidation. An important caveat is that the number of transplanted patients is quite small in both series, and these retrospective analyses are clearly underpowered to address this question. Accordingly, the role of stem cell transplant consolidation in first remission for DHL remains undefined. What is clear, is that a high proportion of DHL patients will never achieve complete response (CR) in the first place and subsequently have low rates of success with second-line therapy. Indeed the most dominant predictor of outcome in DHL has been the ability to achieve a CR to upfront therapy, regardless of what that first-line therapy is.[3,4,20] This finding does, however, reinforce the desire to employ regimens that have produced the highest CR rates in published analyses. In the MDACC study, the complete remission rate in the entire cohort was 55%, and was highest in patients treated with DA-EPOCH-R or R-hyperCVAD/MA, both at 68%, compared with R-CHOP at 40%.[3] In the multicenter study, DA-EPOCH-R was associated with the highest rate of CR of approximately 65%, followed by R-hyperCVAD.[4] These retrospective data suggest that intensified chemoimmunotherapy protocols should be preferred in the majority of patients with DHL. Supporting these findings, is a subset analysis of an interim evaluation of an ongoing multicenter phase II clinical trial of dose DA-EPOCH-R in MYC-rearranged DLBCL. Among 52 subjects reported, 14 also had a translocation of BCL-2 detected by FISH, with over 80% of these subjects free from progression at 1 year.[24] Further updates from this ongoing study are eagerly anticipated. Based on these data, DA-EPOCH-R is emerging as the preferred choice among many lymphoma specialists based on the aforementioned evidence of efficacy and the tolerability even in older adults who have excess toxicity associated with regimens such as R-hyperCVAD and R-CODOX-M/R-IVAC. Choice of chemotherapy cannot be a one size fits all approach, however, and it is worth recalling that a small subset of patients will indeed be cured with R-CHOP. Although this represents a distinct minority, rare DHL patients presenting with stage I disease and no IPI risk factors can be considered for R-CHOP followed by involved site radiation therapy with an anticipated excellent outcome. Indeed, given the general risk of chemotherapy resistance in DHL, it would be prudent to include consolidative radiation therapy in all DHL patients who present with localized disease, uncommon though that is, although no prospective data have specifically addressed this question. Given the increased prevalence of CNS disease at diagnosis and high risk of CNS recurrence, treatment directed at the CNS compartment must also be considered. Use of methotrexate-containing CNS prophylaxis, usually by intrathecal administration, has been associated with improved outcome, and should be considered in all but the lowest-risk patients.[4] Use of systemic methotrexate for CNS prophylaxis is a component of the R-hyperCVAD/MA regimen, and has long been used in concert with R-CHOP for high-risk DLBCL, where it has demonstrated safety and evidence of efficacy.[25] DA-EPOCH-R, however, has uniformly been studied with intrathecal methotrexate prophylaxis, and so no safety or efficacy data exist for the intercalation of systemic methotrexate with this particular chemoimmunotherapy platform.

MANAGEMENT OF MYC/BCL2 DOUBLE-EXPRESSING LYMPHOMAS

Coexpression of MYC and BCL2 is an adverse prognostic feature in DLBCL, but is still far more favorable than true DHL. Among DELs, the 4-year OS with R-CHOP therapy is approximately 55%, similar to what one would expect in a high-risk IPI patient.[5] Both MYC and BCL2 expression are required to confer an adverse prognosis, as neither MYC nor BCL2 immunohistochemical expression alone confers a worse outcome.[5,19]

Unlike DHL, no retrospective or prospective data exist to suggest that intensified treatment approaches offer any value compared with standard R-CHOP. Although it may be tempting to extrapolate from the limited DHL literature in favor of more intensified strategies, such an extrapolation ignores that DHL and DEL are quite different diseases at both biologic and clinical levels. DEL cases usually have a non-GCB origin, and these patients appear to garner less benefit from DA-EPOCH-R compared with GCB DLBCL.[26] Accordingly, R-CHOP remains the standard therapy in DEL by which future treatments should be compared, and at present there are no data to recommend alternative approaches in the front-line setting outside of a clinical trial.

RELAPSED DISEASE AND FUTURE DIRECTIONS

Patients with DHL with primary refractory or relapsed disease have an extremely poor prognosis with few long-term survivors.[3,4] Options in second-line therapy include a high-dose cytarabine-based regimen such as R-DHAP (rituximab, dexamethasone, high-dose cytarabine, cisplatin) or R-ESHAP (rituximab, etoposide, methylprednisolone, high-dose cytarabine, cisplatin), gemcitabine-based regimens such as R-GDP (rituximab, gemcitabine, dexamethasone, cisplatin), or the high-dose ifosfamide-based regimen R-ICE (rituximab, ifosfamide, carboplatin, etoposide). None of these traditional chemoimmunotherapy regimens, however, would be expected to produce a significant rate of complete or sustained remissions. Accordingly, optimal therapy for relapsed or refractory DHL should ideally be performed in the context of a clinical trial incorporating novel treatment strategies. Appealing options for novel therapies include emerging small molecule inhibitors that decrease MYC expression, including BET (bromodomain and extra-terminal proteins) inhibitors and histone deacetylase inhibitors.[27–30] The BCL-2 inhibitor venetoclax is also extremely appealing based on DHL and DEL biology, and has shown responses in heavily pretreated DLBCL in a phase I study.[31] Several emerging treatment strategies are in development that may work independently of cell of origin or MYC and BCL expression. These include antibody drug conjugates (ADCs) as well as novel immunotherapy approaches including PD-1/PD-L1 inhibition, bispecific T-cell engaging antibodies (BiTE), and chimeric antigen receptor (CAR) T-cells targeting CD19.[32–35] All of these strategies have shown promise in relapsed/refractory DLBCL, and warrant investigation in DHL and DEL. Novel agents with preferential activity in the ABC subset of DLBCL would also be of interest specifically in DEL patients, so subset analyses of ongoing studies incorporating lenalidomide and ibrutinib will be of interest.[36,37]

Presently, DHL remains an unmet medical need. Advances have been made since this entity was initially described, including an improved understanding of biologic and pathologic features, and prognostic factors that can identify a small subgroup of DHL patients with a favorable prognosis. For the majority of patients, intensified induction treatment strategies such as DA-EPOCH-R, including intrathecal methotrexate should be considered, as well as consolidative radiation in cases of localized disease. Ongoing evaluation should further assess different treatment strategies based on underlying risk factors, as well as the role of both autologous and allogeneic stem cell transplantation. Ultimately, the next great steps forward in this field will emerge from incorporating novel targeted therapies to overcome discrete biologic and molecular liabilities in this high-risk disease.

REFERENCES

1. Aukema SM, Siebert R, Schuuring E, et al. Double-hit B-cell lymphomas. Blood 2011;117:2319–31.

2. Barrans S, Crouch S, Smith A, et al. Rearrangement of MYC is associated with poor prognosis in patients with diffuse large B-cell lymphoma treated in the era of rituximab. J Clin Oncol 2010;28:3360–5.

3. Oki Y, Noorani M, Lin P, et al. Double hit lymphoma: the MD Anderson Cancer Center clinical experience. Br J Haematol 2014;166:891–901.

4. Petrich AM, Gandhi M, Jovanovic B, et al. Impact of induction regimen and stem cell transplantation on outcomes in double-hit lymphoma: a multicenter retrospective analysis. Blood 2014;124:2354–61.

5. Johnson NA, Savage KJ, Ludkovski O, et al. Lymphomas with concurrent BCL2 and MYC translocations: the critical factors associated with survival. Blood 2009;114:2273–9.

6. Snuderl M, Kolman OK, Chen YB, et al. B-cell lymphomas with concurrent IGH-BCL2 and MYC rearrangements are aggressive neoplasms with clinical and pathologic features distinct from Burkitt lymphoma and diffuse large B-cell lymphoma. Am J Surg Pathol 2010;34:327–40.

7. Tomita N, Tokunaka M, Nakamura N, et al. Clinicopathological features of lymphoma/leukemia patients carrying both BCL2 and MYC translocations. Haematologica 2009;94:935–43.

8. Macpherson N, Lesack D, Klasa R, et al. Small noncleaved, non-Burkitt's (Burkit-Like) lymphoma: cytogenetics predict outcome and reflect clinical presentation. J Clin Oncol 1999;17:1558–67.

9. Li S, Lin P, Fayad LE, et al. B-cell lymphomas with MYC/8q24 rearrangements and IGH@BCL2/t(14;18)(q32;q21): an aggressive disease with heterogeneous histology, germinal center B-cell immunophenotype and poor outcome. Mod Pathol 2012;25:145–56.

10. Swerdlow SH, Campo E, Harris NL, et al. WHO classification of tumours of hematopoietic and lymphoid tissues. 4th edition. Lyon (France): WHO; 2008.

11. Foot NJ, Dunn RG, Geoghegan H, et al. Fluorescence in situ hybridisation analysis of formalin-fixed paraffin-embedded tissue sections in the diagnostic work-up of non-Burkitt high grade B-cell non-Hodgkin's lymphoma: a single centre's experience. J Clin Pathol 2011;64:802–8.

12. Lin P, Dickason TJ, Fayad LE, et al. Prognostic value of MYC rearrangement in cases of B-cell lymphoma, unclassifiable, with features intermediate between diffuse large B-cell lymphoma and Burkitt lymphoma. Cancer 2012;118:1566–73.

13. Swerdlow SH, Campo E, Pileri SA, et al. The 2016 revision of the World Health Organization (WHO) classification of lymphoid neoplasms. Blood 2016;127(20):2375–90.

14. Meyer PN, Fu K, Greiner TC, et al. Immunohistochemical methods for predicting cell of origin and survival in patients with diffuse large B-cell lymphoma treated with rituximab. J Clin Oncol 2010;29:200–7.

15. Green TM, Nielsen O, de Stricker K, et al. High levels of nuclear MYC protein predict the presence of MYC rearrangement in diffuse large B-cell lymphoma. Am J Surg Pathol 2012;36:612–9.

16. Landsburg DJ, Petrich AM, Abramson JS, et al. Impact of oncogene rearrangement patterns on outcomes in patients with double-hit non-Hodgkin lymphoma. Cancer 2016;122:559–64.

17. Le Gouill S, Talmant P, Touzeau C, et al. The clinical presentation and prognosis of diffuse large B-cell lymphoma with t(14;18) and 8q24/c-MYC rearrangement. Haematologica 2007;92:1335–42.

18. Niitsu N, Okamoto M, Miura I, et al. Clinical features and prognosis of de novo diffuse large B-cell lymphoma with t(14;18) and 8q24/c-MYC translocations. Leukemia 2009;23:777–83.

19. Green TM, Young KH, Visco C, et al. Immunohistochemical double-hit score is a strong predictor of outcome in patients with diffuse large B-cell lymphoma treated with rituximab plus cyclophosphamide, doxorubicin, vincristine, and prednisone. J Clin Oncol 2012;30:3460–7.

20. Cohen JB, Geyer SM, Lozanski G, et al. Complete response to induction therapy in patients with Myc-positive and double-hit non-Hodgkin lymphoma is associated with prolonged progression-free survival. Cancer 2014;120:1677–85.

21. Abramson JS, Barnes JA, Feng Y, et al. Double hit lymphomas: evaluation of prognostic factors and impact of therapy. Blood 2012;120:1619.

22. Copie-Bergman C, Cuilliere-Dartigues P, Baia M, et al. MYC-IG rearrangements are negative predictors of survival in DLBCL patients treated with immunochemotherapy: a GELA/LYSA study. Blood 2015;126:2466–74.

23. Longo DL, Young RC, Wesley M, et al. Twenty years of MOPP therapy for Hodgkin's disease. J Clin Oncol 1986;4:1295–306.

24. Dunleavy K, Fanale M, LaCasce A, et al. Preliminary report of a multicenter prospective phase II study of DA-EPOCH-R in MYC-rearranged aggressive B-Cell lymphoma. Blood 2014;124:395.

25. Abramson JS, Hellmann M, Barnes JA, et al. Intravenous methotrexate as CNS prophylaxis is associated with a low risk of CNS recurrence in high risk patients with diffuse large B-cell lymphoma. Cancer 2010;116(18):4283–90.

26. Wilson WH, Dunleavy K, Pittaluga S, et al. Phase II study of dose-adjusted EPOCH and rituximab in untreated diffuse large B-cell lymphoma with analysis of germinal center and post-germinal center biomarkers. J Clin Oncol 2008;26: 2717–24.

27. Abramson JS, Blum KA, Flinn IW, et al. BET inhibitor CPI-0610 is well tolerated and induces responses in diffuse large B-Cell lymphoma and follicular lymphoma: preliminary analysis of an ongoing phase 1 study. Blood 2015;126: 1491.

28. Delmore JE, Issa GC, Lemieux ME, et al. BET bromodomain inhibition as a therapeutic strategy to target c-Myc. Cell 2011;146:904–17.

29. Barnes JA, Redd RA, Jacobsen ED, et al. Panobinostat in combination with rituximab in heavily pretreated diffuse large B-cell lymphoma: results of a phase II study. Blood 2014;124:3055.

30. Bhadury J, Nilsson LM, Muralidharan SV, et al. BET and HDAC inhibitors induce similar genes and biological effects and synergize to kill in Myc-induced murine lymphoma. Proc Natl Acad Sci U S A 2014;111:E2721–30.

31. Davids M, Seymour J, Gerecitano J. Phase I study of ABT-199 (GDC-0199) in patients with relapsed/refractory non-Hodgkin lymphoma: responses observed in diffuse large B-cell (DLBCL) and follicular lymphoma (FL) at higher cohort doses. Haematologica 2014;99 [abstract: S1348].

32. Palanca-Wessels MC, Czuczman M, Salles G, et al. Safety and activity of the anti-CD79B antibody-drug conjugate polatuzumab vedotin in relapsed or refractory B-cell non-Hodgkin lymphoma and chronic lymphocytic leukaemia: a phase 1 study. Lancet Oncol 2015;16:704–15.

33. Goebeler ME, Knop S, Viardot A, et al. Bispecific T-cell engager (BiTE) antibody construct blinatumomab for the treatment of patients with relapsed/refractory non-Hodgkin lymphoma: final results from a phase I study. J Clin Oncol 2016; 34(10):1104–11.

34. Kochenderfer JN, Dudley ME, Kassim SH, et al. Chemotherapy-refractory diffuse large B-cell lymphoma and indolent B-cell malignancies can be effectively treated with autologous T cells expressing an anti-CD19 chimeric antigen receptor. J Clin Oncol 2015;33(6):540–9.
35. Lesokhin AM, Ansell SM, Armand P, et al. Preliminary results of a phase I study of Nivolumab (BMS-936558) in patients with relapsed or refractory lymphoid malignancies. Blood 2014;124:291.
36. Wilson WH, Young RM, Schmitz R, et al. Targeting B cell receptor signaling with ibrutinib in diffuse large B cell lymphoma. Nat Med 2015;21:922–6.
37. Hernandez-Ilizaliturri FJ, Deeb G, Zinzani PL, et al. Higher response to lenalidomide in relapsed/refractory diffuse large B-cell lymphoma in nongerminal center B-cell-like than in germinal center B-cell-like phenotype. Cancer 2011;117: 5058–66.

Gray Zone Lymphoma
Current Diagnosis and Treatment Options

Monika Pilichowska, MD[a], Athena Kritharis, MD[b],
Andrew M. Evens, DO, MSc[b],*

KEYWORDS

- Gray zone lymphoma • B-cell • Classical Hodgkin lymphoma
- Diffuse large B-cell lymphoma • Biology • Prognosis • Treatment

KEY POINTS

- The WHO recognizes a distinct category of B-cell lymphoma, unclassifiable, with features intermediate between diffuse large B-cell lymphoma (DLBCL) and classical Hodgkin lymphoma (cHL), also known as gray zone lymphoma (GZL).
- The immunophenotype of GZL is frequently discordant with tumor cells morphologically resembling DLBCL, but immunophenotypically being more consistent with cHL, and vice versa.
- Clinically, the initial case descriptions of GZL were primarily with mediastinal presentation; however, a nonmediastinal (systemic) clinical subtype is now fully recognized.
- Regardless of clinical presentation, patients with GZL have relatively high relapse rates, especially compared with primary mediastinal DLBCL and cHL.
- Off of a clinical trial, we advocate treating GZL with a DLBCL-directed regimen (eg, R-CHOP or DA-EPOCH-R) with consideration for consolidative radiotherapy for bulk disease.

INTRODUCTION

Gray zone lymphoma (GZL) is a rare neoplasm initially described in 2005 based on the recognition of an aggressive subset of primary mediastinal B-cell lymphoma (PMBCL) with poor prognosis.[1] GZL was officially first recognized in the World Health Organization classification as a distinct entity in 2008 as a B-cell lymphoma, unclassifiable, with features intermediate between diffuse large B-cell lymphoma (DLBCL) and classical Hodgkin lymphoma (cHL).[2] Since this time, there has been more insight into the

[a] Department of Pathology and Laboratory Medicine, Tufts Medical Center, 800 Washington Street, Boston, MA 02111, USA; [b] Division of Hematology/Oncology, Tufts Medical Center, 800 Washington Street, Boston, MA 02111, USA
* Corresponding author.
E-mail address: AEvens@tuftsmedicalcenter.org

pathologic diagnosis, biology, and clinical outcomes for patients with GZL. Although initially clinically described as primarily involving the mediastinum,[1,3,4] further analyses have elucidated primary mediastinal and nonmediastinal (systemic) clinical disease presentations.[5,6] Notably, this article does not include discussion of the gray zone entity of lymphoma with features of intermediate DLBCL and Burkitt lymphoma.

GZL with mediastinal presentation (MGZL) is similar in presentation to cHL in part as it typically occurs in young adults in the third and fourth decade. Conversely, patients with GZL without mediastinal presentation (NMGZL) are typically older and more often present with advanced-stage disease. Furthermore, unlike cHL and PMBCL, both MGZL and NMGZL have a more aggressive clinical course with comparatively inferior outcomes. Given its newer recognition and relative paucity of associated clinical data, continued description of this unique disease entity is warranted. The following is a detailed review of the current literature and descriptions of the diagnosis, biology, prognosis, and treatment of GZL.

CASE STUDY

A 26-year-old Middle Eastern man was seen for second opinion of a new diagnosis of stage IIBXE cHL. On initial presentation, he experienced several weeks of nonproductive cough and drenching night sweats. A chest radiograph showed left upper lobe consolidation and he was started on antibiotics for a presumed pneumonia. His symptoms did not abate. Computerized tomography of the chest indicated multiple soft tissue masses that filled the upper mediastinum including an 11 cm × 14 cm anterior mediastinal mass with hilar adenopathy. Bronchoscopy at outside hospital with left anterior mediastinoscopy was performed. Based on morphology and positivity for CD15 and CD30, an initial diagnosis of nodular sclerosis Hodgkin lymphoma was made. The laboratory data were notable for a mild anemia, with hemoglobin 12 g/dL and hematocrit of 36% without further abnormalities. There was no evidence of bone marrow involvement on staging biopsy.

Additional pathologic review conducted at our institution and the National Institutes of Health (NIH) noted unusual morphology and immunophenotype. In addition to areas of cHL, the tumor exhibited extensive syncytial sheets of large cells, Reed-Sternberg cells, and variants. The neoplastic cells showed strong positivity for CD20 and CD15 with strong to variable positivity for CD30 (**Fig. 1**). The final diagnosis was B-cell lymphoma, unclassifiable, with features intermediate between DLBCL and cHL (ie, GZL). The patient was treated with cyclophosphamide, doxorubicin, oncovin, and prednisone and rituximab (CHOP-R) for six cycles. The patient had a Deauville score of 3 after two cycles and was Deauville score 2 at end of chemotherapy; he subsequently received mediastinal involved-node radiation therapy (3000 cGy). The patient currently remains disease-free 34 months following initial diagnosis.

BIOLOGY

GZL is known to arise from an altered B cell. In GZL, the putative cell of origin is thymic B cell, which is also a common precursor for cHL and PMBCL. This common precursor hypothesis explains why cHL, PMBCL, or GZL may relapse as the other related entity and why they are found as synchronous neoplasms.[7] The notion of a common cell of origin is supported by data examining gene expression signatures of GZL, PMBCL, and cHL being similar as were numerous genetic abnormalities, such as gains in chromosome 9p and 2p.[8] However, because GZL may differentiate in either direction (eg, Reed-Sternberg cell/variant or DLBCL), epigenetic changes as opposed

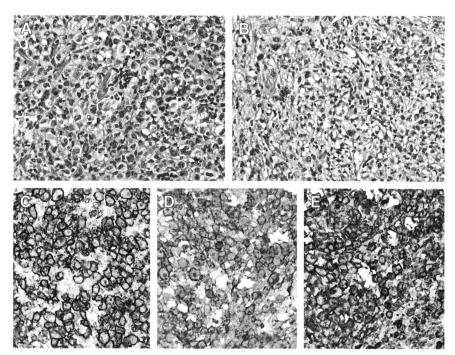

Fig. 1. Gray zone lymphoma: World Health Organization B-cell lymphoma, unclassifiable, with features intermediate between DLBCL and cHL. A 26-year-old man presenting with bulky mediastinal mass. (*A*) The tumor is composed of large pleomorphic cells, some resembling Reed-Sternberg cells and variants occurring in sheets as seen in DLBCL (hematoxylin-eosin, original magnification ×200). (*B*) In some areas, the morphology resembles cHL with infrequent Reed-Sternberg cells occurring on inflammatory background with small lymphocytes, histiocytes, and eosinophils (hematoxylin-eosin, original magnification ×200). The neoplastic cells in DLBCL-like and cHL-like areas are strongly positive for CD20 (*C*), CD15 (*D*), and CD30 (*E*) (immunoperoxidase, original magnification ×200).

to genetic aberrations may more strongly influence the final morphology and immunophenotype.

Eberle and colleagues[9] performed a DNA methylation analyses of 30 cases including cHL, PMBCL, and GZL. They demonstrated a close relationship between the three diseases but with unique signatures that distinguished GZL from HL and PMBCL. These included lack of de novo hypomethylation in cHL, hypomethylation of *HOXA5* in GZL, and hypermethylation of *EPHA7* and *DAPK1* in PMBCL. In addition, the nuclear factor-κB pathway was highly enriched and was important to the pathogenesis of all three disease entities. Notably, most of the aforementioned biologic studies have been conducted among patients with MGZL; it is not known if NMGZL has similar or distinct biology.

DIAGNOSIS

The diagnosis of GZL should be made by expert pathologic evaluation of the involved tissue preferably obtained by an excisional or incisional biopsy. GZL is highly variable with each tumor displaying a unique set of features. A spectrum of morphologies known with cHL and DLBCL can occur and divergent morphologic areas are seen within the same tumor necessitating extensive sampling for the correct diagnosis.

The neoplastic cells are usually large with centroblastic or immunoblastic appearance, high degree of pleomorphism, and can include bona fide Reed-Sternberg cells and variants. Mummified cells can be present. In cases resembling PMBCL the neoplastic cells occur in sheets. In cases resembling cHL the neoplastic cells are sparse and occur on mixed inflammatory background with small lymphocytes, histiocytes, and eosinophils. These cases can exhibit significant degree of fibrosis and distinction from true cHL is difficult. Necrosis can be present and be extensive. Neutrophilic infiltrates, however, are not a usual feature.

Similar to morphologic findings, the immunophenotype of GZL is variable and has transitional features between cHL and DLBCL (**Table 1**). Tumors resembling cHL can show prominent CD20, weaker/absent CD30, and absent CD15, whereas tumors resembling DLBCL may be strongly positive for CD30 and CD15 with negative CD20 and CD79a. Because the B-cell program is preserved, B-cell transcription factors, such as PAX5, OCT2, and BOB1, are positive in neoplastic cells.[7] In comparison with a cohort of 51 patients with PMBCL, patients with MGZL were more often male, expressed CD15, and had lower expression of CD20.[7]

In a retrospective multicenter study of 112 patients with GZL studied by Evens and colleagues,[6] the immunophenotype of GZL seemed concordant with prior studies. In addition, there was no apparent significant difference in immunophenotype between MGZL and NMGZL. The most prevalent immunophenotypes were CD20[+] (93%), CD30[+] (89%), CD79a[+] (78%), Pax5[+] (98%), Oct2[+] (96%), and MUM1[+] (100%).

Table 1
Morphologic and immunophenotypic features of GZL and related pathologic spectrum

Feature	PMLBCL	DLBCL	cHL	GZL
Morphology				
RS cells and variants	Rare	Rare	Yes	Yes in areas
HL background	No	No	Yes	Yes in areas
Sheets of large cells	Yes	Yes	Syncytial variant	Yes in areas
Fibrous bands	No	No	Yes	Uncommon
"Alveolar" fibrosis	Yes	No	No	Sometimes
Necrosis	Yes	Yes	Common	Common
Neutrophilic infiltrates	No	No	Yes	No
Immunophenotype				
CD20	+	+	−/+	−/+ or +
CD30	+ weak, variable	−/+	+	+ or +/−
CD15	−/+	−	+/−	+/−
CD79a	+	+	−/+	−/+ or +
PAX5	+	+	+ (weak)	−/+ or +
Bcl6	+/−	+/−	+/− (weak)	+/− variable
OCT2	+	+	−/+	+/− or +
MUM1/IRF4	+/−	+ ABC type	+	+
CD45	+	+	−	+/− or +
EBV (EBER)	−	−/+	−/+	−/+

Abbreviations: +, all cases positive; +/−, most cases positive; −/+, some cases positive; −, all cases negative; ABC, activated B-cell type; cHL, classical Hodgkin lymphoma; DLBCL, diffuse large B-cell lymphoma; EBER, Epstein-Barr virus–encoded small mRNAs (by in situ hybridization); EBV, Epstein-Barr virus; HL, Hodgkin lymphoma; RS, Reed-Sternberg.

CD15 (46%) and CD45 (67%) staining were more variable, whereas only 11% and 28% of patients had CD10 and Epstein-Barr virus positivity, respectively (the latter by EBER in situ hybridization staining). It should be highlighted, however, that central pathologic review was not performed for this retrospective multicenter study; pathologic work-up and diagnoses were completed at the local academic centers.

Altogether, diagnosis of GZL remains challenging; work-up and/or consultation at a center with hematopathology expertise of this particular entity is highly recommended. We advocate detailed review of B-cell markers (eg, CD20, PAX5, CD79a, BCL6, BOB1, OCT2) along with CD30, CD15, and MUM1 when GZL is suspected. In situ hybridization for Epstein-Barr virus should also be included. Collectively, the diagnosis of GZL should be entertained in cases with transitional morphology and discordant immunophenotype if strong expression of CD20 is identified in cHL or strong CD15 expression is seen in an otherwise typical DLBCL.

CLINICAL PRESENTATION

The original reports describing GZL contained patients primarily with mediastinal disease presenting clinically similarly to PMBCL (**Table 2**).[1,10–12] Subsequent reports of GZL have shown a distinctive nonmediastinal systemic presentation.[6,9] Wilson and colleagues[13] recently reported outcomes among 24 patients with MGZL diagnosed and treated over an approximate 20-year period at the NIH. The median age of these patients was 33 years and approximately two-thirds were male. Of these patients, nearly half had a bulky mediastinal mass greater than 10 cm, whereas a minority of patients had extranodal involvement and only 13% had stage IV disease.

In terms of comparison of MGZL with NMGZL, patients with NMGZL presented significantly less often with bulk disease, but they were significantly older and presented more often with extranodal involvement and advanced-stage disease in the series by Evens and colleagues.[6] In part because of these latter features, patients with NMGZL had significantly worse prognostic scores (International Prognostic Scoring system and International Prognostic Index [IPI]) compared with patients with MGZL.

PRIMARY MANAGEMENT

There are no standard management guidelines for GZL. In part this is because of the small number of analyses examining therapeutic approaches for GZL and challenges in diagnosis. From the aforementioned prospective NIH study, 24 patients with MGZL were treated with dose-adjusted etoposide, prednisone, oncovin, cyclophosphamide, doxorubicin, and rituximab (DA-EPOCH-R) and outcomes were compared with similarly treated patients with PMBCL.[13] Patients with MGZL had significantly inferior outcomes compared with PMBCL (5-year event-free survival 62% vs 93%, and 5-year overall survival [OS] 74% vs 97%, respectively).[13,14]

Among the 112 patients with GZL reported by Evens and colleagues treated across 19 North American centers, the two most common treatment approaches were CHOP-R and doxorubicin, bleomycin, vinblastine, and dacarbazine (ADVD) ± rituximab with a handful of patients treated with DA-EPOCH-R. Approximately two-thirds of patients received rituximab as part of frontline therapy. The overall response rates and complete remission rates for all patients were 71% and 59%, respectively, with 33% of patients having primary refractory disease (no differences between MGZL and NMGZL). The overall response rates and complete remission rates for patients who received rituximab as part of front-line therapy were 82% and 73%, respectively, versus 59% and 43%, respectively, without rituximab ($P = .02$ and $P = .008$, respectively).

Table 2
Clinical characteristics from GZL series

Author, Year	No. Pts	Median Age, y (Range)	M:F	Mediastinal Disease, %	B Symptoms, %	Advanced Stage, %	Bulky Disease, %	PFS/EFS, %
Traverse-Glehen et al,[1] 2005[a]	21	31 (13–62)	0.90	100	NR	NR	NR	NR
Oschlies et al,[10] 2011	4	14 (11–18)	3.0	100	50	100[c]	NR	0
Eberle et al,[9] 2011[a]	18	29 (16–51)	2.0	100	NR	NR	NR	NR
Eberle et al,[9] 2011[a]	9	55 (26–91)	0.50	0	NR	NR	NR	NR
Gualco et al,[11] 2012	10	34 (15–85)	1.22	80	NR	20	NR	50
Wilson et al,[13] 2014[a]	24	33 (14–59)	1.67	100	NR	13	46	62
Evens et al,[6] 2015[b]	48	37 (60–93)	1.4	100	45	13	44	46
Evens et al,[6] 2015[b]	64	51 (60–84)	2.37	0	63	81	8	36

Minimum four patients.

Abbreviations: EFS, event-free survival; NR, not reported; OS, overall survival; PFS, progression-free survival.

[a] There is some overlap of patients studied in these series.

[b] Mediastinal and nonmediastinal GZL cases from the same series are separated to highlight differences among these clinical entities.

[c] St. Jude's stage of disease.

At 31-month median follow-up, the 2-year progression-free survival (PFS) and OS for all patients were 40% and 88%, respectively (**Fig. 2**). Two-year PFS rates for patients with stage I/II versus III/IV disease were 54% versus 30%, respectively, and the corresponding OS rates were 94% versus 76%, respectively. Interestingly, despite a comparative preponderance of early stage disease and lower IPI, the survival rates were not statistically different for MGZL versus NMGZL patients (see **Fig. 2**). In terms of frontline chemotherapy regimens in this retrospective series, PFS rate seemed significantly inferior for patients treated with ABVD ± rituximab versus treatment with a DLBCL-based regimen (ie, CHOP ± R and DA-EPOCH-R) with corresponding 2-year rates of 23% versus 52%, respectively (see **Fig. 2**). This finding persisted on multivariable Cox regression, including controlling for IPI and use of rituximab.

ROLE OF RADIOTHERAPY

There are minimal prospective and no randomized data regarding the benefit of radiotherapy in GZL. In the MGZL DA-EPOCH-R series by Wilson and colleagues,[13] use of radiotherapy is not standard practice with this therapeutic regimen for PMBCL patients.[15] Treatment paradigms for GZL in the study by Evens and colleagues[6] more often used adjunctive consolidative radiotherapy with early stage and/or bulky disease; improved outcomes were not seen in patients who received radiotherapy. However, caution should be applied to this finding given the retrospective nature and relatively small patient numbers. Notably, relapses localized in the mediastinum treated with radiotherapy may be curative. Wilson and colleagues[13] demonstrated that 44% (four of nine) of patients achieved continuous remission with salvage radiation therapy alone. It is not known if outcomes would be improved for MGZL if adjuvant radiotherapy were more routinely used in conjunction following DA-EPOCH chemotherapy.

PROGNOSTICATION

The prospective DA-EPOCH-R study by Wilson and colleagues[13] identified PMBL-like tumor morphology, expression of CD15 on malignant cells, and presence of CD68+ tumor-infiltrating dendritic cells as makers for poor prognosis in MGZL. The gene signature encoding for dendritic cell–specific intracellular adhesion molecule-3-grabbing nonintegrin (DC-SIGN) is a marker of dendritic cells and activated macrophages[16]; in this series, cases with greater than or equal to one positive tumor associated-dendritic/activated macrophage cells by immunohistochemistry was associated with markedly inferior outcomes (ie, OS of 52% vs 100%; $P = .0025$). Similarly to cHL low peripheral blood absolute lymphocyte count in MGZL was associated with inferior event-free survival and OS, whereas tumor mass size and expression of CD20 were not prognostic.

Prognostic factors associated with inferior PFS on univariable analyses in the Evens and colleagues[6] series included poor performance status, increased lactate dehydrogenase, anemia, and advanced stage disease, whereas only stage was prognostic for OS. Both the IPI and International Prognostic Scoring system were prognostic for PFS and OS (as categorical and continuous variables). On multivariable analyses, performance status was the most dominant prognostic factor for PFS, whereas increased lactate dehydrogenase was borderline. For OS, advanced stage disease was the only significant prognostic factor (hazard ratio, 4.89; $P<.05$). Interestingly, CD20 positivity in malignant cells also independently predicted PFS on Cox regression controlling for rituximab treatment (ie, 88% of CD20-negative patients with GZL experienced progressive disease).

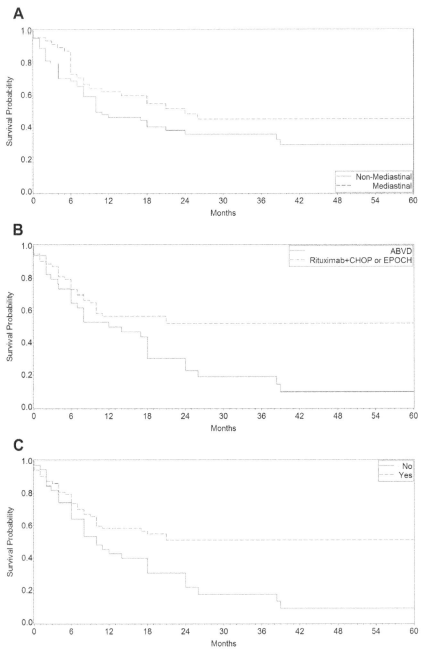

Fig. 2. GZL outcomes. The 2-year (A) PFS and OS rates for patients with mediastinal versus nonmediastinal (systemic) GZL from a recently reported multicenter retrospective series.[6] The outcomes (B) based on frontline therapeutic regimen; 2-year PFS for patients who received a standard frontline DLBCL regimen (ie, CHOP ± R and DA-EPOCH-R) versus ABVD ± R were 52% versus 23%, P = .03. Kaplan-Meier curves (C) for patients who received rituximab as a part of frontline therapy versus not; 2-year PFS were 51% versus 22%, respectively, P = .01. (*Adapted from* Evens AM, Kanakry JA, Sehn LH, et al. Gray zone lymphoma with features intermediate between classical Hodgkin lymphoma and diffuse large B-cell lymphoma: characteristics, outcomes, and prognostication among a large multicenter cohort. Am J Hematol 2015;90(9):781; with permission.)

RELAPSED/REFRACTORY DISEASE

Among available data, the ability to salvage patients with GZL with relapsed/refractory disease seems good. In the series by Evens and colleagues,[6] the median time to relapse for patients with GZL was 7 months (range, 1–64 months); most patients were treated with standard combination chemotherapy salvage regimens. Furthermore, most patients underwent hematopoietic stem cell transplantation (HSCT), usually autologous. The 2-year OS rate for patients with relapsed/refractory GZL who underwent HSCT was 88% versus 67% for patients who did not. This finding persisted on multivariable analyses controlling for IPI and response to pre-HSCT salvage therapy.[6] This improvement likely reflected in part that fit patients with chemotherapy-sensitive disease underwent SCT. Nevertheless, given these findings, there should be consideration for salvage combination chemotherapy followed by autologous HSCT for patients with relapsed/refractory GZL. Additionally, as described before for select cases with localized relapse in the mediastinum, there may be consideration for radiotherapy (± chemotherapy) without HSCT.[13]

SUMMARY

Since its original description in 2005[1] and its inclusion in the World Health Organization in 2008,[2] there has been important biologic and clinical knowledge gained about GZL. Despite the increased recognition of this disease as a pathologic and clinical entity, it is important to highlight that diagnosis is difficult and requires involvement of hematopathology with disease expertise in this area. Furthermore, there remains a critical need for pathologic harmonization and consensus diagnostic criteria.

It is also fully recognized that patients with GZL may present with primary mediastinal localization or with systemic disease. Pathology or biology differences between these varied clinical presentations remains to be defined. Regardless of clinical presentation, patients with GZL have high relapse rates, especially compared with patients with PMLCL and cHL. Patients with GZL seem to be salvaged fairly successfully with salvage therapy, especially when including HSCT. Further examination toward defining the most optimal chemotherapy regimen and the appropriate timing of HSCT is essential.

Off of a clinical trial, we recommend DLBCL-directed therapy (eg, R-CHOP or DA-EPOCH-R) for frontline GZL therapy with consideration for use of adjunctive radiotherapy for patients with localized and/or bulky disease. Finally, there should be continued exploration toward the use and integration of novel targeted therapeutic agents (eg, brentuximab vedotin, new-generation CD20 antibodies, PD-1 inhibitors) into the treatment paradigm of GZL.

REFERENCES

1. Traverse-Glehen A, Pittaluga S, Gaulard P, et al. Mediastinal gray zone lymphoma: the missing link between classic Hodgkin's lymphoma and mediastinal large B-cell lymphoma. Am J Surg Pathol 2005;29(11):1411–21.
2. Swerdlow SH, Campo E, Harris NL, et al. WHO classification of tumours of haematopoietic and lymphoid tissues. 4th edition. Lyon (France): International Agency for Research on Cancer; 2008.
3. Grant C, Dunleavy K, Eberle FC, et al. Primary mediastinal large B-cell lymphoma, classic Hodgkin lymphoma presenting in the mediastinum, and mediastinal gray zone lymphoma: what is the oncologist to do? Curr Hematol Malig Rep 2011;6(3):157–63.

4. García J, Mollejo M, Fraga M, et al. Large B-cell lymphoma with Hodgkin features. Histopathology 2005;47(1):101–10.

5. Eberle FC, Salaverria I, Steidl C, et al. Gray zone lymphoma: chromosomal aberrations with immunophenotypic and clinical correlations. Mod Pathol 2011;24(12): 1586–97.

6. Evens AM, Kanakry JA, Sehn LH, et al. Gray zone lymphoma with features intermediate between classical Hodgkin lymphoma and diffuse large B-cell lymphoma: characteristics, outcomes, and prognostication among a large multicenter cohort. Am J Hematol 2015;90(9):778–83.

7. Dunleavy K, Wilson WH. Primary mediastinal B-cell lymphoma and mediastinal gray zone lymphoma: do they require a unique therapeutic approach? Blood 2015;125(1):33–9.

8. Eberle FC, Jaffe ES. XII. Gray zone lymphomas: a biological experiment, and a challenge for diagnosis and management. Ann Oncol 2011;22(Suppl 4):iv64–6.

9. Eberle FC, Rodriguez-Canales J, Wei L, et al. Methylation profiling of mediastinal gray zone lymphoma reveals a distinctive signature with elements shared by classical Hodgkin's lymphoma and primary mediastinal large B-cell lymphoma. Haematologica 2011;96(4):558–66.

10. Oschlies I, Burkhardt B, Salaverria I, et al. Clinical, pathological and genetic features of primary mediastinal large B-cell lymphomas and mediastinal gray zone lymphomas in children. Haematologica 2011;96(2):262–8.

11. Gualco G, Natkunam Y, Bacchi CE. The spectrum of B-cell lymphoma, unclassifiable, with features intermediate between diffuse large B-cell lymphoma and classical Hodgkin lymphoma: a description of 10 cases. Mod Pathol 2012; 25(5):661–74.

12. Minami J, Dobashi N, Asai O, et al. Two cases of mediastinal gray zone lymphoma. J Clin Exp Hematop 2010;50(2):143–9.

13. Wilson WH, Pittaluga S, Nicolae A, et al. A prospective study of mediastinal gray-zone lymphoma. Blood 2014;124(10):1563–9.

14. Dunleavy K, Pittaluga S, Shovlin M, et al. Untreated primary mediastinal B-cell (PMBL) and mediastinal grey zone (MGZL) lymphomas: comparison of biological features and clinical outcome following DA-EPOCH-R without radiation. Ann Oncol 2011;134(22).

15. Dunleavy K, Pittaluga S, Maeda LS, et al. Dose-adjusted EPOCH-rituximab therapy in primary mediastinal B-cell lymphoma. N Engl J Med 2013;368(15): 1408–16.

16. Geijtenbeek TB, Krooshoop DJ, Bleijs DA, et al. DC-SIGN-ICAM-2 interaction mediates dendritic cell trafficking. Nat Immunol 2000;1(4):353–7.

Optimizing Outcomes in Primary Mediastinal B-cell Lymphoma

Pier Luigi Zinzani, MD, PhD*, Alessandro Broccoli, MD

KEYWORDS

- Anti-PD-1 • Brentuximab vedotin
- Fluorodeoxyglucose positron emission tomography
- Methotrexate, doxorubicin, cyclophosphamide, vincristine, bleomycin, prednisone
- Primary mediastinal B-cell lymphoma • Radiotherapy • Rituximab • Ruxolitinib

KEY POINTS

- Applying the most effective chemoimmunotherapy regimen will induce the highest rate of complete responses after first-line treatment.
- Determining which patients will benefit from consolidation radiotherapy is a key strategy to optimize outcomes.
- Minimization of long-term treatment-related toxic effects is necessary, as most patients are likely to be cured and will enjoy long periods free of disease.
- In patients with relapsed or refractory disease, the use of new drugs, with mechanisms of action based on peculiar biologic features of the tumor, will impact the ability to obtain disease control and enhance survival.

INTRODUCTION

Primary mediastinal B-cell lymphoma (PMBCL) is a rather infrequent aggressive lymphoma, putatively arising from a transformed thymic B cell. It accounts for less than 5% of all non-Hodgkin lymphomas, and typically affects adolescents and young women in their third or fourth decade.[1] It clinically presents with bulky mediastinal masses, usually exerting compressive effects on nearby vessels and airways (**Fig. 1**), giving rise to the possible abrupt onset of dyspnea; dysphagia; thoracic pain; and facial, neck, breast, and arm edema (**Fig. 2**), or infiltrating the adjacent lung parenchyma. It should be often regarded as a hematological emergency and promptly treated; the initial treatment decision is crucial for the management of this disease.

Disclosure Statement: The authors have nothing to disclose.
Institute of Hematology L. e A. Seràgnoli, University of Bologna, Via Massarenti, 9, Bologna 40138, Italy
* Corresponding author.
E-mail address: pierluigi.zinzani@unibo.it

Hematol Oncol Clin N Am 30 (2016) 1261–1275
http://dx.doi.org/10.1016/j.hoc.2016.07.011
0889-8588/16/© 2016 Elsevier Inc. All rights reserved.

hemonc.theclinics.com

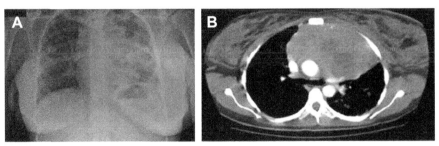

Fig. 1. Conventional radiological appearance of a massive mediastinal mass that roughly alters the mediastinal RX profile (*A*). The same adenopathic bulk as it appears on contrast-enhanced CT scan of the chest (*B*).

PMBCL was originally recognized as a subtype of diffuse large B-cell lymphoma (DLBCL) since the 1994 Revised European American Lymphoma (REAL) classification, and it has been regarded as a unique clinical and biological entity since the 2001 World Health Organization classification. Apart from its peculiar clinical presentation and pathologic features, this disease also displays a unique molecular fingerprint, which clearly distinguishes it from the rest of DLBCL. That same fingerprint, however, partly overlaps with the molecular profile of nodular sclerosis Hodgkin disease,[2,3] with which it shares at least a third of its genes, abnormalities on chromosome 9p (in nearly three-quarters of cases),[4] and CD30 expression (although weaker).[5]

In the last 20 years, several studies—mostly retrospective in their fashion due to the rarity of the disease and to the difficulty of designing randomized clinical trials specifically addressed to these patients—have tried to provide answers to several issues regarding the optimal treatment and management of patients. Above all, although

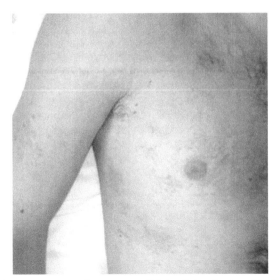

Fig. 2. The superior vena cava syndrome: superficial collateral veins at both the upper limbs and at the upper thoracic quadrants become evident as a consequence of the compression or obstruction of the superior vena cava.

the necessity of an anthracycline-based induction is understood,[6,7] the choice of the initial chemotherapy approach is still debated, including the value of the addition of rituximab. Although most of institutions have agreed to adopt an R-CHOP (cyclophosphamide, doxorubicin, vincristine, and prednisone) induction (as they would do for any other subtypes of DLBCL)[8,9] others prefer a more intense approach, either based on weekly administered third-generation regimens or on more aggressive strategies.[10]

Apart from the debate on which first-line approach seems more suitable, there are other aspects that require clarification:

The actual role of external beam radiotherapy (RT), recognized as an adjuvant strategy consolidates the a response to chemotherapy, and the possibility of its omission in certain categories of patients to reduce the likelihood of radiation-induced long-term toxicity

The value of fluorodeoxyglucose (FDG) positron emission tomography (PET) scan and the way in which its results are interpreted in this peculiar context, either when performed at disease staging or after induction treatment

If PET itself can be regarded as a possible guide to the administration of a subsequent consolidation treatment, whether based on external RT or on a high-dose approach and autotransplant

The treatment of refractory and relapsing patients, for whom standard approaches have shown rather unsatisfactory results[11]

Some new drugs are now emerging as potentially active agents in the setting of recurrent disease, as their mechanisms of action are based on specific biologic features of PMBCL.

Purpose of this article is to review the currently adopted strategies in the first-line treatment of PMBCL, to analyze the risks and benefits of postinduction RT consolidation, and to discuss the potential role of PET in helping physicians optimize the approach to their patients. A preview to some new agents on the horizon is also provided. A patient evaluation overview is provided in **Box 1**.

Box 1
Patient evaluation overview

- Histologically confirmed diagnosis of PMBCL made by an expert hematopathologist (excisional biopsy of a suspect mediastinal mass in a compatible clinical context)

- Full patient history, collection of concomitant medications, and complete physical examination (seek for superficial lymph nodes enlargement, jugular vein distension, thoracic edema, collateral veins, pleural effusion; inspect the oral cavity; listen to heart sounds and murmurs)

- Laboratory: full blood counts, creatinine, lactate dehydrogenase (LDH), transaminases, blood proteins with electrophoresis; serology for hepatitis B and C viruses and human immunodeficiency virus

- CT scan of neck, thorax, abdomen and pelvis (with contrast) and fluorodeoxyglucose PET scan

- Bone marrow biopsy (can be omitted in the event that an urgent treatment is required because of severe dyspnea, dysphagia, or superior vena cava syndrome)

- Transthoracic echocardiogram, to evaluate the fitness of the patient in receiving anthracyclines and to rule out the presence of pericardial effusion or possible cardiac tamponade

- PET scan is to be repeated 6 to 8 weeks after the end of the induction treatment, along with a full-body CT scan; interim PET scan evaluation is encouraged but not mandatory, as it is still considered investigational

FIRST-LINE CHEMOTHERAPY COMBINATIONS IN PRERITUXIMAB ERA: DIFFERENT PERSPECTIVES

Since prerituximab era, the first-line chemotherapy schedule has represented a matter of controversy. Although the CHOP regimen was mainly adopted by US centers,[7] the European experience has carried out evidence that MACOP-B (methotrexate, doxorubicin, cyclophosphamide, vincristine, bleomycin, prednisone) or VACOP-B (etoposide, doxorubicin, cyclophosphamide, vincristine, bleomycin, prednisone), both weekly dosed third-generation dose-dense regimens, could be superior to CHOP.[12–14] As a consequence of the application of dose-dense regimens, in fact, remission rates and survival functions have appeared to be at least as good as—or probably even better than—those observed for DLBCL patients, thus retracting the initial impression that PMBCL was per se a prognostically unfavorable subset of DLBCL.

However, this conclusion was only drawn from existing reports, since no randomized clinical trial has been carried on so far, and prospective studies are also lacking (**Table 1**). Overall it is clear that an anthracycline-containing regimen should be regarded as the first approach to PMBCL.[6,7]

Lazzarino and colleagues[15,16] first showed the MACOP-B/VACOP-B superiority on CHOP both in terms of complete response (CR) rates and relapse-free survival (RFS), with a 73% CR rate for the former treatment versus 36% for the latter treatment, and a 3-year RFS of 58% versus 38%. The same issue was confirmed by a subsequent retrospective multicenter Italian experience of 138 patients. Patients on MACOP-B/VACOP-B achieved better results than those on CHOP, both with CR and event-free survival (EFS) rates, with a statistically significant difference in low

Table 1
Summary of the published experience with primary mediastinal B-cell lymphoma patients in the prerituximab era

Author, Year	Treatment	Patients	CR, %	PFS or RFS, %
Zinzani et al,[14] 1996	(F)-MAC(H)OP-B + RT	22	95	89 (62 mo)
Lazzarino et al,[16] 1997	—	106	—	—
	CHOP ± RT	—	36	38 (36 mo)
	M(V)ACOP-B ± RT	—	73	58 (36 mo)
Zinzani et al,[19] 1999	MACOP-B + RT	50	86	93 (96 mo)
Zinzani et al,[20] 2001	MACOP-B + RT	89	88	91 (108 mo)
Zinzani et al,[18] 2002	—	426	—	—
	CHOP ± RT	105	61	35 (120 mo)
	Third-generation[a] ± RT	277	79	67 (120 mo)
	High-dose/autoSCT ± RT	44	75	78 (120 mo)
Todeschini et al,[17] 2004	—	138	—	—
	CHOP ± RT	43	51	40 (120 mo)
	M(V)ACOP-B ± RT	95	80	76 (120 mo)
Savage et al,[7] 2006	CHOP, CHOP-like ± RT	63	n.r.	71 (60 mo)
	M(V)ACOP-B ± RT	47	n.r.	87 (60 mo)[b]
Mazzarotto et al,[21] 2007	Third-generation[a] ± RT	53	89	85 (94 mo)
De Sanctis et al,[22] 2008	MACOP-B + RT	92	87	81 (160 mo)

Abbreviations: autoSCT, autologous stem cell transplantation; n.r., not reported; RT, external beam radiation therapy.
[a] Third-generation treatments include: MACOP-B, VACOP-B and ProMACE-CytaBOM.
[b] Figures indicate overall survival.

and low–intermediate International Prognostic Index (IPI) risk groups (into which most patients with PMBCL generally fall), although lacking significance in high–intermediate-risk and high-risk disease.[17]

The results of a multinational retrospective analysis published in 2002 by the International Extranodal Lymphoma Study Group (IELSG) clearly showed that patients treated with third-generation regimens or high-dose therapy performed better than those who received a first-generation approach (ie, CHOP, **Fig. 3**), and that RT (delivered to 90% of the enrolled patients) played a pivotal role in the consolidation of response,[18] as it was able to convert partial responses into CR, as documented with a gallium (^{67}Ga) scan.[19,20]

On the basis of these results, MACOP-B or VACOP-B induction, followed by mediastinal RT, was thus suggested to be a suitable induction strategy for PMBCL patients.[21,22] Nevertheless, the effective superiority of third-generation treatments over CHOP and CHOP-like regimens has never been validated, either in larger phase 3 studies or in randomized trials. Alternative strategies, such as the application of high-dose methotrexate,[23] have yielded similar response rates, although with a significantly higher incidence of toxic events and hospitalization rates.

INDUCTION THERAPY IN THE RITUXIMAB ERA

The role of rituximab added to CHOP in patients with DLBCL is now unarguably defined[8,9]; its value in patients with PMBCL is less well established, as available data are mainly from retrospective experiences and do not rely on appropriately powered randomized trials.

Data extrapolated from the Mabthera International (MInT) study regarding a subgroup of 87 PMBCL patients (all with an age-adjusted IPI $\leq$1) defined the statistically significant superiority of those treated with R-CHOP/R-CHOP-like over those who received CHOP in terms of CR (84% vs 54%) and EFS (78% vs 52%), whereas overall survival (OS) rates were comparable (89% vs 78%).[24] Moreover, rituximab added to CHOP in 76 patients has demonstrated better EFS and OS rates compared with

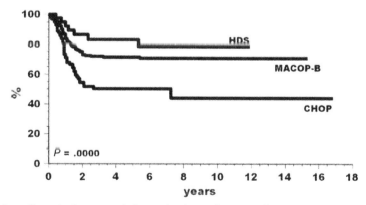

Fig. 3. Overall survival curves of the main chemotherapy subgroups applied as first-line treatment in the prerituximab era. (*From* Zinzani PL, Martelli M, Bertini M, et al. Induction chemotherapy strategies for primary mediastinal large B-cell lymphoma with sclerosis: a retrospective multinational study on 426 previously untreated patients. Haematologica 2002;87:1261; with permission.)

historical controls who received CHOP (80% and 89% vs 47% and 69% at 5 years, respectively). Additionally, there was a lower rate of early treatment failure (9% vs 30%) as well as higher CR rates and significant reduction of disease progression,[25] irrespective of consolidation RT.

On the other hand, in a retrospective study from British Columbia, a comparison of R-CHOP and CHOP alone in PMBCL patients, failed to show any statistically significant survival advantage of the former regimen.[7] A short follow-up period and a small number of patients in the R-containing group may be a possible explanation. In addition, patients treated with MACOP-B/VACOP-B showed superior outcomes over CHOP-type treatments in terms of OS (87%, 82%, and 71% for patients treated with M[V]ACOP-B, R-CHOP, and CHOP, respectively). Data from a recent experience have also shown that in a subset of 63 PMBCL patients treated with R-CHOP, with or without radiation, a primary induction failure unacceptably occurred in 21% of the treated patients, particularly in those with increased IPI score (33% of patients with IPI $\geq$ 2), advanced age and stage (21% of patients), bulky mediastinal disease (71% of patients), or multiple extranodal localizations.[26]

A multicenter Italian experience has demonstrated that the combination of rituximab with a third-generation regimen is not significantly different from R-CHOP or M[V] ACOP-B alone in terms of EFS.[27] This means that the addition of rituximab may improve outcomes if a CHOP-like regimen is used as induction therapy (as also suggested by other reports[28]), but it confers little or no benefit if it is added to a more intense treatment strategy (**Table 2**).

Table 2
Summary of the published experience with primary mediastinal B-cell lymphoma patients with chemoimmunotherapy combinations

Author, Year	Treatment	Patients	CR, %	PFS or RFS, %
Savage et al,[7] 2006	R-CHOP ± RT	18	n.r.	82 (60 mo)[a]
Zinzani et al,[27] 2009	R-M(V)ACOP-B	45	80	88 (60 mo)
Moskowitz et al,[40] 2010	R-CHOP/ICE	54	n.r.	78 (36 mo)
Rieger et al,[24] 2011	R-CHOP	44	52	78 (78 mo)
Vassilakopoulos et al,[25] 2012	CHOP ± RT	45	n.r.	47 (60 mo)
	R-CHOP ± RT	76	n.r.	80 (60 mo)
Dunleavy et al,[29] 2013	DA-EPOCH-R	51	96	93 (60 mo)
Soumerai et al,[26] 2014	R-CHOP	63	71	68 (60 mo)
Savage et al,[43] 2012	R-CHOP ± RT	59	—	—
	• R-CHOP[b]	33	n.r.	78% (60 mo)
	• R-CHOP + RT[c]	26	n.r.	83% (60 mo)
Zinzani et al,[44] 2015	R-MACOP-B ± RT	74	82	91 (113 mo)
	• R-MACOP-B[b]	23	100	90 (68 mo)
	• R-MACOP-B + RT[c]	51	75	91 (113 mo)
Martelli et al,[41] 2014	R-CHOP/M(V)ACOP-B ± RT	115	—	—
	• Negative PET[d]		100	98 (60 mo)
	• PET > Deauville 2		82	82 (60 mo)
	• PET > Deauville 3		68	68 (60 mo)

Abbreviations: n.r., not reported; R, rituximab; RT, external beam radiation therapy.
[a] Figures indicate overall survival.
[b] If PET negative at the end of treatment.
[c] If PET positive at the end of treatment.
[d] End-of-treatment PET evaluation. Negative PET refers to a Deauville score of 1 and 2.

Recently, Dunleavy and colleagues[29] demonstrated in a phase 2 prospective trial involving 51 patients, that the use of a dose-adjusted chemotherapy based on etoposide, doxorubicin, cyclophosphamide, vincristine, and prednisone (DA-EPOCH) and containing rituximab, yielded 5-year EFS and OS rates of 93% and 97%, respectively. These results appeared better than DA-EPOCH alone,[30] suggesting that the addition of rituximab significantly improved the outcomes of chemotherapy in this subset of patients. More importantly, this study also pointed out that the use of DA-EPOCH-R could obviate the need for RT in 96% of the cases, with no relapsing patients over a median follow-up of more than 5 years. Half of the patients treated, in fact, had a maximum standardized uptake value (SUVmax) at the end-of-chemotherapy PET scan that was no more than the value of mediastinal blood pool, whereas among those with a higher value, a residual disease was clearly documented in just 17% of the cases. The excellent cure rates obtained with this approach and without RT may therefore suggest that radiation can be safely omitted in carefully selected patients.

RADIATION THERAPY CONSOLIDATION APPROACH: IS MORE ALWAYS BETTER?

External RT, conceived as the delivery of radiation on residues of bulky masses at the end of chemotherapy, has shown great efficacy when incorporated after a chemotherapy-based induction, particularly in converting partial response (PR) into CR and in rendering active residual masses negative at ^{67}Ga-scan or PET.[17–22]

Recently, the role of RT was retrospectively assessed in 37 patients treated with R-VACOP-B and R-CHOP,[31] whose response after induction chemoimmunotherapy was documented by PET scan using the Deauville five-points scale (5-PS).[32] RT was delivered to all patients, independent of the 5-PS score at the end of induction. All patients with a score of 3 and 4 could obtain PET negativity (ie, 5-PS score 1–2) after RT, whereas just 25% of patients with score 5 could achieve a continuous CR. Moreover, patients with 5-PS score of 1 to 3 showed a significantly increased OS rate if compared with those with score 4 to 5 after chemoimmunotherapy (100% vs 77%), although without a statistically significant difference in progression-free survival (PFS) at 3 years (94% vs 83%, respectively; $P = .3$). This experience indicates that patients with a 5-PS score of 5 are at higher risk of failure even after RT than those with a lower score, although RT still remains a valuable option for patients with PET positivity after induction.

A review conducted by Jackson and colleagues[33] on 250 patients with stage I and II PMBCL from the Surveillance, Epidemiology, and End Results (SEER) database has demonstrated that the use of RT was associated with a significant improvement in 5-year OS (90% for irradiated patients vs 79%), thus showing that the 11% absolute survival benefit corresponds to 9 patients needed-to-treat with RT to prevent 1 death at 5 years. However, a trend toward the reduction of RT use in the United States was also described, with half of patients being spared RT from 2006 and 2011, probably indicating increased concerns of treating physicians about the risk of RT-induced cardiopulmonary events and secondary neoplasms.[34–37] The same authors ended up to similar findings in another registry-based review (National Cancer Database), in which they found a significant 10% increase in 5-year OS for PMBCL patients treated with combined-modality treatment (systemic + RT) with no stage limitations.[38]

These data appear conflicting with those shown by Giri and colleagues[39] on 258 patients, again from the SEER database, which indicated no significant difference in OS between patients treated with or without RT (82.5% vs 78.6%), although it was evident that irradiated patients had a more favorable trend. The disparity seen in these similar reviews[33,39] mainly depends on the disease stage they considered. The former study included patients who could have taken greater advantage from mediastinal irradiation, whereas the latter study also included at least 30% of patients with stage III-IV disease.

The concept of omitting RT in patients receiving a dose-intense induction and, in general, in those cases in whom a rituximab-based first-line treatment is contemplated has been suggested by some contemporary studies, such as the aforementioned study from Dunleavy and colleagues[29] with DA-EPOCH-R, and in a study from Memorial Sloan Kettering Cancer Center,[40] in which a sequential intervention with R-CHOP plus ICE (ifosfamide, carboplatin, etoposide) without RT yielded OS and PFS rates of 88% and 78%, respectively, with patients failing this program being salvaged in half of cases with an RT-based transplantation. RT should be still regarded as a powerful consolidation strategy after a rituximab plus chemotherapy induction in patients with PMBCL. However, the identification of patients for whom RT can be safely omitted is an issue of paramount importance. Moreover, a thorough radiographic evaluation at the end of chemoimmunotherapy, along with the application of modern RT techniques, is mandatory to identify volumes to be irradiated, minimizing exposure to nearby organs at risk.

HOW WILL POSITRON EMISSION TOMOGRAPHY ASSIST PHYSICIANS IN CHOOSING TREATMENTS WISELY?

Because of the large amount of fibrous tissue within tumor masses and the large bulks often encountered at disease onset, residual lumps are commonly present after treatment and may persist during follow-up. For this reason, response assessment by computed tomography (CT) scan may not be accurate enough, and PET scan appears useful in discriminating between viable neoplastic and necrotic or fibrotic tissue.

Although PET is used empirically in PMBCL, and no formal evaluation regarding its prognostic impact in this context has been performed so far, its high negative-predictive value after induction has been demonstrated. Its positive predictive value in PMBCL is poor, given that PET-avid inflammatory components within masses otherwise negative for cancer cells can be easily detected.[29,41] Therefore, end-treatment PET-positive scans require a cautious interpretation in terms of persistent disease, and inconclusive cases need to be solved by biopsy whenever possible.[42]

Data on the role of PET after chemoimmunotherapy indicate that metabolic CR (5-PS score 1–2) can be achieved in less than half of patients. However, patients with a positive PET scan after induction, whose uptake is higher than mediastinal blood pool but lower than liver (5-PS score 3), do not show worse OS and PFS than patients with 5-PS 1 to 2. A 5-PS score 3 is considered an effective threshold to discriminate between patients with lower or higher risk of failure (OS 100% vs 83%, PFS 99% vs 68% at 5 years).[41]

On the basis of these observations, it can be postulated that postchemotherapy PET evaluation may represent a tool to guide RT usage, reasonably sparing mediastinal irradiation in PET-negative cases. The ongoing phase 3, randomized IELSG-37 trial will prospectively evaluate RT in patients with a negative PET scan at the end of chemoimmunotherapy, trying to formally demonstrate that PFS in the observation arm is not worse than in the RT arm.

Savage and colleagues[43] applied a PET-guided RT approach in 59 patients treated with R-CHOP; patients with a PET-documented CR were observed, whereas those with a positive PET-scan received RT. Ninety-six percent of patients with a positive PET scan and 6% of patients with a negative PET scan were irradiated. Time to progression and OS at 5 years were comparable for PET-negative and PET-positive patients (78% vs 83% and 88% vs 95%, respectively). Similarly, the authors' group published an experience in 74 patients, all treated with an R-MACOP-B induction.[44] Again, PET-negative cases (defined according to the International Harmonization Project criteria[45]) were only observed, and PET-positive patients received RT. OS and DFS rates were 82% and 91% at 10 years, respectively, without differences between patients who were or were not irradiated (**Fig. 4**).

More recently, Vassilakopoulos and colleagues[46] reported their experience with PET/CT in 106 PMBCL patients responding to R-CHOP. Responses were categorized according to Deauville 5-PS, and RT was applied after chemoimmunotherapy at the discretion of the treating physician. Among the 63 PET-negative patients, nonirradiated patients (51% of the total) had no statistically significant inferior outcomes than those who received RT in terms of freedom from progression (FFP, 91% vs 100%). In the remaining 43 PET-positive cases (88% received RT), patients with a 5-PS score of 3 had similar failure rates to those with a negative PET; therefore, a score of 4 to 5 allowed a more precise discrimination between PET positivity or negativity and correlated with FFP at 3 years (96% vs 61% for patients with scores 1–3 and 4–5, respectively) as also reported elsewhere.[41,47] Importantly, RT permitted disease control in most of cases, with clinical relapses seen in 26% of patients, particularly among those who remained PET-positive after RT.

THE TREATMENT OF REFRACTORY AND RELAPSING PATIENTS: A THERAPEUTIC DILEMMA

Relapses tend to occur early during the course of post-treatment follow-up, mostly within the first 18 months. Overall, unsatisfactory responses to induction roughly involve 15% to 20% of patients. Disease at relapse generally behaves aggressively; it may remain confined to the mediastinum or spread to subdiaphragmatic organs, such as adrenals, kidneys, ovaries, pancreas, or to the central nervous system.

Outcomes for patients with relapsed or refractory PMBCL are generally dismal, as disease is often refractory to salvage chemotherapy. The optimal disease management in this context is represented by the application of an appropriate salvage regimen (platinum-based or other intensive regimens), followed by autologous stem cell transplantation (SCT), as it is generally accepted for patients with DLBCL.

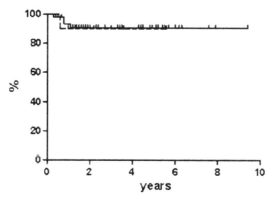

Fig. 4. Progression-free survival curves for patients treated with consolidative mediastinal radiation (PET-positive after induction, *solid line*) or just observed without radiotherapy (PET-negative after induction, *dotted line*). (*From* Zinzani PL, Broccoli A, Casadei B, et al. The role of rituximab and positron emission tomography in the treatment of primary mediastinal large B-cell lymphoma: experience on 74 patients. Hematol Oncol 2015;33:148; with permission.)

Kuruvilla and colleagues[11] have described that survival rates in PMBCL patients were poorer than what was observed for a matched population of DLBCL patients, with OS rates at 2 years after progression that just halved those of DLBCL. On the contrary, a previously reported retrospective analysis[48] has pointed out that PFS survival rates for primarily refractory and relapsed patients (58% and 27% at 5 years for each category, respectively) could be even better than what was seen in aggressive lymphomas when high-dose treatments and autologous SCT were properly used. Chemotherapy-responsive disease before transplant was regarded as the most relevant predictor of treatment success, as demonstrated by a significant increase in 5-year PFS (75% vs 33% observed in chemotherapy-nonresponsive patients, $P = .007$).[48] A possibility of cure in 40% to 80% of patients with disease that favorably responds to salvage treatment and to autologous SCT has also been confirmed in several other series.[10,49,50] Finally, a recent retrospective study from Japan has further elucidated the role of SCT in the relapsed and refractory setting, as it documented a significantly higher OS for transplanted versus not-transplanted patients (67% and 31% respectively).[51]

Because of the paucity of data regarding allogeneic SCT in PMBCL patients, this procedure should be still considered experimental, and its role needs to be further clarified in the era of new drugs.

INVESTIGATIONAL APPROACHES FOR REFRACTORY AND RELAPSING PATIENTS

Some peculiar molecular and biologic features of PMBCL[4,5] suggest a possible role of novel agents in PMBCL patients, especially in chemorefractory patients. Anti-programmed death 1 (PD1) antibodies, Janus kinase (JAK2) inhibitors, and the anti-CD30 antibody-drug conjugate brentuximab vedotin are now being explored in clinical trials, as their use is supported by in vitro data,[52] by their application in other PD1 and CD30-expressing lymphoid malignancies,[53,54] and by preliminary reports.[55]

The CD30 antigen is present in the majority of cases of PMBCL, although it is expressed weakly and heterogeneously.[1,5] A recently published phase 2 trial of brentuximab vedotin in patients with relapsed/refractory DLBCL also included 6 patients with PMBCL; a 17% CR rate was observed, and half of patients maintained a disease stability. Responses did not correlate with the quantitative CD30 expression on tumor cells.[54] Brentuximab vedotin is currently being investigated in a trial from the Italian Cooperative Study Group on Lymphomas (http://clinicaltrials.gov/ct2/show/NCT02423291) as a single-agent salvage treatment (1.8 mg/kg every 21 days) in patients with PMBCL relapsed after or refractory to at least 1 previous line. It is also applied in combination with R-CHOP as frontline approach in patients with CD30-positive PMBCL, DLBCL, and grey-zone lymphoma (http://clinicaltrials.gov/ct2/show/NCT01994850).

The amplification of chromosome 9p24.1 in both nodular sclerosis Hodgkin disease and PMBCL induces the overexpression of the immunoregulatory genes programmed death ligand 1 (PD-L1) and PD-L2 (both ligands of PD1, expressed on tumor-infiltrating lymphocytes), as well as of JAK2, which in turn induces PD-L1 transcription.[4] The effectiveness of anti-PD1 inhibition in classic Hodgkin disease[53] provides a rationale for the exploitation of an extensive PD-1/PD-L1 axis blockade as a therapeutic strategy for patients with relapsed or refractory PMBCL. A preliminary report of a phase 1b study with the anti-PD1 antibody pembrolizumab applied as a single agent in this context showed an overall response rate of 40%.[55] Pembrolizumab is now being investigated in a phase 2 trial involving patients with relapsed and refractory disease (http://clinicaltrials.gov/ct2/show/NCT02576990), as it is expected that this treatment will induce a meaningful clinical response.

The aberrant activation of the JAK2 and Signal Transducer and Activator of Transcription (STAT) pathway also represents a potentially relevant therapeutic target. The JAK1/JAK2 inhibitor ruxolitinib has demonstrated antiproliferative effects in a dose-dependent manner in both Hodgkin and PMBCL cell lines,[52] and is currently under investigation in a pilot study for patients with relapsed or refractory Hodgkin disease and PMBCL (http://clinicaltrials.gov/ct2/show/NCT01965119).

SUMMARY

The clinical and pathologic peculiarities of PMBCL, the high chances of cure documented in literature in more than 20 years of international experience, and the long disease-free life expectancy of cured patients have always drawn attention in finding out the most suitable first-line approach and the most convenient combination of treatment modalities, on the one hand trying to maximize the long-term clinical outcomes, while on the other hand reducing the potential harmful consequences of highly toxic combined treatments.

An anthracycline-containing chemoimmunotherapy-based first-line approach, either with a third-generation regimen or with R-CHOP, is considered the optimal strategy to induce a high rate of responses, which can be further consolidated by the application of mediastinal RT. An end-of-chemotherapy negative PET scan can help treating physicians in individuating those patients in whom RT can be safely omitted, thus avoiding unnecessary overtreatment and possible long-term toxicities. Conversely, a positive PET scan should be interpreted very carefully, especially if the patient is asymptomatic, as the risk of false positivity does exist. This is why any suspicion of relapse should be thoroughly ruled out by performing a biopsy of the PET-positive tissue (**Fig. 5**). Alternatively, infusional DA-EPOCH applied since

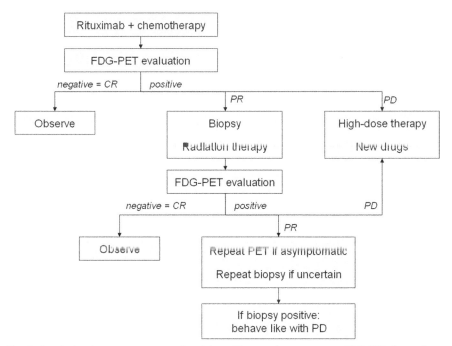

Fig. 5. Postinduction management algorithm. CR, complete response; FDG-PET, fluorodeoxyglucose positron emission tomography; PD, progressive disease; PR, partial response.

the beginning, or a sequential R-CHOP/ICE strategy, may induce favorable outcomes with the avoidance of routinely administered RT.

The treatment of relapsed or refractory disease mainly rests upon high-dose treatments and autologous SCT; however, many patients fail to attain a good response to salvage treatment, thus displaying a significantly poor prognosis. New drugs, whose mechanisms of action are based on peculiar biologic features of the tumor, are worth investigating in this context, as they may impact on a patient's ability to obtain better disease control and possibly benefit from transplant procedures.

REFERENCES

1. Gaulard P, Harris NL, Pileri SA, et al. Primary mediastinal (thymic) large B-cell lymphoma. In: Swerdlow SH, Campo E, Harris NL, et al, editors. World Health Organization classification of tumors of haematopoietic and lymphoid tissues. 4th edition. Lyon (France): IARC Press; 2008. p. 250–1.
2. Rosenwald A, Wright G, Leroy K, et al. Molecular diagnosis of primary mediastinal B cell lymphoma identifies a clinically favourable subgroup of diffuse large B cell lymphoma related to Hodgkin lymphoma. J Exp Med 2003;198:851–62.
3. Savage KJ, Monti S, Kutok JL, et al. The molecular signature of mediastinal large B-cell lymphoma differs from that of other diffuse large B-cell lymphomas and shares features with classical Hodgkin lymphoma. Blood 2003;102:3871–9.
4. Twa DD, Chan FC, Ben-Neriah S, et al. Genomic rearrangements involving programmed death ligands are recurrent in primary mediastinal large B-cell lymphoma. Blood 2014;123:2062–5.
5. Steidl C, Gascoyne RD. The molecular pathogenesis of primary mediastinal large B-cell lymphoma. Blood 2011;118:2659–69.
6. Zinzani PL, Martelli M, Poletti V, et al. Practice guidelines for the management of extranodal non-Hodgkin's lymphomas of adult non-immunodeficient patients. Part I: primary lung and mediastinal lymphomas. A project of the Italian Society of Hematology, the Italian Society of experimental Hematology and the Italian Group for Bone Marrow Transplantation. Haematologica 2008;93:1364–71.
7. Savage KJ, Al-Rajhi N, Voss N, et al. Favorable outcome of primary mediastinal large B-cell lymphoma in a single institution: the British Columbia experience. Ann Oncol 2006;17:123–30.
8. Pfreundschuh M, Trümper L, Osterborg A, et al. CHOP-like chemotherapy plus rituximab compared with CHOP-like chemotherapy alone in young patients with good-prognosis diffuse large B-cell lymphoma: a randomized controlled trial by the Mabthera International Trial (MInT) Group. Lancet Oncol 2006;7:379–91.
9. Coiffier B, Lepage E, Briere J, et al. CHOP chemotherapy plus rituximab compared with CHOP alone in elderly patients with diffuse large B-cell lymphoma. N Engl J Med 2002;346:235–42.
10. Rodríguez J, Conde E, Gutiérrez A, et al. Primary mediastinal large cell lymphoma (PMBL): frontline treatment with autologous stem cell transplantation (ASCT). The GEL-TAMO experience. Hematol Oncol 2008;26:171–8.
11. Kuruvilla J, Pintilie M, Tsang R, et al. Salvage chemotherapy and autologous stem cell transplantation are inferior for relapsed or refractory primary mediastinal large B-cell lymphoma compared with diffuse large B-cell lymphoma. Leuk Lymphoma 2008;49:1329–36.
12. Klimo P, Connors JM. MACOP-B chemotherapy for the treatment of diffuse large B-cell lymphoma. Ann Intern Med 1985;102:596–601.

13. Bertini M, Orsucci L, Vitolo U, et al. Stage II large B-cell lymphoma with sclerosis treated with MACOP-B. Ann Oncol 1991;2:733–7.

14. Zinzani PL, Bendandi M, Frezza G, et al. Primary mediastinal B-cell lymphoma with sclerosis: clinical and therapeutic evaluation of 22 patients. Leuk Lymphoma 1996;21:311–6.

15. Lazzarino M, Orlandi E, Paulli M, et al. Primary mediastinal B-cell lymphoma with sclerosis: an aggressive tumor with distinctive clinical and pathologic features. J Clin Oncol 1993;11:2306–13.

16. Lazzarino M, Orlandi E, Paulli M. Treatment outcome and prognostic factors for primary mediastinal (thymic) B-cell lymphoma: a multicenter study of 106 patients. J Clin Oncol 1997;15:1646–53.

17. Todeschini G, Secchi S, Morra E, et al. Primary mediastinal large B-cell lymphoma (PMLBCL): long term results from a retrospective multicenter Italian experience in 138 patients treated with CHOP or MACOP-B/VACOP-B. Br J Cancer 2004;90:372–6.

18. Zinzani PL, Martelli M, Bertini M, et al. Induction chemotherapy strategies for primary mediastinal large B-cell lymphoma with sclerosis: a retrospective multinational study on 426 previously untreated patients. Haematologica 2002;87: 1258–64.

19. Zinzani PL, Martelli M, Magagnoli M, et al. Treatment and clinical management of primary mediastinal large B-cell lymphoma with sclerosis: MACOP-B regimen and mediastinal radiotherapy monitored by (67)Gallium scan in 50 patients. Blood 1999;94:3289–93.

20. Zinzani PL, Martelli M, Bendandi M, et al. Primary mediastinal large B-cell lymphoma with sclerosis: a clinical study of 89 patients treated with MACOP-B chemotherapy and radiation therapy. Haematologica 2001;86:187–91.

21. Mazzarotto R, Boso C, Vianello F, et al. Primary mediastinal large B-cell lymphoma: results of intensive chemotherapy regimens (MACOP-B/VACOP-B) plus involved field radiotherapy on 53 patients. A single institution experience. Int J Radiat Oncol Biol Phys 2007;68:823–9.

22. De Sanctis V, Finolezzi E, Osti MF, et al. MACOP-B and involved-field radiotherapy is an effective and safe therapy for primary mediastinal large B cell lymphoma. Int J Radiat Oncol Biol Phys 2008;72:1154–60.

23. Fietz T, Knauf U, Hänel M, et al. Treatment of primary mediastinal large B cell lymphoma with an alternating chemotherapy regimen based on high-dose methotrexate. Ann Hematol 2009;88:433–9.

24. Rieger M, Österborg A, Pettengell R, et al. Primary mediastinal B-cell lymphoma treated with CHOP-like chemotherapy with or without rituximab: results of the Mabthera International Trial Group study. Ann Oncol 2011;22:664–70.

25. Vassilakopoulos TP, Pangalis GA, Katsigiannis A, et al. Rituximab, cyclophosphamide, doxorubicin, vincristine, and prednisone with or without radiotherapy in primary mediastinal large B-cell lymphoma: the emerging standard of care. Oncologist 2012;17:239–49.

26. Soumerai JD, Hellmann MD, Feng Y, et al. Treatment of primary mediastinal B-cell lymphoma with rituximab, cyclophosphamide, doxorubicin, vincristine and prednisone is associated with a high rate of primary refractory disease. Leuk Lymphoma 2014;55:538–43.

27. Zinzani PL, Stefoni V, Finolezzi E, et al. Rituximab combined with MACOP-B or VACOP-B and radiation therapy in primary mediastinal large B-cell lymphoma: a retrospective study. Clin Lymphoma Myeloma 2009;9:381–5.

28. Avigdor A, Sirotkin T, Kedmi M, et al. The impact of R-VACOP-B and interim FDG-PET/CT on outcome in primary mediastinal large B cell lymphoma. Ann Hematol 2014;93:1297–304.

29. Dunleavy K, Pittaluga S, Maeda LS, et al. Dose-adjusted EPOCH-rituximab therapy in primary mediastinal B-cell lymphoma. N Engl J Med 2013;368:1408–16.

30. Wilson WH, Grossbard ML, Pittaluga S, et al. Dose-adjusted EPOCH chemotherapy for untreated large B-cell lymphomas: a pharmacodynamic approach with high efficacy. Blood 2002;99:2685–93.

31. Filippi AR, Piva C, Giunta F, et al. Radiation therapy in primari mediastinal B-cell lymphoma with positron emission tomography positivity after rituximab chemotherapy. Int J Radiat Oncol Biol Phys 2013;87:311–6.

32. Meignan M, Barrington S, Itti E, et al. Report on the 4th International Workshop on positron emission tomography in lymphoma held in Menton, France, 3-5 October 2012. Leuk Lymphoma 2014;55:31–7.

33. Jackson MW, Rusthoven CG, Jones BL, et al. Improved survival with radiation therapy in stage I-II primary mediastinal B cell lymphoma: a Surveillance, Epidemiology, and End Results database analysis. Int J Radiat Oncol Biol Phys 2016; 94:126–32.

34. van Nimwegen FA, Schaapveld M, Cutter DJ, et al. Radiation dose-response relationship for risk of coronary heart disease in survivors of Hodgkin lymphoma. J Clin Oncol 2016;34:235–43.

35. Gujral DM, Lloyd G, Bhattacharyya S. Radiation-induced valvular heart disease. Heart 2015. http://dx.doi.org/10.1136/heartjnl-2015–308765.

36. Pinnix CC, Smith GL, Milgrom S, et al. Predictors of radiation pneumonitis in patients receiving intensity modulated radiation therapy for Hodgkin and non-Hodgkin lymphoma. Int J Radiat Oncol Biol Phys 2015;92:175–82.

37. Berrington de Gonzalez A, Gilbert E, Curtis R, et al. Second solid cancers after radiation therapy: a systematic review of the epidemiologic studies of the radiation dose-response relationship. Int J Radiat Oncol Biol Phys 2013;86:224–33.

38. Jackson MW, Rusthoven CG, Jones BL, et al. Improved survival with combined modality therapy in the modern era for primary mediastinal B-cell lymphoma. Am J Hematol 2016;91(5):476–80.

39. Giri S, Bhatt VR, Pathak R, et al. Role of radiation therapy in primary mediastinal large B-cell lymphoma in rituximab era: a US population-based analysis. Am J Hematol 2015;90:1052–4.

40. Moskowitz C, Hamlin PA, Maragulia J, et al. Sequential dose-dense RCHOP followed by ICE consolidation (MSKCC protocol 01-142) without radireportapy for patients with primary mediastinal large B cell lymphoma. In: 52nd ASH Annual Meeting Abstracts. Orlando, December 4-7, 2010. [abstract: 420].

41. Martelli M, Ceriani L, Zucca E, et al. [18F]fluorodeoxyglucose positron emission tomography predicts survival after chemoimmunotherapy for primary mediastinal large B-cell lymphoma: results of the International Extranodal Lymphoma Study Group IELSG-26 Study. J Clin Oncol 2014;32:1769–75.

42. Zinzani PL, Tani M, Trisolini R, et al. Histological verification of positive positron emission tomography findings in the follow-up of patients with mediastinal lymphoma. Haematologica 2007;92:771–7.

43. Savage K, Yenson PR, Shenkier T, et al. The outcome of primary mediastinal large B-cell lymphoma (PMBCL) in the R-CHOP treatment era. In: 54th ASH Annual Meeting Abstracts. Atlanta, December 8-11, 2012. [abstract: 303].

44. Zinzani PL, Broccoli A, Casadei B, et al. The role of rituximab and positron emission tomography in the treatment of primary mediastinal large B-cell lymphoma: experience on 74 patients. Hematol Oncol 2015;33:145–50.
45. Juweid ME, Stroobants S, Hoekstra OS, et al. Use of positron emission tomography for response assessment of lymphoma: consensus of the Imaging Subcommittee of International Harmonization Project in Lymphoma. J Clin Oncol 2007;25: 571–8.
46. Vassilakopoulos TP, Pangalis GA, Chatziioannou S, et al. PET/CT in primary mediastinal large B-cell lymphoma responding to rituximab-CHOP: an analysis of 106 patients regarding prognostic significance and implications for subsequent radiotherapy. Leukemia 2016;30:238–42.
47. Nagle SJ, Chong EA, Chekol S, et al. The role of FDG-PET imaging as a prognostic marker of outcome in primary mediastinal B-cell lymphoma. Cancer Med 2015;4:7–15.
48. Sehn LH, Antin JH, Shulman LN, et al. Primary diffuse large B-cell lymphoma of the mediastinum: outcome following high-dose chemotherapy and autologous hematopoietic cell transplantation. Blood 1998;91:717–23.
49. Hamlin PA, Portlock CS, Straus DJ, et al. Primary mediastinal large B-cell lymphoma: optimal therapy and prognostic factor analysis in 141 consecutive patients treated at Memorial Sloan Kettering from 1980 to 1999. Br J Haematol 2005;130:691–9.
50. Aoki T, Shimada K, Suzuki R, et al. High-dose chemotherapy followed by autologous stem cell transplantation for relapsed/refractory primary mediastinal large B-cell lymphoma. Blood Cancer J 2015;5:e372.
51. Aoki T, Izutsu K, Suzuki R, et al. Novel prognostic model of primary mediastinal large B-cell lymphoma (PMBL): a multicenter cooperative retrospective study in Japan. In: 55th ASH Annual Meeting Abstracts. New Orleans, December 7-10, 2013. [abstract: 638].
52. Yin C, Lee S, Ayello J, et al. JAK1/JAK2 inhibitor, ruxolitinib inhibits cell proliferation and induces apoptosis in Hodgkin lymphomas (HL) and primary mediastinal B-cell lymphomas (PMBL). In: 54th ASH Annual Meeting Abstracts. Atlanta, December 8-11, 2012. [abstract: 4886].
53. Ansell SM, Lesokhin AM, Borrello I, et al. PD-1 blockade with nivolumab in relapsed or refractory Hodgkin's lymphoma. N Engl J Med 2015;372:311–9.
54. Jacobsen ED, Sharman JP, Oki Y, et al. Brentuximab vedotin demonstrates objective responses in a phase 2 study of relapsed/refractory DLBCL with variable CD30 expression. Blood 2015;125:1394–402.
55. Zinzani PL, Ribrag V, Moskowitz CH, et al. Phase 1b study of pembrolizumab in patients with relapsed/refractory primary mediastinal large B-cell lymphoma: keynote-013. In: 21st EHA Meeting Abstracts. Copenhagen, June 9-12, 2016. [abstract: S797].

Central Nervous System Prophylaxis for Aggressive B-cell Lymphoma
Who, What, and When?

Norbert Schmitz, MD, PhD[a],*, Maike Nickelsen, MD[a],
Kerry J. Savage, MD, MSc[b],*

KEYWORDS

- B-cell lymphoma • Central nervous system • Prophylaxis

KEY POINTS

- Central nervous system (CNS) relapse of aggressive B-cell lymphoma is a rare but serious complication with a short median survival.
- Different approaches have been used to define risks factors for CNS relapse and to establish efficient prophylactic measures.
- The CNS International Prognostic Index was established on patients treated in clinical trials of the German Aggressive non-Hodgkin Lymphoma Study Group (DSHNHL) and in the Mabthera International Trial, and was validated on patients treated in British Columbia (British Columbia Cancer Agency).
- Although patients with low or intermediate risk of CNS relapse should not undergo special diagnostic or therapeutic measures, the authors suggest CNS MRI as well as cytology and flow cytometry of the cerebrospinal fluid for high-risk patients (and patients with testicular involvement) at diagnosis and to consider prophylactic high-dose methotrexate treatment of patients without proven CNS involvement.
- Future risk and treatment models may include molecular features (BCL2/MYK) and new treatment options like ibrutinib and lenalidomide.

INTRODUCTION

Secondary involvement of the central nervous system (CNS) in patients with aggressive B-cell lymphoma is a serious complication with a median survival of only few

Contributions: All authors participated in collecting and reviewing the data and writing the article.

Conflicts of Interest: The authors declare no competing financial interests

[a] Department of Hematology, Oncology and Stem Cell Transplantation, Asklepios Hospital St. Georg, Lohmuehlenstrasse 5, Hamburg D-20099, Germany; [b] Department of Medical Oncology, British Columbia Cancer Agency, 600 West 10th Avenue, Vancouver, British Columbia V5Z 4E6, Canada

* Corresponding author.

E-mail addresses: n.schmitz@asklepios.com; ksavage@bccancer.bc.ca

Hematol Oncol Clin N Am 30 (2016) 1277–1291
http://dx.doi.org/10.1016/j.hoc.2016.07.008
0889-8588/16/© 2016 Elsevier Inc. All rights reserved.

months to less than 1 year.[1,8] However, it is a rare event, with a recent meta-analysis of almost 5000 patients with diffuse large B-cell lymphoma (DLBCL) treated with rituximab, cyclophosphamide, doxorubicin, vincristine, and prednisone (R-CHOP) or equivalent anthracycline-based chemotherapy showing a risk of CNS recurrence of only ≈5%.[4] Thus, it is not rational to support prophylaxis in all patients. However, the risk is considerably greater in those with high-risk features at diagnosis, and identifying a high-risk group is key to guiding prophylactic strategies. In addition, the optimal type of CNS prophylaxis remains unknown. Intrathecal chemotherapy is commonly administered; however, most studies fail to show a protective effect (**Table 1**); parenchymal relapse remains the predominant site in the rituximab era.[11] Extrapolating from treatment paradigms in primary CNS lymphoma, high-dose methotrexate (HDMTX) has been explored for use in primary prophylaxis with encouraging results,[12,13] but toxicities remain problematic and its use is restricted to younger patients. Further, systemic relapse also remains problematic in this high-risk group.[11] This article reviews risk factors for CNS relapse with a focus on studies evaluating patients with DLBCL treated in the rituximab era as well as studies evaluating specific prophylaxis strategies. In addition, it discusses the role of further risk factors for CNS disease as well as the potential of novel therapies such as ibrutinib and lenalidomide in combination with R-CHOP.

WHO: RISK OF CENTRAL NERVOUS SYSTEM DISEASE

There have been several studies evaluating potential risk factors for CNS recurrence in DLBCL. Originally, risk estimates were largely based on early experience of small studies from single institutions[14,15] or cooperative groups.[16] These series published decades ago do not reflect modern diagnostic and therapeutic standards and are now of limited value. In the last decade, there have been several studies evaluating the risk of CNS recurrence in patients with DLBCL treated with R-CHOP or an equivalent regimen either as post hoc analyses of prospective randomized studies[2,5,17] or retrospective analyses performed on population-based cohorts of patients with aggressive B-cell lymphoma, primarily DLBCL.[7,10,18–22] Some of these studies compared the incidence and type of CNS disease in patients treated with R-CHOP or cyclophosphamide, doxorubicin, vincristine, and prednisone (CHOP).[2,17,19] Taken together, at best there has been a modest impact of rituximab on reducing the risk of CNS relapse. The RICOVER-60 trial evaluated 1112 patients with aggressive B-cell lymphoma, primarily DLBCL (81.6%) and found that the 2-year incidence of CNS disease was 6.9% after CHOP14 (biweekly cyclophosphamide, doxorubicin, vincristine, prednisone) and 4.1% after R-CHOP14 ($P = .046$). A retrospective analysis from the British Columbia Cancer Agency (BCCA) found a similar trend in a higher risk population (3-year risk, 9.7% R-CHOP vs 6.4% CHOP; $P = .085$) and receiving rituximab was associated with a protective effect in multivariate analysis (hazard ratio = 0.045; $P = .034$); the impact of rituximab was more profound in patients in complete remission (3-year risk, 5.8% vs 2.2%; $P = .009$), suggesting that the predominant impact is in systemic disease control with secondary reduction in CNS disease.[19] In 2016, only studies in patients treated with R-CHOP or combinations of rituximab with alternative chemotherapy regimens reflect current standard of care.

Before summarizing and discussing the key findings of recent studies investigating the risk of secondary CNS disease it is important to note the degree of heterogeneity across studies with regard to the definition of high-risk patients, CNS-directed diagnostic investigations used, and recommendations and type of CNS prophylaxis

Table 1
Studies evaluating the impact of IT CNS prophylaxis in high-risk patients with DLBCL treated with R-CHOP

Study	Number of Patients	Systemic/IT Treatment	CNS Prophylaxis Indications	CNS Relapse (%)	P Value
Schmitz et al,[5] 2012	2196 (1576 w/o R, 620 with R)	(R)-CHOEP[a] IT MTX	BM, testis, head, sinuses, orbits, oral cavity, tongue, and salivary glands	2.6 (all pt)	.386
Boehme et al,[2] 2009	1222 (612 w/o R, 610 with R)	(R)-CHOP IT. MTX	BM, testis, head, sinuses, orbits, oral cavity, tongue, and salivary glands	2.5 (w/o prophylaxis) 4.4 (with prophylaxis)	NS
Kumar et al,[6] 2012	989 (all with R)	R-CHOP IT MTX ± IT Ara-C, IV MTX (28%)	At the discretion of investigator	2.1 (w/o prophylaxis) 10.9 (with prophylaxis)	.007
Tai et al,[7] 2011	499 (179 w/o R, 320 with R)	(R)-CHOP IT. MTX	>1 ENS, orbits, sinuses, breast, testis, bone, BM	5 (w/o prophylaxis) 11 (with prophylaxis)	NR
Tomita[8]	322 (all with R)	R-CHOP IT. MTX	↑ LDH, bulk >10 cm, PS ≥2, BM, nasal, bone, breast, skin, testis	2.8 (w/o prophylaxis) 7.5 (with prophylaxis)	.14
Arkenau et al,[9] 2007	259 (77 w/o R, 62 with R)	(R)-CHOP (R)-PmitCEBO IT. MTX ± Ara-C	BM, testis, sinuses, orbits, bone, blood	1.1 (CI, 0%–2.5%) 2 pt w/o prophylaxis 1 pt with prophylaxis	NR
Guirguis et al,[10] 2012	214 (all with R)	R-CHOP IT MTX (25 pt), IV MTX (17 pt)	↑ LDH, >1 ENS, testis, epidural, sinuses, or skull	2 (w/o prophylaxis) 1.9 (with prophylaxis)	NR

Abbreviations: Ara-c, cytarabine; BM, bone marrow; CI, confidence interval; E, etoposide; ENS, extranodal site; IT, intrathecal; IV, intravenous; LDH, lactate dehydrogenase; MTX, methotrexate; NR, not reported; NS, not significant; ps, performance status; pt, patients; R, rituximab; R-PmitCEBO, rituximab, prednisolone, mitoxantrone cyclophosphamide, etoposide, bleomycin, vincristine; w/o, without.
[a] Includes patients treated with sequential high dose therapy and rituximab.

incorporated into first-line treatment. These differences may affect the proportion of patients diagnosed with CNS relapse and the identification of risk factors, and may also affect the evaluation of CNS prophylaxis.

Most importantly, proposals for future strategies (ie, who, what, and at which time) should take into account that the availability and more strict implementation of state-of-the-art diagnostic approaches like brain MRI[23] and fluorescence-activated cell sorting (FACS) analysis of the cerebrospinal fluid (CSF)[24] detect CNS disease at diagnosis in a greater but unknown proportion of patients who previously went undetected, leaving behind a remnant CNS-negative population with a risk of CNS disease that will be overestimated by applying current risk models. The dynamics of CNS relapse imply that a substantial proportion of patients already harbor lymphoma in the CNS at the time of diagnosis, rather than developing de novo CNS involvement after a remission in other compartments has been achieved.

Another limitation is that most information on CNS disease is restricted to patients with DLBCL treated with R-CHOP and may not apply to other aggressive B-cell lymphomas or alternative treatment regimens. For instance, the (R)-ACVBP (adriamycin, cyclophosphamide, vindesine, bleomycin, prednisolone) regimen used in International Prognostic Index (IPI) high-intermediate or high-risk DLBCL is combined with an intensive consolidation phase including intravenous (IV) methotrexate (MTX), etoposide, ifosfamide, and cytosine-arabinoside. These drugs, all of which cross the BBB, likely contribute to the low frequency of CNS disease (<1%) seen in patients treated with this regimen even before rituximab was introduced into first-line therapy for DLBCL.[25] Studies using the (R)-ACVBP regimen[26] therefore should not be used to define risk groups or prophylactic strategies for patients treated with the standard R-CHOP regimen. Whether rates of CNS recurrences seen in patients treated with R-CHOEP[27] or DA-EPOCH-R[28] differ from those observed in R-CHOP–treated patients is unknown. The phase 3 study comparing DA-EPOCH-R with R-CHOP (ClinicalTrial.gov number NCT00118209) has been completed and the results are eagerly awaited, including impact on the risk of CNS relapse. Etoposide crosses the BBB and earlier studies without rituximab showed that the addition of etoposide reduced the frequency of CNS relapse[29]; however, with the addition of rituximab, the effect is no longer apparent.[30]

For reasons mentioned earlier, this article focuses on risk factor analyses and prophylactic strategies reported for patients with DLBCL treated with R-CHOP. Patients with rare subtypes of DLBCL (primary cutaneous DLBCL, leg type; Epstein-Barr virus–positive DLBCL of the elderly; intravascular large B-cell lymphoma) or patients who are HIV positive[31] may have different (higher) incidences of CNS relapse. **Table 2** summarizes risk factors for CNS relapse found in larger studies (>200 patients) of patients with aggressive B-cell lymphoma. Some of these studies compared R-CHOP or CHOP[2,17,19]; for these studies, only patients treated with R-CHOP and the risk factors identified in R-CHOP–treated patients by multivariate analysis are reported. Altogether, the data confirm that secondary CNS involvement is a fairly rare complication of DLBCL, occurring in 2.3% to 8.4% of patients analyzed (with 2-year rates of 2.8%–4.8%). The overall variation in frequencies of CNS disease reported by different investigators reflects the differing patient populations studied and possibly prophylactic strategies used. Identified risk factors include the individual IPI risk factors (age >60 years, high lactate dehydrogenase [LDH] level, poor performance status, advanced stage, and >1 extranodal site). In addition, involvement of kidney, adrenals, female reproductive organs, testis, and bone have been reported to increase the risk of CNS disease. Bone marrow involvement has also been reported to be associated with increased risk of CNS recurrence, although studies do not always specify whether it is caused by involvement of DLBCL. In the largest study

Table 2
Risk factors for CNS disease in patients with DLBCL[a] using (R)-CHOP

Study	Patients[b]	IPI	↑ LDH[c]	>1 ENS	Advanced Stage	Extranodal Site		Other
Schmitz et al[30]	64 out of 2164 (3.0%)	S	S	NS	S	Kidney/adrenal Skin	2.8 7.5	—
Savage et al,[32] 2014	71 out of 1597 (4.4%)	S	S	S	S	Kidney/adrenal Marrow Testis	2.9 1.7 6.6	—
Tomita et al[7]	82 out of 1221 (6.7%)	NS	NS	NS	NS	Breast Adrenal Bone	10.5 4.6 2.0	Aged >60 y, 2.1
Schmitz et al,[5] 2012	14 out of 620 (2.3%)	Not applicable	3.8	NS	5.4	NS		R 0.3, not in high-risk patients
Boehme et al[2]	22 out of 608 (3.6%)	NR	S	S	NS	NR		ECOG scale >1
Tai et al[7]	19 out of 320 (6.0%)	NS	NS	NS	NS	Kidney Testis Breast	20.1 6.7 6.1	ECOG scale >1, 2.0 Non-CR, 3.3
Villa et al[19]	19 out of 309 (6.1%)	NS	NS	NS	Stage IV 8.0	Kidney	3.3	—
Shimazu et al[20]	20 out of 238 (8.4%)	NR	2.4	2.0	NS	Marrow	2.1	Aged >60 y, 2.5
Guirguis et al[10]	8 out of 214 (3.7%)	NS	NS	NS	NS	Testis	33.5	None
Yamamoto et al[21]	8 out of 203 (3.9%)	NS	NS	NS	NS	NS		—
Chihara et al[22]	9 out of 203 (4.4%)	NS	NS	Any EN 2.9	NS	NS		Bulk >7.5 cm, 3.34 ALC <1.0 × 10⁹/L, 2.38
Feugier et al[17]	11 out of 202 (5.4%)	S	S	NS	NS	NS		ECOG scale, >1

Abbreviations: ALC, absolute leucocyte count; CR, complete remission; ENS, extranodal site; ns, not significant; S, significant.
[a] Studies by Schmitz and colleagues[5] and by Boehme and colleagues[2] contain about 15% of patients with other aggressive B-cell lymphomas (blastoid mantle cell lymphoma, follicular lymphoma grade 3).
[b] Patients with CNS disease/patients on study.
[c] Numbers in columns ↑ LDH, >1 ENS, Advanced Stage, >1 ENS, and Other are hazard ratios reported from multivariate analyses.

published so far, including 2164 patients treated with R-CHOP or R-CHOE(etopo-side)P, of prospective trials conducted by the German High-grade Lymphoma Study Group (DSHNHL),[30] a CNS risk model was developed, including all five IPI-factors and kidneys/adrenals (CNS-IPI). Patients were stratified as low risk (0, 1 factors), intermediate risk (2, 3 factors), or high risk (≥4 factors). Notably, the 12% of patients forming the high-risk group had a 2-year-rate of CNS disease of ≈10% (**Table 3**). This clinical risk model has been validated in an independent data set of 1597 patients with DLBCL treated with R-CHOP from the BCCA (**Fig. 1**).[30] Meanwhile, other studies of PET-staged patients with DLBCL also applied this model and confirmed its validity (Gleeson and colleagues, personal communication, 2016). Although the CNS-IPI is a robust, reproducible model and serves as a useful benchmark to evaluate other risk factors, including biomarkers, a very-high-risk group was not identified.

Of note, testes involvement has been associated with a high risk of CNS relapse in some studies in the rituximab treatment era. The BCCA validation cohort did identify testes as a risk factor for CNS relapse and very few patients received CNS prophylaxis.[32] In contrast, the German cohort did not identify it as a risk factor, possibly because of the inclusion of lower risk patients in a clinical trial setting and/or the impact of intrathecal (IT) prophylaxis. Similarly, the retrospective study from the Danish group of PET-staged patients and the prospective study from the International Extranodal Study group showed a lower risk of CNS relapse in PET-staged patients with DLBCL and testicular involvement but these patients also received CNS prophylaxis.[33] Collectively, these studies support that testes should be considered a high-risk site and prophylaxis may be protective. Further, sinus involvement has been associated with CNS relapse[34] in the prerituximab era; however, it seems that this risk disappears with the integration of rituximab.[35]

In retrospective series, the presence of an *MYC* translocation,[36] and in particular *MYC* translocations occurring together with BCL2 and/or BCL6 breaks (double-hit [DHIT] or triple-hit lymphomas), have been associated with an increased risk for CNS disease.[37–39] As a result, it is recommended that all patients should undergo CNS-directed diagnostic evaluation, and primary treatment, typically with a dose-intensive regimen, should include CNS prophylaxis strategies.[40] Of note, fluorescence in situ hybridization (FISH) studies were undertaken specifically in patients with clinical or pathological high-risk features, which may overestimate CNS risk compared with an unselected population. Furthermore, there is limited information on the risk of secondary CNS relapse in double hit patients without CNS involvement at diagnosis. In a study from the MD Anderson center, the cumulative risk of CNS relapse was 13% at 2 years but interpretation is challenging because several patients had involvement at diagnosis and a spectrum of therapies, including those with CNS-penetrant agents, were used.[38] More recently, a study from the BCCA

Table 3				
CNS risk estimates by the CNS-IPI				
Study	**Number of Patients**	**Low-risk n (%) 2-y CNS Risk (%)**	**Intermediate-risk n (%) 2-y CNS Risk (%)**	**High-risk n (%) 2-y CNS Risk (%)**
Schmitz et al,[30] 2016	2164 (1735 DLBCL)	1002 (46.3) 0.8	896 (41.4) 2.9	263 (12.3) 10
Savage et al,[32] 2014	1597	463 (30.8) 0.8	694 (46.2) 3.9	344 (23) 12

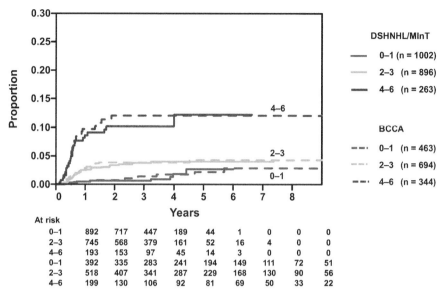

Fig. 1. Risk of CNS relapse according to the CNS-IPI. MInT, Mabthera International Trial. (*From* Schmitz N, Zeynalova S, Nickelsen M, et al. The central nervous system international prognostic index (CNS-IPI) — A risk model for CNS relapse in patients with diffuse large B-cell lymphoma (DLBCL) treated with R-CHOP. J Clin Oncol 2016; with permission.)

showed that the poor prognosis observed in dual expressers of MYC and BCL2 by immunohistochemistry is in part caused by an increased risk for CNS relapse. The dual expressers were reported to have a cumulative risk of CNS relapse of 9.7% compared with 2.2% in non–dual expressers.[41] Although activated B-cell (defined by Lymph2Cx[42]) or non-GCB (germinal center B-cell like) DLBCL (defined by the Hans algorithm[43]) subtype was also associated with a high risk of CNS relapse, only dual expresser MYC+BCL2+ status and the CNS-IPI[44] were associated with CNS relapse in multivariate analysis. Within the high-risk CNS-IPI, dual expresser MYC+BCL2+ identified a subset with a 2- year risk of CNS relapse of 22.7% compared with 2.3% (*P* = .02).[39] Similarly, within the CNS-IPI intermediate-risk group, dual expresser MYC+BCL2+ identified a group with a higher risk of CNS relapse (11% vs 3.2%; *P* = .049). These data suggest that combining clinical risk factor analysis with dual expression MYC+BCL2+ may help to optimize CNS risk assessment. Validation of this and other objective biomarkers would be of great value in defining which patients should undergo CNS-directed strategies and be considered for prophylactic strategies.

WHAT: PROPHYLAXIS OF CENTRAL NERVOUS SYSTEM DISEASE

The appropriate type of CNS prophylaxis for patients identified at high risk remains unknown. In contrast with treatment of primary DLBCL of the CNS, there is limited experience with radiotherapy to the brain and/or spinal axis for the prevention of secondary CNS disease in patients with aggressive B-cell lymphoma. It is potentially neurotoxic and would have limited value in protecting against leptomeningeal relapse. The type of CNS prophylaxis should also take into account the spectrum of CNS recurrence. A retrospective series from the BCCA evaluated the site of relapse by the CNS-IPI in

1732 patients with DLBCL treated with R-CHOP. For the high-risk CNS-IPI, a group on which prophylaxis strategies may be focused, 55% of CNS relapses were isolated and the remainder occurred in the setting of systemic disease.[11] For the CNS relapses, 70% involved the CNS parenchyma and 30% were isolated to the leptomeningeal compartment. These data support that prophylaxis strategies must consider drugs that deeply penetrate into the brain.

Primary prophylaxis of CNS disease in DLBCL traditionally consisted of IT MTX, IT cytosine-arabinoside (Ara-C), IT hydrocortisone, or combinations of these drugs. Liposomal Ara-C has also been used because of its long-acting formulation, but significant evidence that liposomal Ara-C is better than Ara-C is lacking.[45] Although comparative studies with regard to timing and frequency of IT injections are unavailable, a minimum of 4 IT injections early between systemic treatment courses has been recommended. Simultaneous IT administration of cytotoxic drugs and hydrocortisone may reduce side effects, including arachnoiditis, but whether it has an additional protective effect is unknown. Current practice is based on positive experience in patients with acute lymphoblastic leukemia and other lymphomas, in which CNS involvement was more frequent than in DLBCL and mostly restricted to the CSF. IT chemotherapy does not reach measurable concentrations in the brain parenchyma except for areas directly adjacent to the brain. In practical terms, and particularly for patients treated with R-CHOP, there is increasing evidence from recent studies (summarized in **Table 1**) that IT prophylaxis is not protective. Paradoxically, in some studies the CNS relapse rate is higher in patients who received IT prophylaxis.[6,46] However, this must be considered an artifact because the patient cohorts that received prophylaxis were enriched for patients deemed at high risk for CNS disease. Given the lack of evidence showing a protective effect and the potential for patient discomfort and toxicities (leukopenia, arachnoiditis, post–lumbar puncture headache, infections, mucositis) seen with IT injections of cytotoxic drugs,[47,48] definitive recommendations cannot be endorsed. Note that IT prophylaxis is the only type of CNS protection integrated into dose adjusted etoposide, prednisolone, vincristine, cyclophosphamide, doxorubicin and rituximab (DA-EPOCH-R), which is used with high efficacy in Burkitt lymphoma.[46] Whether this represents selection of a lower risk population entered into a clinical trial or a truly protective effect is unknown. Further, it is possible that etoposide also provides additional protection because it does penetrate the BBB.

Of note, historically, IT prophylaxis in patients with sinus involvement seemed to reduce the risk of CNS relapse, presumably because of a different mechanism of spread through the cribriform plate.[34] However, as described, in the rituximab era, CNS relapse in patients with DLBCL with sinus involvement is uncommon and, thus, IT prophylaxis is no longer endorsed.[35]

Given the limitations of IT CNS prophylaxis, systemic therapy, typically in the form of HDMTX, has also been explored. Unlike IT chemotherapy, in which great variation of drug level in the subarachnoid space can occur, HDMTX can potentially result in an even distribution of therapeutic drug levels throughout all CNS compartments.[49] The results of a French study comparing ACVBP, which incorporates 2 infusions of HDMTX (3 g/m^2), with CHOP showed fewer CNS recurrences in the dose-intensive regimen (2.7% vs 8%).[26] Similarly, a phase 2 trial evaluating dose-intensive R-CHOP–like chemotherapy followed by systemic CNS prophylaxis in the form of high-dose cytarabine (3 g/m^2 IV twice daily for 2 days) and HDMTX (3 g/m^2) in aaIPI 2 to 3 patients showed a CNS relapse rate of 4.4%, all occurring within 6 months, suggesting that earlier integration of systemic prophylaxis would be of value.[12] Additional retrospective studies also support the use of systemic prophylaxis with high-dose antimetabolites.[13,50,51] A retrospective study from Massachusetts General Hospital evaluating a treatment program of R-CHOP with integration of HDMTX (3–3.5 g/m^2) for 3 cycles in patients deemed to be at high risk based on specific extranodal site involvement, 2 or more extranodal sites and increased LDH level or the Hollender 5-point criteria[52] showed a risk of CNS relapse of only 3%, which compares favorably with historical estimates.[13] Currently available studies support 3 to 4 cycles of HDMTX integrated on days 10 to 15 with R-CHOP. The National Comprehensive Cancer Network guidelines[53] recommend CNS prophylaxis in patients at high risk by the CNS-IPI ($\geq$4 factors), in addition to those with testicular involvement or with DHIT lymphoma. Given the uncertainty as to the optimal type of CNS prophylaxis, HDMTX 3 to 3.5 g/m^2 (preferred) or IT MTX/Ara-C for 4 to 8 cycles are potential options. The European Society of Medical Oncology (ESMO) guidelines endorse HDMTX as the preferred type of CNS prophylaxis in high-risk patients defined as high-intermediate/high-risk IPI (especially with >1 extranodal site or increased LDH level) and for those with testicular or adrenal/renal involvement.[54] From the available evidence, and given the predominance of parenchymal involvement, the authors endorse HDMTX; studies correlating systemic dose and CSF levels support 3 to 3.5 g/m^2 as the preferred CNS prophylaxis because 1.5 g/m^2 may not achieve adequate CSF drug levels.[55] In particular, in elderly patients (>60 years old) such doses may be too toxic and MTX at 1 to 2 g/m^2 may be used. Such prophylaxis should be considered in patients with high-risk CNS-IPI (>4 risk factors) particularly if accompanied by immunohistochemistry (IHC) dual expression of MYC and BCL2. Patients with testicular, renal, or adrenal[30] involvement should receive prophylaxis regardless of their CNS-IPI.

Recent publications have shown that small molecule therapeutics such as the Bruton tyrosine kinase inhibitor ibrutinib[56] and the immunomodulator lenalidomide[57] cross the BBB, and limited studies show efficacy in primary CNS lymphoma[58,59] or mantle lymphoma with CNS involvement. A phase I study was initiated in patients with untreated or relapsed primary CNS lymphoma evaluating the combination of Chemotherapeutic agents that cross the BBB with ibrutinib (TEDDI-R [temozolomide, etoposide, Doxil, dexamethasone, ibrutinib, rituximab]); early results support that ibrutinib does achieve meaningful CSF concentrations and early efficacy analyses are promising.[60]

Available data support selective activity of ibrutinib and lenalidomide in activated B-cell (ABC) (or non-GCB) DLBCL and, as such, there are ongoing phase 3 studies comparing R-CHOP plus ibrutinib or R-CHOP pus lenalidomide versus standard R-CHOP. Given that CNS relapse is higher in ABC/non-GCB,[41] it will be of interest to learn whether integration of these agents reduces this risk and would ultimately improve outcome.

Further, the DSHNHL will start a phase II study using R-CHOEP plus ibrutinib in young high-risk patients (age-adjusted IPI 2 or 3) with DLBCL.

WHEN: TIMING OF PROPHYLAXIS

CNS relapse in DLBCL is an early event, typically occurring within the first 6 to 9 months after diagnosis; late recurrences are rare with the exception of patients with testicular involvement. Therefore, any prophylactic measure should be administered as soon as possible after diagnosis. Delaying CNS prophylaxis until systemic first-line therapy has been completed probably is not the optimal strategy. Ongoing studies are evaluating the integration of systemic MTX either before starting R-CHOP or early between courses. Prophylaxis of CNS disease should not compromise systemic therapy.

DISCUSSION

Secondary involvement of the CNS is an early and mostly fatal complication for patients with DLBCL. The addition of rituximab to CHOP or CHOP like regimens has only modestly affected the risk of CNS relapse. However, with an overall incidence of only 5%, CNS recurrence is not frequent enough to justify specific diagnostic and prophylactic measures in every patient. Therefore, the challenge remains to better define risk factors and develop focused prophylactic strategies in target high-risk populations to avoid this usually fatal outcome. Recent international efforts to better define the risk profile of individual patients has resulted in the highly robust and reproducible CNS-IPI.[31] Identification of a very-high-risk group can be further refined by incorporating other biomarkers, such as dual expression of MYC ($\geq$40%) and BCL2 ($\geq$50%) by IHC (dual expresser lymphomas), which, when coupled with high-risk CNS-IPI, identifies a group with a CNS relapse risk of greater than 20%.[41] It is anticipated that additional studies will validate this as a relevant biomarker and other molecular factors will be elucidated to target high-risk patients. Of note, true DHIT or triple-hit disease by FISH is outside this risk stratification. Although there may be lower risk patients within this subtype,[61] there is currently no reliable way to identify them and CNS prophylaxis should be integrated into treatment regimens.

Patients with low-risk or intermediate-risk CNS-IPI have a risk of CNS relapse of less than 5% and can be spared any diagnostic and prophylactic measures, the exception being those with primary testicular DLBCL.

The appropriate management of identified high-risk patients remains a challenge. Patients in the high-risk group have an approximately 10% or greater risk of experiencing CNS relapse and should be considered for CNS-directed investigations and prophylaxis strategies. The number of extranodal sites may also be relevant, with patients with 3 and particularly 4 or more sites having a significantly increased risk,[62] although these patients are typically in the high risk CNS-IPI group regardless.

Rigorous application of modern diagnostic tools like MRI of the brain and FACS analysis of the CSF in this high-risk group of patients will identify more patients with CNS involvement at diagnosis. Although it remains uncertain whether FACS positive CSF is always associated with CNS relapse,[63] given the implications, patients should receive CNS-specific protocols using drugs crossing the BBB, and recent studies support the integration of systemic antimetabolite chemotherapy and consolidative high-dose therapy with CNS-penetrant agents and autologous stem cell transplant.[64] For the remaining CNS-negative patients, the risk of CNS disease may be lower than anticipated because an undefined percentage of patients with previously undetected CNS involvement at diagnosis has been shown by modern technology to harbor lymphoma in the CNS.

Given the limitations of IT prophylaxis, and the high proportion of CNS relapses that include the brain parenchyma,[11] high-risk patients should be considered for prophylaxis with HDMTX if they are without significant comorbidities. Of note, in the rare scenario of a patient with kidney/adrenal involvement but in the low or intermediate CNS-IPI risk group, CNS prophylaxis should be administered. Similarly, patients with testicular involvement should be considered for CNS diagnostic procedures and prophylaxis, preferably with HDMTX. If a case is identified as a dual expresser, CNS-directed work-up can also be considered in the intermediate-risk CNS-IPI group; however, further recommendations regarding CNS prophylaxis should follow confirmation in a separate data set of these findings. Whenever possible, patients should be encouraged to participate in prospective clinical trials. Until more definitive data are available, a management approach is outlined in **Fig. 2** and similar algorithms have also been proposed by recent reviews and guidelines.[65–67]

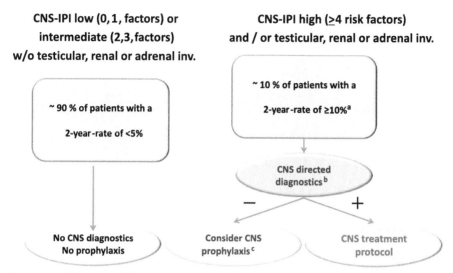

Fig. 2. Possible approach for diagnosis and prophylaxis of CNS involvement in patients with DLBCL. [a] Patients with CNS-IPI high and BCL2 and MYC positive by immunohistochemistry have a 2-year rate of CNS relapse of 22%.[41] [b] Computed tomography head or MRI head (preferred), CSF analysis (cytology and flow cytometry). [c] Especially if dual expresser MYC+BCL2+ and/or more than 2 extranodal sites.

In summary, despite improvements in outcomes in the rituximab treatment era, CNS relapse continues to pose a considerable management problem. Further studies identifying objective biomarkers that can be integrated with clinical risk models like the CNS-IPI will more accurately identify patients who should undergo detailed CNS-directed investigations and be considered for CNS prophylaxis. Studies are ongoing integrating small molecules crossing the BBB (eg, ibrutinib, lenalidomide) with R-CHOP and may ultimately improve the risk of CNS relapse.

REFERENCES

1. Bernstein SH, Unger JM, Leblanc M, et al. Natural history of CNS relapse inpatients with aggressive non Hodgkin's lymphoma: a 20 year follow up analysis of SWOG 8516- the Southwest Oncology Group. J Clin Oncol 2009;27:114–9.
2. Boehme V, Schmitz N, Zeynalova S, et al. CNS events in elderly patients with aggressive lymphoma treated with modern chemotherapy (CHOP-14) with or without rituximab: an analysis of patients treated in the RICOVER-60 trial of the German High-Grade Non-Hodgkin Lymphoma Study Group (DSHNHL). Blood 2009;113:3896–902.
3. Kridel R, Dietrich PY. Prevention of CNS relapse in diffuse large B cell lymphoma. Lancet Oncol 2011;12:1258–66.
4. Ghose A, Elias HK, Guha G. Influence of rituximab on central nervous system relapse in diffuse large B-cell lymphoma and role of prophylaxis – a systematic review of prospective studies. Clin Lymphoma Myeloma Leuk 2015;15:451–7.
5. Schmitz N, Zeynalova S, Glass B, et al. CNS disease in younger patients with aggressive B-cell lymphoma: an analysis of patients treated on the Mabthera International Trial and trials of the German High-Grade Non-Hodgkin Lymphoma Study Group. Ann Oncol 2012;23:1267–73.

6. Kumar A, Vanderplas A, LaCasce AS, et al. Lack of benefit of central nervous system prophylaxis for diffuse large B-cell lymphoma in the rituximab era: findings from a large national database. Cancer 2012;118:2944–51.

7. Tai WM, Chung J, Tang PL, et al. Central nervous system (CNS) relapse in diffuse large B cell lymphoma (DLBCL): pre- and post-rituximab. Ann Hematol 2011;90: 809–18.

8. Tomita N, Takasaki H, Ishiyama Y, et al. Intrathecal methotrexate prophylaxis and central nervous system relapse in diffuse large B-cell lymphoma patients following R-CHOP. Leuk Lymphoma 2014;10:1–20.

9. Arkenau HT, Chong G, Cunningham D, et al. The role of intrathecal chemotherapy prophylaxis in patients with diffuse large B-cell lymphoma. Ann Oncol 2007;18: 541–5.

10. Guirguis HR, Cheung MC, Mahrous M, et al. Impact of central nervous system (CNS) prophylaxis on the incidence and risk factors for CNS relapse in patients with diffuse large B-cell lymphoma treated in the rituximab era: a single centre experience and review of the literature. Br J Haematol 2012;159:39–49.

11. Kansara R, villa D, Gerrie AS, et al. Evaluation of the site of central nervous system (CNS) relapse in patients with diffuse large B-cell lymphoma (DLBCL) by the CNS Risk Model. Hematol Oncol 2015;33:212.

12. Holte H, Leppä S, Björkholm M, et al. Dose-densified chemoimmunotherapy followed by systemic central nervous system prophylaxis for younger high-risk diffuse large B-cell/follicular grade 3 lymphoma patients: results of a phase II Nordic Lymphoma Group study. Ann Oncol 2013;24:1385–92.

13. Abramson JS, Hellmann M, Barnes JA, et al. Intravenous methotrexate as central nervous system (CNS) prophylaxis is associated with a low risk of CNS recurrence in high-risk patients with diffuse large B-cell lymphoma. Cancer 2010; 116:4283–90.

14. MacKintosh FR, Colby TV, Podolsky WJ, et al. Central nervous system involvement in non-Hodgkin's lymphoma: an analysis of 105 cases. Cancer 1982;49: 586–95.

15. van Besien K, Ha CS, Murphy S, et al. Risk factors, treatment, and outcome of central nervous system recurrence in adults with intermediate-grade and immunoblastic lymphoma. Blood 1998;91:1178–84.

16. Johnson GJ, Oken MM, Anderson JR, et al. Central nervous system relapse in unfavourable-histology non-Hodgkin's lymphoma: is prophylaxis indicated? Lancet 1984;2:685–7.

17. Feugier P, Virion JM, Tilly H, et al. Incidence and risk factors for central nervous system occurrence in elderly patients with diffuse large-B-cell lymphoma: influence of Rituximab. Ann Oncol 2004;15:129–33.

18. Tomita N, Yokoyama M, Yamamoto W, et al. Central nervous system event in patients with diffuse large B-cell lymphoma in the rituximab era. Cancer Sci 2012; 103:245–51.

19. Villa D, Connors JM, Shenkier TN, et al. Incidence and risk factors for central nervous system relapse in patients with diffuse large B-cell lymphoma: the impact of the addition of rituximab to CHOP chemotherapy. Ann Oncol 2010;21:1046–52.

20. Shimazu Y, Notohara K, Ueda Y. Diffuse large B-cell lymphoma with central nervous system relapse: prognosis and risk factors according to retrospective analysis from a single-center experience. Int J Hematol 2009;89:577–83.

21. Yamamoto W, Tomita N, Watanabe R, et al. Central nervous system involvement in diffuse large B-cell lymphoma. Eur J Haematol 2010;85:6–10.

22. Chihara D, Oki Y, Matsuo K, et al. Incidence and risk factors for central nervous system relapse in patients with diffuse large B-cell lymphoma: analyses with competing risk regression model. Leuk Lymphoma 2011;52(12):2270–5.

23. Baraniskin A, Deckert M, Schulte-Altedorneburg G, et al. Current strategies in the diagnosis of diffuse large B-cell lymphoma of the central nervous system. Br J Haematol 2012;156:421–32.

24. Wilson WH, Bromberg JE, Stetler-Stevenson M, et al. Detection and outcome of occult leptomeningeal disease in diffuse large B-cell lymphoma and Burkitt lymphoma. Haematologica 2014;99:1228–35.

25. Tilly H, Lepage E, Coiffier B, et al. Intensive conventional chemotherapy (ACVBP regimen) compared with standard CHOP for poor-prognosis aggressive non-Hodgkin lymphoma. Blood 2003;102:4284–9.

26. Récher C, Coiffier B, Haioun C, et al. Intensified chemotherapy with ACVBP plus rituximab versus standard CHOP plus rituximab for the treatment of diffuse large B-cell lymphoma (LNH03-2B): an open-label randomised phase 3 trial. Lancet 2011;378:1858–67.

27. Schmitz N, Nickelsen M, Ziepert M, et al. Conventional chemotherapy (CHOEP-14) with rituximab or high-dose chemotherapy (MegaCHOEP) with rituximab for young, high-risk patients with aggressive B-cell lymphoma: an open-label, randomised, phase 3 trial (DSHNHL 2002-1). Lancet Oncol 2012;13:1250–9.

28. Wilson WH, Dunleavy K, Pittaluga S, et al. Phase II study of dose adjusted EPOCH and rituximab in untreated diffuse large B-cell lymphoma with analysis of germinal center and post-germinal center biomarkers. J Clin Oncol 2008;26:2717–24.

29. Boehme V, Zeynalova S, Kloess M, et al. Incidence and risk factors of central nervous system recurrence in aggressive lymphoma – a survey of 1693 patients treated in protocols of the German High-Grade Non-Hodgkin's Lymphoma Study Group (DSHNHL). Ann Oncol 2007;18:149–57.

30. Schmitz N, Zeynalova S, Nickelsen M, et al. The central nervous system international prognostic index (CNS-IPI) — A risk model for CNS relapse in patients with diffuse large B-cell lymphoma (DLBCL) treated with R-CHOP. J Clin Oncol 2016. [Epub ahead of print].

31. Sarker D, Thirlwell C, Nelson M, et al. Leptomeningeal disease in AIDS-related non-Hodgkin's lymphoma. AIDS 2003;17:861–5.

32. Savage KJ, Zeynalova S, Kansara R, et al. Validation of a prognostic model to assess the risk of CNS disease in patients with aggressive B-cell lymphoma [abstract: 394]. Blood 2014;134(21).

33. El –Galaly TC, Cheah CY, Hutchings M, et al. Female patients with DLBCL and involvement of the reproductive organs have poor outcomes and markedly increased risk of CNS relapse with R-CHOP (-like) therapy [abstract: 211]. Hematol Oncol 2015;33(209).

34. Laskin JJ, Savage KJ, Voss N, et al. Primary paranasal sinus lymphoma: natural history and improved outcome with central nervous system chemoprophylaxis. Leuk Lymphoma 2005;46(12):1721–7.

35. Murawski N, Held G, Ziepert M, et al. The role of radiotherapy and intrathecal CNS prophylaxis in extralymphatic craniofacial aggressive B-cell lymphomas. Blood 2014;124:720–8.

36. Savage KJ, Johnson NA, Ben-Neriah S, et al. MYC gene rearrangements are associated with a poor prognosis in diffuse large B-cell lymphoma patients treated with R-CHOP chemotherapy. Blood 2009;114:3533–7.

37. Aukema SM, Siebert R, Schuuring E, et al. Double-hit B-cell lymphomas. Blood 2011;117:2319–31.

38. Oki Y, Noorani M, Lin P, et al. Double hit lymphoma: the MD Anderson Cancer Center clinical experience. Br J Haematol 2014;166:891–901.

39. Li S, Lin P, Fayad LE, et al. B-cell lymphomas with MYC/8q24 rearrangements and IGH@BCL2/t(14;18)(q32/;q21): an aggressive disease with heterogenous histology, germinal center B-cell immunophenotype and poor outcome. Mod Pathol 2012;25:145–56.

40. Petrich AM, Gandhi M, Jovanovic B, et al. Impact of induction regimen and stem cell transplantation on outcomes in double-hit lymphoma: a multicenter retrospective analysis. Blood 2014;124:2354–61.

41. Savage K, Slack GW, Mottok A, et al. The impact of dual expression of MYC and BCL2 by immunohistochemistry on the risk of CNS relapse in DLBCL. Blood 2016;127(18):2182–8.

42. Scott DW, Wright GW, Williams PM, et al. Determining cell-of-origin subtypes of diffuse large B-cell lymphoma using gene expression in formalin-fixed paraffin-embedded tissue. Blood 2014;123:1214–7.

43. Hans CP, Weisenburger DD, Greiner TC, et al. Confirmation of the molecular classification of diffuse large B-cell lymphoma by immunohistochemistry using tissue microarray. Blood 2004;103:275–82.

44. Savage KJ, Sehn LH, Villa D, et al. The impact of concurrent MYC BCL2 protein expression on the risk of secondary central nervous system relapse in diffuse large B-cell lymphoma (DLBCL). Blood 2014;124(21):495.

45. Glantz M, LaFollette S, Jaeckle KA, et al. Randomized trial of a slow-release versus a standard formulation of cytarabine for the intrathecal treatment of lymphomatous meningitis. J Clin Oncol 1999;17:3110–6.

46. Dunleavy K, Pittaluga S, Shovlin M, et al. Low intensity therapy in adults with Burkitt's lymphoma. N Engl J Med 2013;369(20):1915–25.

47. Dietrich PY. Intrathecal MTX for DLBCL: from an inappropriate prophylactic tradition to a medical error? Blood 2009;114:1999.

48. Schmitz N, Zeynalova S, Loeffler M, et al. Response: Intrathecal methotrexate and central nervous system events. Blood 2009;114:1999–2000.

49. Shapiro WR, Young DF, Mehta BM. Methotrexate: distribution in cerebrospinal fluid after intravenous, ventricular and lumbar injections. N Engl J Med 1975; 293:161–6.

50. Cheah CY, Herbert KE, Rourke KO, et al. A multicentre retrospective comparison of central nervous system prophylaxis strategies among patients with high-risk diffuse large B-cell lymphoma. Br J Cancer 2014;111:1072–9.

51. Ferreri AJM, Bruno-Ventre M, Donadoni G. Risk-tailored CNS prophylaxis in a mono-institutional series of 200 patients with diffuse large B-cell lymphoma treated in the rituximab era. Br J Haematol 2015;168:654–62.

52. Hollender A, Kvaloy S, Nome O, et al. Central nervous system involvement following diagnosis of non-Hodgkin's lymphoma: a risk model. Ann Oncol 2001; 13:1099–107.

53. National Comprehensive Cancer Network guidelines version 2.216 Diffuse large B-cell lymphoma. Available at: www.nccn.org.

54. Tilly H, Gomes da Silva M, Vitolo U, et al. Diffuse large B-cell lymphoma (DLBCL): ESMO Clinical Practice Guidelines for diagnosis, treatment and follow up. Ann Oncol 2015;26(Suppl 5):v116–25.

55. Gilchrist NL, Caldwell J, Watson ID, et al. Comparison of serum and cerebrospinal fluid levels of methotrexate in man during high-dose chemotherapy for

aggressive non-Hodgkin's lymphoma. Cancer Chemother Pharmacol 1985;15: 290–4.

56. Bernard S, Goldwirt L, Amorim S, et al. Activity of ibrutinib in mantle cell lymphoma patients with central nervous system relapse. Blood 2015;126:1695–8.

57. Houillier C, Choquet S, Toitou V, et al. Lenalidomide monotherapy as salvage treatment for recurrent primary CNS lymphoma. Neurology 2015;84:325–6.

58. Roubenstein JL, Treseler PA, Stewart PJ. Regression of refractory intraocular large B-cell lymphoma with lenalidomide monotherapy. J Clin Oncol 2011;29: 595–7.

59. Warrren KE, Goldman S, Pollack IF, et al. Phase I trial of lenalidomide in pediatric patients with recurrent, refractory of progressive primary CNS tumors: pediatric brain tumor consortium study PBTC-018. J Clin Oncol 2011;29:324–9.

60. Dunleavy K, Lai C, Roschewski M, et al. Phase I/II study of TEDDI-R with ibrutinib in untreated and relapsed/refractory primary CNS lymphoma. Hematol Oncol 2015;33(Suppl 1):174.

61. Copie-Bergman C, Cuilière-Dartigues P, Baia M, et al. MYC-IG rearrangements are negative predictors of survival in DLBCL patients treated with immunochemotherapy: a GELA/LYSA study. Blood 2015;126:2466–74.

62. Cheah CY, Hutchings M, Rady K, et al. The absolute number of extranodal sites detected by PET-CT is a powerful predictor of secondary central nervous system involvement in patients with diffuse large B-cell lymphoma treated with R-CHOP. Blood 2015;126:3905.

63. Alvarez R, Dupuis J, Plonquet A, et al. Clinical relevance of flow cytometric immunophenotyping of the cerebrospinal fluid in patients with diffuse large B-cell lymphoma. Ann Oncol 2012;23:1274–9.

64. Korfel A, Elter T, Thiel E, et al. Phase II study of central nervous system (CNS)-directed chemotherapy including high-dose chemotherapy with autologous stem cell transplantation for CNS relapse of aggressive lymphomas. Haematologica 2013;98:364–70.

65. Siegal T, Goldschmidt N. CNS prophylaxis in diffuse large B-cell lymphoma: if, when, how and for whom? Blood Rev 2012;26:97–106.

66. Fletcher CD, Kahl BS. Central nervous system involvement in diffuse large B-cell lymphoma: an analysis of risks and prevention strategies in the post-rituximab era. Leuk Lymphoma 2014;55:2228–40.

67. Ghose A, Kundu R, Latif T. Prophylactic CNS directed therapy in systemic diffuse large B cell lymphoma. Crit Rev Oncol Hematol 2014;91:202–303.

The Challenge of Primary Central Nervous System Lymphoma

Julia Carnevale, MD[a], James L. Rubenstein, MD, PhD[b],*

KEYWORDS

- Aggressive lymphoma • Primary CNS lymphoma • Brain tumor • NF-κB
- High-dose chemotherapy

KEY POINTS

- Long-term survival and cure is feasible in primary central nervous system lymphoma (PCNSL) without whole brain radiotherapy (WBRT).
- WBRT consolidation is associated with severe neurotoxicity, particularly in patients older than 60.
- High-dose chemotherapy is currently under investigation as first-line consolidation.
- There is a need for novel therapies that target key survival pathways in PCNSL, including activation of nuclear factor-κB survival signaling.

INTRODUCTION

Although primary central nervous system lymphoma (PCNSL) remains a rare neoplasm, representing only 2% to 3% of all cases of non-Hodgkin's lymphoma (NHL), the incidence of PCNSL among immunocompetent patients seems to be increasing, particularly among persons age 65 years and older.[1] The characteristic pathobiology of PCNSL is that of an aggressive lymphoma, localized within the central nervous system (CNS) and often disseminated within brain, cranial nerves, leptomeninges, cerebrospinal fluid (CSF), intraocular structures and spinal cord, without overt systemic disease.[2,3]

PCNSL has long been recognized to be an aggressive brain tumor associated with a poor prognosis.[4] Historically known as reticulum cell sarcoma or microglioma,

Supported by the National Institutes of Health, University of California San Francisco-Gladstone Institute of Virology & Immunology Center for AIDS Research (P30 AI027763), NIH R01CA139-83-01A1, and by the Leukemia and Lymphoma Society (J.L. Rubenstein).
Disclosures: Dr J.L. Rubenstein receives research funding from Genentech and Celgene

[a] Division of Hematology/Oncology, University of California, San Francisco, 505 Parnassus Avenue, San Francisco, CA 94143, USA; [b] Division of Hematology/Oncology, Helen Diller Family Comprehensive Cancer Center, University of California, San Francisco, M1282 Box 1270, San Francisco, CA 94143, USA
* Corresponding author.
E-mail address: jamesr@medicine.ucsf.edu

Hematol Oncol Clin N Am 30 (2016) 1293–1316
http://dx.doi.org/10.1016/j.hoc.2016.07.013
0889-8588/16/© 2016 Elsevier Inc. All rights reserved.

management principles for this disease have emerged slowly. Beginning in the 1960s, in the absence of prospective data, whole brain radiotherapy (WBRT) was used as the first-line intervention as a means to elicit immediate responses in patients faced with a rapidly deteriorating course; WBRT alone typically resulted in median survival of 12 months. To date, the most significant advance in PCNSL has been the recognition, in the 1970s, of the efficacy of high-dose methotrexate (HD-MTX).[5,6] Several recent prospective trials have demonstrated markedly improved outcomes in PCNSL. Our goal is to highlight significant advances in our understanding of disease biology, diagnosis, staging, and therapeutic management.[7–12]

ETIOLOGY

Risk factors for PCNSL include acquired and/or congenital immunodeficiency states. PCNSL is an AIDS-defining illness associated with a low CD4 cell count (<50 cells/mL) and Epstein–Barr virus (EBV) infection. In systemic AIDS-related lymphomas, EBV infection of the lymphoma may be predictive of secondary CNS involvement.[13] Congenital immunodeficiency states such as Wiskott-Aldrich syndrome, severe combined or common variable immunodeficiency, or ataxia-telangiectasia carry an approximately 4% risk of PCNSL. Posttransplant lymphoproliferative disorder (PTLD) involving CNS develops in 1% to 2% of renal transplant recipients and 2% to 7% recipients of liver, cardiac, and lung transplant recipients. CNS PTLD is associated with EBV in the setting of iatrogenic T-cell immunodeficiency induced by immunosuppressive agents such as mycophenolate mofetil (CellCept, Genentech, San Francisco, CA).[14] Among patients with PCNSL without clinically overt immunosuppression, EBV infection of lymphoma is rare.[15]

CLINICAL FEATURES AND PATHOGENESIS

PCNSL is typically a highly infiltrative neoplasm that has been characterized as a "whole brain disease," particularly at relapse.[16] For this reason, its radiographic appearance typically underestimates disease extent, and like malignant gliomas, PCNSL is not amenable to curative resection.[16] One of the archetypical histologic features of PCNSL is angiotropism; the accumulation of lymphoma cells around tumor vessels, a phenotype that likely disrupts the blood–brain barrier and enables radiographic detection of lesions via pathologic contrast enhancement. PCNSL commonly is diagnosed as a solitary mass, typically with vasogenic edema and mass effect. The frequency of multiple lesions is increased among the immunosuppressed[17] (**Fig. 1**).

Although NHL presenting in the brain is typically classified as PCNSL, subclinical tumor-related clones are often detectable in the blood and bone marrow of PCNSL patients, suggesting that the brain microenvironment might promote malignant progression.[18,19]

Intraocular disease is a common manifestation: 20% of PCNSL patients present with involvement of the retina, uvea, and vitreous. An important principle is that apparently localized intraocular lymphoma (IOL) will disseminate within brain in greater than 80% of cases; therefore, detection of IOL mandates staging of the neuroaxis. Therapies for IOL that address this risk should be strongly considered.[20]

Approximately 95% of PCNSL are large B-cell lymphoma; other include T-cell (2%),[21] Burkitt, lymphoblastic, and marginal zone lymphomas. PCNSL is distinguished from dural-based marginal zone lymphomas because these rarely invade brain parenchyma and typically share overlapping radiographic features on MRI with meningioma.[22]

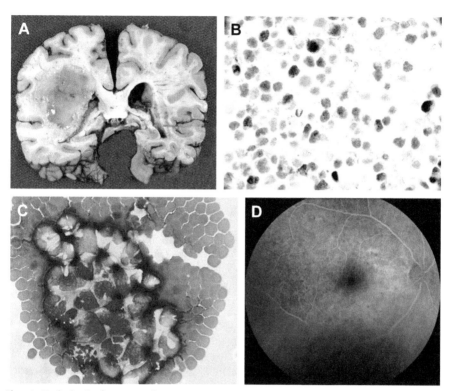

Fig. 1. Pathologic features of primary central nervous system lymphoma (PCNSL). (*A*) Diffuse, large B-cell lymphoma involving the left parietal lobe and basal ganglia with significant mass effect, subependymal spread, and invasion of the lateral ventricle, upon progression with high-dose methotrexate and rituximab-based chemotherapy. (*B*) High expression of MUM1 by diffuse large B-cell lymphoma cells in a diagnostic specimen of PCNSL, as demonstrated by immunohistochemistry. (*C*) Cytology of diffuse large B-cell lymphoma in cerebrospinal fluid in recurrent PCNSL. (*D*) Fluorescein angiography demonstrates classic 'leopard spots' in intraocular lymphoma. (*Courtesy of* Ray Sobel, MD, Stanford University School of Medicine, Stanford, CA.)

MOLECULAR PATHOGENESIS OF PRIMARY CENTRAL NERVOUS SYSTEM LYMPHOMA

Determination of the unique genetic features of PCNSL poses a greater challenge than for systemic diffuse, large B-cell lymphoma, both because of the rarity of this neoplasm and the paucity of material available for investigational studies. Most diagnostic specimens are obtained by stereotactic biopsy or via analysis of the CSF. Most investigations have focused on the elucidation of PCNSL, large cell type. Between 50% and 80% of PCNSL express BCL6 by immunohistochemistry[23]; 95% stain positive for MUM-1 and, therefore, the majority of PCNSL cases are of a late germinal center or an activated B-cell immunophenotype.[15] Immunohistochemical characterization of tumors from patients that participated in CALGB 50202 demonstrated that high BCL6 correlated with refractory disease and shorter progression-free and overall survival, thus representing a potentially useful molecular prognostic biomarker. Although the adverse prognostic significance of high BCL-6 in PCNSL was confirmed recently in an independent large prospective trial,[24] several small retrospective studies provided a conflicting result, namely that BCL-6 correlates with a better prognosis. This discrepancy raises the possibility that the prognostic significance of BCL-6 may depend on treatment-related factors, such as rituximab or whole-brain radiotherapy. Between 56% and 93% of PCNSL express BCL2.[15,23]

Transcriptional analyses of PCNSL identified several candidate mediators of disease pathogenesis, including expression of Pim 1 and *MYC*.[25,26] Increased MYC in PCNSL was confirmed in the recent CALGB 50202 study.[12] Upregulation of microRNAs associated with MYC pathway (miR-17-5p, miR-20a, miR-9) has also been demonstrated.[27] Circulating extracellular microRNAs in CSF such as miR-21were also recently described in PCNSL, suggesting usefulness as clinical biomarkers.[28]

Given that aberrant somatic hypermutation contributes to the pathobiology of diffuse, large B-cell lymphoma, Montesinos-Rongen et al[29] evaluated the potential role of this mechanism in PCNSL. Somatic hypermutation of 4 protooncogenes was identified—*PAX5*, *PIM1*, *c-MYC*, and *RhoH/TTF*—genes that regulate B-cell development, proliferation, and apoptosis. Mutational frequencies for these were 2- to 5-fold higher in PCNSL compared with extraneural diffuse, large B-cell lymphoma.[29] Such high mutation frequencies suggest a prolonged interaction of the tumor cell in the germinal center microenvironment.[30] Whole exome sequencing studies of PCNSL identified protein-coding mutations involving mediators of cell signaling, CARD14, CD79A/B, TLR2, TLR6, and TLR10, regulators of cell cycle, CCND3, and CDK20, and chromatin structure CREBBP, MLL2, ARID1A/B, and SMARCA4.[31]

The $p16^{INK4a}$ gene is commonly inactivated by either homozygous deletion (40%–50%) or 5'-CpG hypermethylation (15%–30%) in PCNSL.[32] Inactivation of $p14^{ARF}$ and $p16^{INK4a}$ genes by homozygous deletion or promoter hypermethylation may represent an important step in the molecular pathogenesis of PCNSL. The $p14^{ARF}$ gene normally induces growth arrest and stabilizes p53 protein in the nucleus. Both $p14^{ARF}$ and $p16^{INK4a}$ genes are frequently codeleted; moreover, mice lacking the murine homolog of $p14^{ARF}$ develop a variety of tumors, including lymphomas, sarcomas, and gliomas.[20,33–35] In contrast, mutations in the *TP53* gene have been observed in only a small proportion of PCNSL.

Comparative genomic hybridization has identified other genetic lesions in PCNSL. Recurrent gains have been detected on chromosome 12 as well as on the long arms of chromosomes 1, 7, and 18; gain on chromosome 12 seems to be the most common chromosomal alteration, specifically in the 12q region harboring STAT6, MDM2, CDK4, and GLI1.[20,34,36]

Another common genomic aberrational hotspot in PCNSL involves losses on chromosome 6p21 that harbor loci for HLA[36–38] as well as broad deletions involving chromosome 6q. Chromosome 6q deletions, in particular 6q21-23, may be most frequent and occur in 40% to 60% of PCNSL.[39] Candidate tumor suppressors linked to chromosome 6q include *PRDM1*, a tumor suppressor and regulator of B-cell differentiation[40]; *PTPRK*, a protein tyrosine phosphatase that participates in cell adhesion signaling events[41]; and *A20* (*TNFAIP3*), a negative regulator of nuclear factor-κB (NF-κB) signaling.[42]

Further evidence for the aberrant activation of NF-κB pathways in PCNSL is supported by a gain in DNA copy number for *MALT1*[43] as well as activating mutations of *CARD11*[44] and *MyD88*. The activating exchange of leucine to proline at position 265 of *MyD88* may be enriched in PCNSL and has been demonstrated to occur in between 38% and 50% of cases[45,46] (**Fig. 2**).

Several lines of investigation support a role for JAK/STAT signaling pathway as a mediator of prosurvival signals in PCNSL. Interleukin (IL)-4, a B-cell growth factor that mediates intracellular signals via JAK/STAT, is upregulated at the transcript and protein levels within the vascular microenvironment in PCNSL tumors.[25] Increased

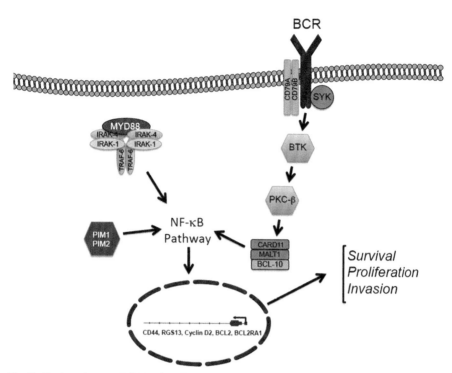

Fig. 2. Nuclear factor-κB (NF-κB) activation in primary CNS lymphoma (PCNSL). NF-κB transcriptional activation is regulated by multiple signals in PCNSL, including the MYD88/IRAK1/4 complex and the B-cell receptor (BCR) complex consisting of CD79A and B and SYK tyrosine kinase. Activation of IRAK1 and 4 kinases via the oncogenic mutation of MYD88 at L265P impacts approximately 50% of PCNSL cases. MYD88 is an adapter protein that mediates toll-like receptor and interleukin-1 receptor signaling. In addition, chronic active signaling via the BCR involving SYK and BTK also potentiates NF-κB activation. Activating mutations involving CD79B, a component of the BCR, as well as CARD11, a mediator of BCR signaling, are each present in approximately 15% of cases and result in NF-κB activation.

concentration of IL-10 (another activator of JAK/STAT) is detectable in the vitreous and CSF in PCNSL and, in independent studies, correlated with adverse prognosis.[47,48] A recent analysis demonstrated upregulated IL-10 transcripts in primary CNS lymphoma tumors compared with secondary CNS lymphomas and nodal lymphomas, with concomitant upregulated IL-10 protein in CSF from cases of PCNSL. In addition, CSF concentration of IL-10 correlated with tumor response and progression in patients treated with rituximab and methotrexate.[49] Finally, intratumoral *JAK1* transcripts are upregulated in PCNSL.[25,50] Importantly, increased IL-10 expression plus activation of JAK/STAT signaling in PCNSL are manifestations of aberrant activation of the MyD88 pathway[51] (see **Fig. 2**; **Figs. 3** and **4**).

In addition, *CD79B*, a component of the B-cell receptor signaling pathway, is mutated in approximately 20% of cases, providing further data that dysregulation of the B-cell receptor and the NF-κB signaling pathway contribute to pathogenesis of PCNSL[52] (see **Fig. 2**). Silencing of *CDKN2A*, a cell cycle regulator, occurs in 50% of cases and is linked with inferior outcomes.[43,45]

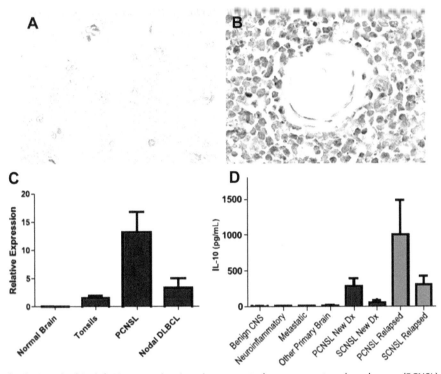

Fig. 3. Interleukin (IL)-10 expression in primary central nervous system lymphomas (PCNSL). Absent expression in normal brain (*A*) with strong expression of IL-10 by lymphoma cells in PCNSL (*B*), as demonstrated by immunohistochemistry (original magnification, ×1000). (*C*) Quantitative reverse transcriptase polymerase chain reaction demonstrates markedly increased expression of IL-10 in diagnostic specimens of PCNSL (n = 23) compared with reactive tonsils and normal brain. The average IL-10 expression was higher in PCNSL compared with 9 cases of nodal diffuse, large B-cell lymphoma (DLBCL), of which 7 were of germinal center phenotype. (*D*) Mean cerebrospinal fluid (CSF) IL-10 protein is 70-fold higher in patients with PCNSL and secondary central nervous system lymphoma compared with neuroinflammatory conditions and other brain tumors ($P<2.3 \times 10^{-5}$). The CSF concentration of IL-10 was highest in relapsed cases. Dx, diagnosis.

TUMOR MICROENVIRONMENT IN PRIMARY CENTRAL NERVOUS SYSTEM LYMPHOMA

The molecular basis for tropism and selective dissemination of lymphoma within the brain are problems that are fundamental to the pathogenesis of PCNSL. In vitro chemotactic responses by large B-cell lymphoma cells isolated from brain lesions have been demonstrated in response to chemokines CXCL12 (SDF-1) and CXCL-13 (B-lymphocyte chemoattractant),[53–55] providing evidence for their role as neurotropic factors. Moreover, high CXCL-13 concentration in CSF from CNS lymphoma patients correlates with adverse prognosis, supporting its role as a prosurvival factor in PCNSL. In addition, determination of the CSF concentration of CXCL-13, as well as IL-10, facilitate diagnosis of CNS lymphoma in that bivariate expression of each molecule has diagnostic sensitivity at least 2-fold greater than cytology or flow cytometry. In a multicenter investigation, the positive predictive value of bivariate increases in IL-10 plus CXCL-13 in CSF was 95% in the identification of untreated PCNSL.[49]

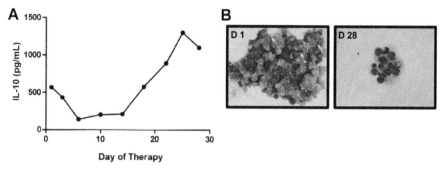

Fig. 4. (A) Interleukin (IL)-10 concentration in the cerebrospinal fluid (CSF) correlates with disease course in patients with recurrent central nervous system lymphomas that are treated with rituximab plus methotrexate (representative of 6 consecutive cases). (B) Cytologic appearance of lymphoma cells in CSF at baseline (day 1) and persistent disease (day 28) at completion of intraventricular therapy with rituximab plus methotrexate. (*From* Rubenstein JL, Wong VS, Kadoch C, et al. CXCL13 plus interleukin 10 is highly specific for the diagnosis of CNS lymphoma. Blood 2013;121:4724; with permission.)

Given that expression of B-cell chemokines CXCL13 and SDF-1 by retinal pigment epithelium has also been demonstrated in primary IOLs, these chemokines may also contribute to lymphoma cell homing to the retinal pigment epithelium from choroidal circulation.[56]

While under physiologic conditions, the brain is believed to be immunologically quiescent, diagnostic specimens of PCNSL often reveal a robust inflammatory response, with infiltrating reactive T cells and activated macrophages. Notably, perivascular T-cell infiltrates in PCNSL may predict a favorable outcome, suggesting that immunotherapeutic interventions that potentiate T-cell–mediated immune surveillance may be effective.[57]

Diagnostic Evaluation of the Patient with a Focal Brain Lesion

Because patients with PCNSL/IOL commonly present with a variety of nonspecific and/or subtle neurologic symptoms, the diagnostic process may be protracted and extend for months to years (**Fig. 5**). The cornerstone of diagnostic testing in suspected PCNSL is MRI of the brain, with gadolinium contrast. In 95% of PCNSL, pathologic enhancement localizes homogeneously to dominant lesions. Among the immunocompetent, lesions are solitary in 65% of PCNSL patients and multifocal in 35%. Involvement of the cerebral hemispheres is most common (38%) followed by the thalamus and basal ganglia (16%), corpus callosum (14%) periventricular loci (12%), and cerebellum (9%).[58]

Although there are insufficient data to recommend newer techniques such as quantitative diffusion-weighted and perfusion MRI as "standard of care," an accumulation of recent data demonstrates the usefulness of these metrics in prognostication as well as diagnosis of CNS lymphomas and related inflammatory and malignant conditions.[10,59–64] Given the quantitative nature of these techniques, and their universal availability in standard MR neuroimaging packages, it is possible that these will be incorporated in future studies.

Although glucocorticoids typically induce radiographic regressions in greater than 40% of patients, steroid-induced responses also increase risk of a nondiagnostic vitreal or brain biopsy.[65] Steroid-induced diagnostic delays may extend for months

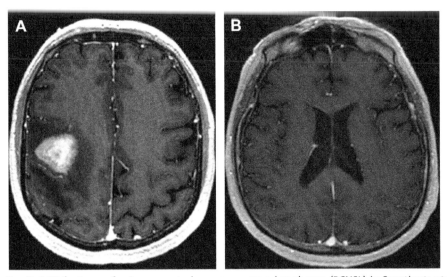

Fig. 5. MRI features of primary central nervous system lymphoma (PCNSL) in 2 patients at diagnosis (*A*). MRI depicts homogeneously enhancing mass with vasogenic edema. (*B*). Normal appearing MRI of patient with progressive neurologic symptoms who was aggressively treated with steroids before a diagnosis could be elicited. Four repeat cerebrospinal fluid (CSF) collections and 1 brain biopsy were nondiagnostic and the diagnosis of disseminated PCNSL was made at autopsy. Notably, the CSF of each patient contained elevated concentrations of CXCL13 and interleukin-10, highly specific biomarkers that facilitate the diagnosis of PCNSL. (*From* Rubenstein JL, Wong VS, Kadoch C, et al. CXCL13 plus interleukin 10 is highly specific for the diagnosis of CNS lymphoma. Blood 2013;121:4745; with permission.)

and, on occasion, steroid-induced regressions of sentinel lesions may delay diagnosis of PCNSL or IOL for years.[66] It is therefore important to emphasize that empiric glucocorticoids such as dexamethasone be tapered rapidly or not administered until a diagnosis is established.

The standard diagnostic approach for PCNSL is stereotactic brain biopsy; in selected cases, a subtotal resection may be appropriate if deemed to be safe. Flow cytometric or cytologic analysis of meningeal lymphoma cells isolated from CSF or vitrectomy may also yield the diagnosis. Notably, although flow cytometry has increased diagnostic yield relative to cytology, CSF needs to be efficiently processed for studies designed to identify, in most cases, a kappa or lambda-restricted B-cell lymphoma. Repeat CSF cytologic or flow cytometric studies infrequently improve diagnostic yield, supporting the development of innovative diagnostic methods based on detection of genomic aberrations, such as detection of oncogenic alleles of MYD88.[67]

Given that approximately 80% of patients with IOL will exhibit CNS dissemination, MRI of the brain with gadolinium may be indicated in the workup of idiopathic uveitis in which lymphoma is a diagnostic consideration. Additional staging tests for IOL include fluorescence angiography and optical coherence tomography, as well as evaluation of mutant L265P MYD88[67]; intraocular concentrations of the cytokines IL-10 and IL-6 may also be useful adjuncts to diagnosis.[68]

Staging evaluation for the patient with presumptive PCNSL includes complete ophthalmologic examination plus systemic staging via computed tomography of chest, abdomen, and pelvis plus bone marrow biopsy; the value of PET in staging of PCNSL is not established,[69] but it may be useful in possible concomitant testicular involvement in men older than 60 (**Fig. 6**).

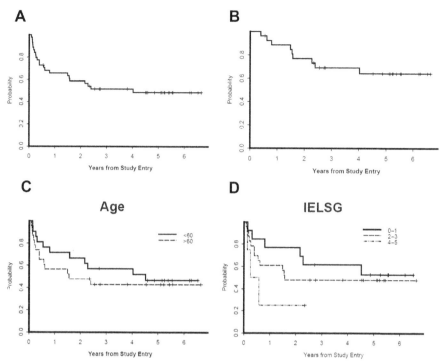

Fig. 6. Outcomes with intensive chemotherapy and immunotherapy in newly diagnosed primary central nervous system lymphoma, without whole brain radiotherapy: CALGB (Alliance 50,202). Outcome for all CALGB 50202 patients; y-axis refers to cumulative probability of event. (A) Progression-free survival (PFS) for all patients. The 2-year PFS was 59%. (B) PFS for those patients who attained a complete response with MT-R (high-dose methotrexate, temozolomide, rituximab) induction and received EA (etoposide cytarabine) consolidation (n = 27). (C) PFS was similar for patients aged greater than 60 years (n = 23) and for younger patients (n = 21; P = .48). (D) There was a trend between shorter PFS and highest International Extranodal Lymphoma Study Group (IELSG) risk score of 4 to 5 (P = .16). (From Rubenstein JL, Hsi ED, Johnson JL, et al. Intensive chemotherapy and immunotherapy in patients with newly diagnosed primary CNS lymphoma: CALGB 50202 (alliance 50202). J Clin Oncol 2013;31:3064 and 3065; with permission.)

CLINICAL PROGNOSTIC DETERMINANTS IN PRIMARY CENTRAL NERVOUS SYSTEM LYMPHOMA

The International Extranodal Lymphoma Study Group identified 5 clinical variables that correlate with prognosis in PCNSL; 3 are shared with systemic NHL: increased lactate dehydrogenase, age greater than 60 years, and performance status of greater than 1; parameters specific to PCNSL include elevated CSF protein as well as tumor location within the deep regions of the brain (periventricular, basal ganglia, brainstem, and/or cerebellum). The presence of 0 to 1, 2 to 3, or 4 to 5 adverse risk factors respectively correlates with 2-year survival rates of 80%, 48%, and 15%, respectively.[70] Historically, age has been the most reliable clinical prognostic factor, however there is disagreement regarding the age cutpoint at which prognosis declines. Although the International Extranodal Lymphoma Study Group considers age 60 years to be the cutpoint above which prognosis declines, the Memorial Sloan-Kettering prognostic index uses a cutpoint of age 50.[11] Notably, in CALGB 50202, which evaluated intensive immunochemotherapy followed by high-dose consolidation, without WBRT, outcomes for PCNSL patients older than 60 was similar to younger patients, a result that suggests that the optimal cutpoint for age as a prognostic variable is strongly linked to the effects of delayed neurotoxicity.[10,12]

PRINCIPLES OF MANAGEMENT IN PRIMARY CENTRAL NERVOUS SYSTEM LYMPHOMA
Surgery: Biopsy Versus Resection

Many authorities recommend against neurosurgical resection of PCNSL, given the scant evidence that surgical cytoreduction provides no survival benefit and increases risk of postoperative neurologic deficit.[72,73] On the other hand, data extracted from the German PCNSL SG-1 Trial provided evidence that aggressive resection of PCNSL correlated with improved progression-free survival (PFS).[74] In many cases, maximum safe resection of lesions provides immediate relief of mass effect, facilitates glucocorticoid taper, and theoretically eliminates drug-resistant tumor clones, without contributing to neurologic deficits, particularly when performed using modern neurosurgical mapping techniques.

Whole Brain Irradiation in Primary Central Nervous System Lymphoma

The positive impact of WBRT in PCNSL is compromised by at least 3 important shortcomings: (1) inadequate local control of lymphoma, (2) subclinical dissemination of radiographically occult lymphoma cells outside of the radiation field, and (3) deleterious delayed effects of radiation on normal brain function. In 1 study, the use of WBRT as the sole intervention in PCNSL yielded a median survival of only 11.6 months, and greater than 60% of patients experienced lymphoma progression within the irradiated field.[75] The archetypical features of the delayed neurotoxicity of WBRT in PCNSL include incontinence, gait, and memory disturbances, toxicities that are most evident in patients older than 60; PCNSL survivors that experience late-delayed neurotoxicity of WBRT may ultimately require custodial care.[76] Although lower doses of WBRT were associated with neurotoxicity that is barely discernable in preliminary studies,[77] additional validation of these results are necessary, and need to be reconciled with the established deleterious neurocognitive effects of prophylactic cranial irradiation at 30 Gy.[78] It seems plausible that the neurotoxicity of WBRT is a continuous variable in terms of its relationship to dose. Importantly, it was recently noted that PCNSL patients older than 60 years of age who received consolidative low-dose WBRT (23.4 Gy) experienced inferior outcome in terms of PFS compared with patients younger than 60 years of age.[79] Given the increasing incidence in PCNSL in older patients, these results substantiate the need for innovative strategies that defer or eliminate WBRT as therapy in PCNSL.

Induction Chemotherapeutic Strategies in Primary Central Nervous System Lymphoma

The feasibility and efficacy of HD-MTX in CNS lymphomas was established in the 1970s[5,6] and led to its incorporation more broadly in induction and salvage regimens. HD-MTX has been identified in multivariate analysis as the most important treatment-related prognostic variable related to survival in CNS lymphomas.[80]

Although the optimal dose of methotrexate has not been defined, systemic doses of 1 g/m^2 or greater mediate lymphocytotoxic effects within brain parenchyma.[6] In a landmark study, Glantz and colleagues[81] demonstrated that intravenous methotrexate administered at 8 g/m^2 over 4 hours yielded higher cytotoxic levels of methotrexate in serum and CSF compared with intrathecal methotrexate (12 mg) at 48 and 72 hours.

Also, investigators at Memorial Sloan-Kettering Cancer Center demonstrated that elimination of intrathecal methotrexate during initial therapy for PCNSL did not affect outcome in patients receiving HD-MTX at doses of at least 3.5 g/m^2.[82] In summary, these studies indicate that high-dose intravenous methotrexate, administered every 2 weeks for a minimum of 6 cycles, can be used to treat large cell lymphoma within brain and leptomeningeal compartments, without intrathecal therapy.[10]

PREVENTION AND MANAGEMENT OF HIGH-DOSE METHOTREXATE TOXICITY

The principal toxicity of HD-MTX is nephropathy, caused by precipitation of methotrexate and its metabolite 7-OH methotrexate within renal tubules. Measures to prevent this life-threatening complication include hydration, urine alkalinization, and avoidance of drugs that interact with MTX such as penicillins, as well as drainage of third space effusions. Additional interventions for delayed methotrexate clearance include carboxypeptidase–G2 (CPDG2, glucarpidase) a recombinant enzyme that rapidly reduces toxic serum methotrexate, via direct hydrolysis of methotrexate[83]; glucarpidase was approved by the US Food and Drug Administration in 2012.

COMBINED MODALITY REGIMENS

Combined modality therapy was pioneered at Memorial Sloan-Kettering Cancer Center and consisted of HD-MTX plus procarbazine and vincristine, followed by WBRT and high-dose cytarabine. Evaluation of this approach in a multicenter Radiation Therapy Oncology Group trial demonstrated a median PFS of 24 months.[84] Because of this encouraging efficacy, combined modality therapy became a widely adopted approach for PCNSL.[85,86] In a multicenter randomized phase II study, Ferreri and colleagues evaluated HD-MTX–based induction, with or without high-dose cytarabine followed by consolidative WBRT; the median failure-free survival in patients receiving HD-Ara-C in combination with HD-MTX was 8 months; in contrast, median failure-free survival for patients treated with HD-MTX without cytarabine was only 4 months.[87] In the SG-1 randomized trial involving 551 PCNSL patients in which one-half received WBRT as first-line consolidation, Thiel and colleagues[88] provided evidence that omission of WBRT from first-line treatment did not impact overall survival. Although the study revealed a modest effect of WBRT on PFS after methotrexate-based induction, this did not translate into improved overall survival, possibly attributable to the neurotoxicity detected in the radiotherapy arm [88]

ALTERNATIVES TO WHOLE BRAIN RADIOTHERAPY CONSOLIDATION: HIGH-DOSE CHEMOTHERAPY

Given the recognition of inadequate efficacy as well as neurotoxicity associated with WBRT, there has been interest in development of strategies that eliminate radiotherapy. One approach has been high-dose chemotherapeutic consolidation, including autologous stem cell transplantation. Regimens that contain CNS-penetrant agents such as carmustine, thiotepa, cyclophosphamide, busulfan, high-dose cytarabine, and etoposide are associated with the best results. However, in 1 early trial, results using the BEAM combination (carmustine, etoposide, cytarabine, and melphalan) followed by autologous stem cell rescue were not encouraging, possibly because a major proportion of patients enrolled in the study had inadequate disease control before myeloablative therapy, likely because of the abbreviated course of HD-MTX administered.[89]

Soussain and colleagues[90] evaluated dose-intensive chemotherapy and autologous stem cell transplant in recurrent CNS lymphomas and IOL. These investigators noted that combination high-dose cytarabine plus etoposide constituted a highly potent salvage regimen for relapsed/refractory CNS lymphomas: 12 of 14 patients attained responses, 8 of which were complete. Responding patients received a myeloablative regimen consisting of thiotepa, busulfan, and cyclophosphamide (TBC) followed by stem cell rescue.[90]

Beginning in 2001, investigators at the University of California, San Francisco began to evaluate dose-intensive chemotherapy in first-line consolidation, without WBRT, after induction immunochemotherapy with rituximab in newly diagnosed PCNSL. The strategy involved a 2-step regimen: the induction phase uses HD-MTX given every 2 weeks with temozolomide and rituximab (MT-R). Intravenous rituximab is administered starting day 3, and weekly for 6 infusions, an interval during which the blood–brain barrier may be most compromised by angiotropic lymphoma.[91] Temozolomide is a lipophilic alkylating agent with activity at relapse in CNS lymphoma, alone and in combination with rituximab.[92–94] Temozolomide yields superior health-related quality of life and toxicity characteristics compared with procarbazine in patients with a brain tumor.[95,96] To consolidate response after induction MT-R, PCNSL patients received intensive consolidation with non–cross-resistant agents with combination "EA": 96-hour infusional etoposide plus 8 doses of cytarabine at 2 g/m^2.[97–99] Notably, infusional etoposide is incorporated within the EPOCH regimen (etoposide, doxorubicin, cyclophosphamide, vincristine, and prednisone), which is highly effective in large B-cell lymphoma.[100,101] Etoposide has demonstrated efficacy in brain tumors, including CNS lymphoid leukemia.[102] Notably, when given with CHOP in patients with aggressive lymphoma, etoposide was associated with a decreased risk of secondary CNS lymphoma.[103]

A key goal of the 2-step MT-R EA program was to develop an induction regimen that incorporates an alkylator, temozolomide[93] as well as rituximab,[104] and yet causes minimal myelosuppression, to enable minimal treatment delays during the first weeks of treatment, the interval at which maximal lymphoma cytoreduction is achieved. Long-term follow-up of the first cohort of PCNSL patients treated with this regimen demonstrates that combination EA is highly effective as consolidation after MT-R in newly diagnosed PCNSL.[10] Based on phase I data, the MT-R plus EA regimen was evaluated in CALGB 50202, demonstrating for the first time the feasibility of high-dose chemotherapy in a multicenter study in newly diagnosed PCNSL. The rate of complete response to MT-R in CALGB 50202 was 66% and the 2-year PFS was 59%. Median time to progression of all 50,202 patients, 4 years, is 2 times longer than achieved with combined modality therapy in multicenter trials using standard dose WBRT and may be similar to or favorable to results of reduced dose WBRT in patients older than 60 years of age.[84,88] Other key findings from CALGB 50202 were that outcomes were similar for PCNSL patients older than 60 years of age compared with younger patients and the observation that the PFS curves reached a stable plateau, supporting the hypothesis that long-term survival can be achieved in PCNSL without brain irradiation (**Fig. 7**).

Given the encouraging results of CALGB 50202, a successor, randomized phase II trial, CALGB 51101, has been activated in the United States, endorsed by the major cooperative groups: Alliance, Eastern Cooperative Oncology Group, and Southwest Oncology Group. In CALGB 51101 after randomization and remission induction therapy with MT-R, patients receive either consolidation with EA or myeloablative therapy with carmustine plus thiotepa.[7]

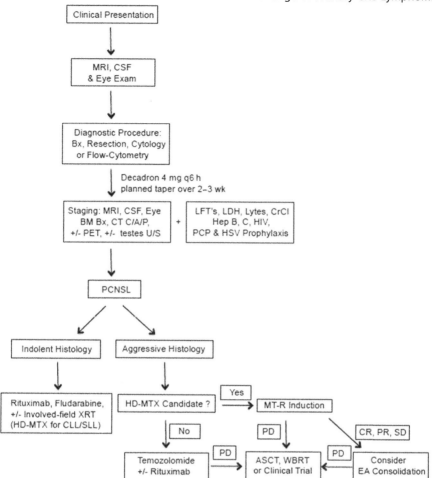

Fig. 7. Approach to treatment of newly diagnosed primary central nervous system (CNS) lymphoma (PCNSL). In the diagnostic workup, an MRI of the spine may be useful if warranted by neurologic symptoms or if analysis of the cerebrospinal fluid (CSF) is contraindicated. Ultrasonography of the testes is indicated for older male patients with CNS involvement of lymphoma in which testes coinvolvement is suspected on clinical and/or radiographic grounds. The value of a PET scan in this setting is not established. Although the schedule of Decadron taper should be individualized, we recommend a planned taper to be completed within 2 to 3 weeks of diagnosis, between the first and second courses of high-dose methotrexate (HD-MTX). Therapeutic options for indolent lymphomas that involve the CNS or dura include rituximab, fludarabine, involved-field irradiation, and HD-MTX for CNS involvement of chronic lymphocytic leukemia/small lymphocytic leukemia. For newly diagnosed patients who are not candidates for HD-MTX, in most cases we recommend a trial of temozolomide and rituximab and/or strategies that use high-dose chemotherapy, before consideration of using whole-brain irradiation. ASCT, autologous stem cell transplantation; BM Bx, bone marrow biopsy; CLL, chronic lymphocytic leukemia; CR, complete response; EA, etoposide-cytarabine; Hep B, C, hepatitis B, C; HIV, human immunodeficiency virus; HSV, herpes simplex virus; LDH, lactate dehydrogenase; LFT, liver function tests; MT-R, combination HD-MTX, temozolomide, and rituximab (rituximab is omitted for T-cell lymphomas); PCP, *Pneumocystis jiroveci* pneumonia; PD, progressive disease; PR, partial response; SD, stable disease; SLL, small lymphocytic lymphoma; WBRT, whole-brain radiotherapy; XRT, x-ray therapy. (*From* Rubenstein JL, Gupta NK, Mannis GN, et al. How I treat CNS lymphomas. Blood 2013;122:2324; with permission. Originally published by the American Society of Hematology.)

The myeloablative approach pioneered by Soussain and colleagues using the TBC conditioning regimen in relapsed CNS lymphoma was also recently evaluated in a phase II investigation performed at Memorial Sloan-Kettering for PCNSL in which newly diagnosed PCNSL patients who responded to induction chemotherapy consisting of rituximab, HD-MTX plus procarbazine, and vincristine received consolidative TBC chemotherapy. Results of this investigation were highly promising with a 2-year PFS of 79%; however, treatment-related mortality among transplanted patients that received the TBC conditioning regimen was substantial at 11.5%.[105]

ALTERNATIVES TO WHOLE BRAIN RADIOTHERAPY: INDUCTION HIGH-DOSE METHOTREXATE THERAPY WITHOUT CONSOLIDATION IN ELDERLY PATIENTS WITH PRIMARY CENTRAL NERVOUS SYSTEM LYMPHOMA

Given the established toxicities of WBRT, as well as concerns regarding the feasibility of high-dose chemotherapy consolidation in patients older than 60, 1 approach has been to apply methotrexate-based induction regimens for newly diagnosed elderly patients and to withhold consolidation, reserving salvage chemotherapy or radiation for disease progression. Results of a recent European intergroup, randomized phase II trial evaluated 2 promising methotrexate-based regimens – HD-MTX (3.5 g/m^2) plus temozolomide versus HD-MTX (3.5 g/m^2) plus procarbazine, vincristine, and high-dose cytarabine; neither regimen included radiotherapy. Remarkably the 1-year PFS (the primary endpoint) was the same with both regimens at 36%; there was, however, a small, but statistically insignificant, trend for improved overall survival in patients that received the 4-drug regimen that contains high-dose cytarabine.[106]

NEUROCOGNITIVE FUNCTION

Given the recent progress in outcomes in PCNSL, the consequences of treatment-related neurotoxicity among survivors has emerged as an increasingly important question. Although reduced-dose brain radiotherapy may be associated with milder cognitive dysfunction among PCNSL survivors compared with standard-dose WBRT,[77] even reduced doses of WBRT as consolidation are associated with impairments of verbal memory and motor speed. By contrast, PCNSL patients treated with HD-MTX without consolidative WBRT do not exhibit severe cognitive dysfunction as determined by neuropsychological testing; PCNSL patients treated with HD-MTX without WBRT nevertheless score lower than normative control subjects in several domains, including motor speed and executive function.[107] Given that PCNSL is an infiltrative brain tumor associated with a spectrum of neurologic symptoms, determination of whether impairments of neurologic function are the consequence of lymphoma versus neurotoxicity of agents such as methotrexate remains a challenge.

TREATMENT OF RECURRENT PRIMARY CENTRAL NERVOUS SYSTEM LYMPHOMA

Several studies have demonstrated that dose-intensive chemotherapy with stem cell rescue can be an effective option in the treatment of relapsed CNS lymphomas and IOL.[8,90,108] In the setting of recurrent disease that is methotrexate-sensitive, one approach is to administer additional cycles of HD-MTX, to achieve maximal cytoreduction, followed by dose-intensive chemotherapy consolidation using non–cross-resistant, CNS-penetrant agents such as thiotepa[9,109,110] High-dose carmustine-based therapy without thiotepa has also been studied[111] (**Table 1**). For CNS lymphomas that have progressed within 6 months of dose-intensive chemotherapeutic consolidation, salvage high-dose chemotherapy may not be an effective

Table 1
Regimens that are active in dose intensive consolidation and myeloablative therapy in central nervous system lymphomas

Intensive Consolidation/Preparative Regimen	Reference
Carmustine, thiotepa, etoposide	Korfel et al,[9] 2013
Infusional etoposide, high-dose cytarabine	Wieduwilt et al,[10] 2012; Rubenstein et al,[12] 2013
Thiotepa, busulfan, cyclophosphamide	Soussain et al,[90] 2002; Soussain et al,[108] 2008; Cote et al,[109] 2012, Omuro et al,[105] 2015
Carmustine, thiotepa	Illerhaus et al,[7] 2008
Cyclophosphamide, carmustine, etoposide	Alvarnas et al,[111] 2000

option. Such patients may be managed with additional HD-MTX, pemetrexed,[112] WBRT, or investigational agents in CNS lymphoma such as lenalidomide or ibrutinib.

RITUXIMAB IN CENTRAL NERVOUS SYSTEM LYMPHOMAS

Although rituximab has become a cornerstone of therapy in systemic B-cell NHL, a number of studies demonstrated that the addition of rituximab to CHOP may not significantly decrease the rate of CNS recurrence of systemic large B-cell lymphoma compared with CHOP alone.[113–115] Nevertheless, intravenous rituximab can induce responses of contrast-enhancing lesions in CNS lymphoma, likely in lesions in which there is substantial disruption of the blood–brain barrier.[104] Further data substantiating the role for rituximab in PCNSL has recently been provided in a randomized phase II study led by Ferreri that evaluated the MATRIX regimen, composed of a methotrexate/cytarabine backbone plus thiotepa and rituximab. Results presented at the 13th International Conference on Malignant Lymphoma, in June 2015 in Lugano, Switzerland, confirm significantly improved outcomes in PCNSL patients who received rituximab.

INTRAVENTRICULAR RITUXIMAB IN CENTRAL NERVOUS SYSTEM LYMPHOMAS

The safety and efficacy of intraventricular rituximab, both as monotherapy and in combination with intraventricular methotrexate, was evaluated recently in the setting of 2 phase I multicenter trials involving patients with recurrent primary and secondary CNS lymphomas.[26,116] These studies demonstrated that, when diluted in preservative-free normal saline and administered into ventricular CSF, 10 and 25-mg doses of rituximab are well-tolerated and elicited responses within leptomeninges, intraocular compartments, and in small parenchymal lesions. The efficacy of intraventricular rituximab was additive or synergistic with methotrexate. One of the key findings was that intraventricular rituximab/methotrexate was particularly active in patients with a high burden of leptomeningeal lymphoma. These studies also suggested that intraventricular rituximab overcomes the problem of the blood–brain barrier, in that CSF responses were documented in patients with baseline serum rituximab concentrations of greater than 15 μg/mL.[26,116] A potential mechanistic explanation for the rapid efficacy of intraventricular rituximab is provided by activation of the complement cascade at C3 as well as the C5b-9 membrane attack complex within CSF upon intra-CSF rituximab administration.[117]

Given the evidence for activity of intravenous rituximab in CNS lymphomas, as monotherapy and in combination with methotrexate-based induction,[118] a number of protocols now incorporate this anti-CD20 monoclonal antibody as a component of induction in PCNSL. Although several studies demonstrate its activity at relapse, intraventricular rituximab remains investigational and the combination of intraventricular plus intravenous rituximab with lenalidomide for recurrent CNS lymphomas is currently being studied in a phase I investigation (NCT01542918).

TREATMENT OF INTRAOCULAR LYMPHOMA

Most cases of IOL involve large B-cell NHL, and are classified as either primary vitreoretinal lymphoma or uveal lymphomas; these are divided into primary neoplasms of the choroid, iris, and ciliary body, or secondary choroidal lymphomas in patients with systemic NHL. Importantly, between 65% and 90% of patients with primary vitreoretinal lymphoma ultimately disseminate throughout the neuroaxis, typically within 30 months. Conversely, IOL impacts 15% to 25% of patients with PCNSL.

Therapies for primary vitreoretinal lymphoma can be divided into local approaches, such as ocular radiation or intravitreal therapy, versus systemic chemotherapy. External beam radiotherapy using opposed lateral beams to the eyes is well-tolerated and associated with low rates of local recurrence. Typical complications of ocular radiotherapy are mild and include dry eye, cataracts, and radiation retinopathy[119] Intravitreal methotrexate and rituximab may be of value in the management of unilateral disease or in the setting of prior ocular radiation.[120,121] Treatment-related complications of intravitreal methotrexate include hemorrhage, endophthalmitis, hypotony, and retinal detachment.[122] Systemic therapeutic options for IOL include HD-MTX,[123] high-dose cytarabine, or trofasfamide.[124,125] Notably, in primary vitreoretinal lymphoma, systemic HD-MTX plus binocular irradiation provides local disease control and addresses the probability of subclinical disease throughout the neuroaxis.[126] Our approach to patients with primary IOL and/or concomitant PCNSL with IOL typically involves 3 steps: (1) HD-MTX–based induction (with rituximab, if disease is CD20+), (2) dose-intensive chemotherapeutic consolidation with EA or autologous stem cell transplantation, and (3) binocular radiotherapy, but not WBRT, if there is persistence and/or recurrence of isolated IOL after completion of dose-intensive consolidation.

PRIMARY CENTRAL NERVOUS SYSTEM LYMPHOMA IN THE IMMUNOCOMPROMISED HOST

Although the incidence of HIV-associated PCNSL declined in incidence with advent of combination antiretroviral therapy, PCNSL remains a significant AIDS-defining illness that represents a major therapeutic challenge. Feasibility and efficacy of HD-MTX in HIV-associated PCNSL has been demonstrated.[127] Similarly, in the setting of CNS PTLD, reconstitution of immune function is a first principle, and is achieved by reduction in immunosuppression. HD-MTX is usually effective but its implementation needs to be balanced with risk of allograft failure.[128] Rituximab is also active in the CNS complications of PTLD, via intravenous as well as intrathecal administration.[129]

CONCLUSIONS AND FUTURE DIRECTIONS

Over the past 50 years, significant progress has been achieved in the treatment of PCNSL, an aggressive variant of large B-cell lymphoma. Between 40% and 50% of PCNSL patients are now likely to exhibit long-term survival and a significant proportion may be cured. However, given that at least 50% of patients develop disease refractory to the established armentarium of agents, it is now imperative that additional studies explore the potential efficacy of selective agents that target candidate resistance mechanisms in high-risk PCNSL patients.[130] For example, pharmacologic agents that evaluate disruption of NF-κB–activating pathways involving the B-cell receptor, Toll-like receptor, and PIM kinases are high priority in early phase investigation in PCNSL. Another key target is MUM-1/IRF-4, targeted by IMiD small molecule agents such as lenalidomide, or CC-122,[131] currently under evaluation in relapsed PCNSL.[132,133] Transformative advances are needed given the predilection of PCNSL for an aging population that often cannot tolerate dose-intensive chemotherapy or WBRT.

REFERENCES

1. Villano JL, Koshy M, Shaikh H, et al. Age, gender, and racial differences in incidence and survival in primary CNS lymphoma. Br J Cancer 2011;105:1414–8.
2. Hochberg FH, Miller DC. Primary central nervous system lymphoma. J Neurosurg 1988;68:835–53.
3. Batchelor T, Loeffler JS. Primary CNS lymphoma. J Clin Oncol 2006;24:1281–8.
4. Norden AD, Drappatz J, Wen PY, et al. Survival among patients with primary central nervous system lymphoma, 1973-2004. J Neurooncol 2011;101:487–93.
5. Ervin T, Canellos GP. Successful treatment of recurrent primary central nervous system lymphoma with high-dose methotrexate. Cancer 1980;45:1556–7.
6. Skarin AI, Zuckerman KS, Pitman SW, et al. High-dose methotrexate with folinic acid in the treatment of advanced non-Hodgkin lymphoma including CNS involvement. Blood 1977;50:1039–47.
7. Illerhaus G, Müller F, Feuerhake F, et al. High-dose chemotherapy and autologous stem-cell transplantation without consolidating radiotherapy as first-line treatment for primary lymphoma of the central nervous system. Haematologica 2008;93:147–8.
8. Bromberg JE, Doorduijn JK, Illerhaus G, et al. Central nervous system recurrence of systemic lymphoma in the era of stem cell transplantation - an International Primary Central Nervous System Lymphoma Study Group project. Haematologica 2013;98:808–13.
9. Korfel A, Elter T, Thiel E, et al. Phase II study of central nervous system (CNS)-directed chemotherapy including high-dose chemotherapy with autologous stem cell transplantation for CNS relapse of aggressive lymphomas. Haematologica 2013;98:364–70.
10. Wieduwilt MJ, Valles F, Issa S, et al. Immunochemotherapy with intensive consolidation for primary CNS lymphoma: a pilot study and prognostic assessment by diffusion-weighted MRI. Clin Cancer Res 2012;18:1146–55.
11. Rubenstein JL, Gupta NK, Mannis GN, et al. How I treat CNS lymphomas. Blood 2013;122:2318–30.
12. Rubenstein JL, Hsi ED, Johnson JL, et al. Intensive chemotherapy and immunotherapy in patients with newly diagnosed primary CNS lymphoma: CALGB 50202 (Alliance 50202). J Clin Oncol 2013;31:3061–8.
13. Cingolani A, Gastaldi R, Fassone L, et al. Epstein-Barr virus infection is predictive of CNS involvement in systemic AIDS-related non-Hodgkin's lymphomas. J Clin Oncol 2000;18:3325–30.
14. Schabet M. Epidemiology of primary CNS lymphoma. J Neurooncol 1999;43:199–201.
15. Camilleri-Broet S, Crinière E, Broët P, et al. A uniform activated B-cell-like immunophenotype might explain the poor prognosis of primary central nervous system lymphomas: analysis of 83 cases. Blood 2006;107:190–6.

16. Lai R, Rosenblum MK, DeAngelis LM. Primary CNS lymphoma: a whole-brain disease? Neurology 2002;59:1557–62.

17. Fine HA, Mayer RJ. Primary central nervous system lymphoma. Ann Intern Med 1993;119:1093–104.

18. McCann KJ, Ashton-Key M, Smith K, et al. Primary central nervous system lymphoma: tumor-related clones exist in the blood and bone marrow with evidence for separate development. Blood 2009;113:4677–80.

19. Jahnke K, Hummel M, Korfel A, et al. Detection of subclinical systemic disease in primary CNS lymphoma by polymerase chain reaction of the rearranged immunoglobulin heavy-chain genes. J Clin Oncol 2006;24:4754–7.

20. Rubenstein JL, Treseler P, O'Brien JM. Pathology and genetics of primary central nervous system and intraocular lymphoma. Hematol Oncol Clin North Am 2005;19:705–17, vii.

21. Shenkier TN, Blay JY, O'Neill BP, et al. Primary CNS lymphoma of T-cell origin: a descriptive analysis from the international primary CNS lymphoma collaborative group. J Clin Oncol 2005;23:2233–9.

22. Tu PH, Giannini C, Judkins AR, et al. Clinicopathologic and genetic profile of intracranial marginal zone lymphoma: a primary low-grade CNS lymphoma that mimics meningioma. J Clin Oncol 2005;23:5718–27.

23. Braaten KM, Betensky RA, de Leval L, et al. BCL-6 expression predicts improved survival in patients with primary central nervous system lymphoma. Clin Cancer Res 2003;9:1063–9.

24. Kreher S, Jöhrens K, Strehlow F, et al. Prognostic impact of B-cell lymphoma 6 in primary CNS lymphoma. Neuro Oncol 2015;17(7):1016–21.

25. Rubenstein JL, Fridlyand J, Shen A, et al. Gene expression and angiotropism in primary CNS lymphoma. Blood 2006;107:3716–23.

26. Rubenstein JL, Fridlyand J, Abrey L, et al. Phase I study of intraventricular administration of rituximab in patients with recurrent CNS and intraocular lymphoma. J Clin Oncol 2007;25:1350–6.

27. Fischer L, Hummel M, Korfel A, et al. Differential micro-RNA expression in primary CNS and nodal diffuse large B-cell lymphomas. Neuro Oncol 2011;13:1090–8.

28. Baraniskin A, Kuhnhenn J, Schlegel U, et al. Identification of microRNAs in the cerebrospinal fluid as marker for primary diffuse large B-cell lymphoma of the central nervous system. Blood 2011;117:3140–6.

29. Montesinos-Rongen M, Roost DV, Schaller C, et al. Primary diffuse large B-cell lymphomas of the central nervous system are targeted by aberrant somatic hypermutation. Blood 2004;103:1869–75.

30. Montesinos-Rongen M, Küppers R, Schlüter D, et al. Primary central nervous system lymphomas are derived from germinal-center B cells and show a preferential usage of the V4-34 gene segment. Am J Pathol 1999;155:2077–86.

31. Vater I, Montesinos-Rongen M, Schlesner M, et al. The mutational pattern of primary lymphoma of the central nervous system determined by whole-exome sequencing. Leukemia 2015;29:677–85.

32. Nakamura M, Sakaki T, Hashimoto H, et al. Frequent alterations of the p14(ARF) and p16(INK4a) genes in primary central nervous system lymphomas. Cancer Res 2001;61:6335–9.

33. Kamijo T, Bodner S, van de Kamp E, et al. Tumor spectrum in ARF-deficient mice. Cancer Res 1999;59:2217–22.

34. Nakamura M, Shimada K, Ishida E, et al. Histopathology, pathogenesis and molecular genetics in primary central nervous system lymphomas. Histol Histopathol 2004;19:211–9.

35. Mrugala MM, Rubenstein JL, Ponzoni M, et al. Insights into the biology of primary central nervous system lymphoma. Curr Oncol Rep 2009;11:73–80.

36. Harada K, Nishizaki T, Kubota H, et al. Distinct primary central nervous system lymphoma defined by comparative genomic hybridization and laser scanning cytometry. Cancer Genet Cytogenet 2001;125:147–50.

37. Cady FM, O'Neill BP, Law ME, et al. Del(6)(q22) and BCL6 rearrangements in primary CNS lymphoma are indicators of an aggressive clinical course. J Clin Oncol 2008;26:4814–9.

38. Boonstra R, Koning A, Mastik M, et al. Analysis of chromosomal copy number changes and oncoprotein expression in primary central nervous system lymphomas: frequent loss of chromosome arm 6q. Virchows Arch 2003;443:164–9.

39. Weber T, Weber RG, Kaulich K, et al. Characteristic chromosomal imbalances in primary central nervous system lymphomas of the diffuse large B-cell type. Brain Pathol 2000;10:73–84.

40. Courts C, Montesinos-Rongen M, Brunn A, et al. Recurrent inactivation of the PRDM1 gene in primary central nervous system lymphoma. J Neuropathol Exp Neurol 2008;67:720–7.

41. Nakamura M, Kishi M, Sakaki T, et al. Novel tumor suppressor loci on 6q22-23 in primary central nervous system lymphomas. Cancer Res 2003;63:737–41.

42. Braggio E, McPhail ER, Macon W, et al. Primary central nervous system lymphomas: a validation study of array-based comparative genomic hybridization in formalin-fixed paraffin-embedded tumor specimens. Clin Cancer Res 2011;17:4245–53.

43. Schwindt H, Vater I, Kreuz M, et al. Chromosomal imbalances and partial uniparental disomies in primary central nervous system lymphoma. Leukemia 2009;23:1875–84.

44. Montesinos-Rongen M, Schmitz R, Brunn A, et al. Mutations of CARD11 but not TNFAIP3 may activate the NF-kappaB pathway in primary CNS lymphoma. Acta Neuropathol 2010;120:529–35.

45. Gonzalez-Aguilar A, Idbaih A, Boisselier B, et al. Recurrent mutations of MYD88 and TBL1XR1 in primary central nervous system lymphomas. Clin Cancer Res 2012;18:5203–11.

46. Montesinos-Rongen M, Godlewska E, Brunn A, et al. Activating L265P mutations of the MYD88 gene are common in primary central nervous system lymphoma. Acta Neuropathol 2011;122:791–2.

47. Roy S, Josephson SA, Fridlyand J, et al. Protein biomarker identification in the CSF of patients with CNS lymphoma. J Clin Oncol 2008;26:96–105.

48. Sasayama T, Nakamizo S, Nishihara M, et al. Cerebrospinal fluid interleukin-10 is a potentially useful biomarker in immunocompetent primary central nervous system lymphoma (PCNSL). Neuro Oncol 2012;14:368–80.

49. Rubenstein JL, Wong VS, Kadoch C, et al. CXCL13 plus interleukin 10 is highly specific for the diagnosis of CNS lymphoma. Blood 2013;121:4740–8.

50. Sung CO, Kim SC, Karnan S, et al. Genomic profiling combined with gene expression profiling in primary central nervous system lymphoma. Blood 2011;117:1291–300.

51. Ngo VN, Young RM, Schmitz R, et al. Oncogenically active MYD88 mutations in human lymphoma. Nature 2011;470:115–9.

52. Montesinos-Rongen M, Schafer E, Siebert R, et al. Genes regulating the B cell receptor pathway are recurrently mutated in primary central nervous system lymphoma. Acta Neuropathol 2012;124:905–6.

53. Fischer L, Kortel A, Pfeiffer S, et al. CXCL13 and CXCL12 in central nervous system lymphoma patients. Clin Cancer Res 2009;15:5968–73.

54. Smith JR, Braziel RM, Paoletti S, et al. Expression of B-cell-attracting chemokine 1 (CXCL13) by malignant lymphocytes and vascular endothelium in primary central nervous system lymphoma. Blood 2003;101:815–21.

55. Smith JR, Falkenhagen KM, Coupland SE, et al. Malignant B cells from patients with primary central nervous system lymphoma express stromal cell-derived factor-1. Am J Clin Pathol 2007;127:633–41.

56. Falkenhagen KM, Braziel RM, Fraunfelder FW, et al. B-Cells in ocular adnexal lymphoproliferative lesions express B-cell attracting chemokine 1 (CXCL13). Am J Ophthalmol 2005;140:335–7.

57. Ponzoni M, Berger F, Chassagne-Clement C, et al. Reactive perivascular T-cell infiltrate predicts survival in primary central nervous system B-cell lymphomas. Br J Haematol 2007;138:316–23.

58. Kuker W, Nägele T, Korfel A, et al. Primary central nervous system lymphomas (PCNSL): MRI features at presentation in 100 patients. J Neurooncol 2005;72: 169–77.

59. Mabray MC, Cohen BA, Villanueva-Meyer JE, et al. Performance of apparent diffusion coefficient values and conventional MRI features in differentiating tumefactive demyelinating lesions from primary brain neoplasms. AJR Am J Roentgenol 2015;205:1075–85.

60. Mabray MC, Barajas RF, Villanueva-Meyer JE, et al. The Combined Performance of ADC, CSF CXC Chemokine Ligand 13, and CSF Interleukin 10 in the Diagnosis of Central Nervous System Lymphoma. AJNR Am J Neuroradiol 2016; 37:74–9.

61. Valles FE, Perez-Valles CL, Regalado S, et al. Combined diffusion and perfusion MR imaging as biomarkers of prognosis in immunocompetent patients with primary central nervous system lymphoma. AJNR Am J Neuroradiol 2013;34: 35–40.

62. Barajas RF Jr, Rubenstein JL, Chang JS, et al. Diffusion-weighted MR imaging derived apparent diffusion coefficient is predictive of clinical outcome in primary central nervous system lymphoma. AJNR Am J Neuroradiol 2010;31:60–6.

63. Fischer L, Koch A, Schlegel U, et al. Non-enhancing relapse of a primary CNS lymphoma with multiple diffusion-restricted lesions. J Neurooncol 2011;102: 163–6.

64. Reiche W, Hagen T, Schuchardt V, et al. Diffusion-weighted MR imaging improves diagnosis of CNS lymphomas. A report of four cases with common and uncommon imaging features. Clin Neurol Neurosurg 2007;109:92–101.

65. Porter AB, Giannini C, Kaufmann T, et al. Primary central nervous system lymphoma can be histologically diagnosed after previous corticosteroid use: a pilot study to determine whether corticosteroids prevent the diagnosis of primary central nervous system lymphoma. Ann Neurol 2008;63:662–7.

66. Pirotte B, Levivier M, Goldman S, et al. Glucocorticoid-induced long-term remission in primary cerebral lymphoma: case report and review of the literature. J Neurooncol 1997;32:63–9.

67. Bonzheim I, Giese S, Deuter C, et al. High frequency of MYD88 mutations in vitreoretinal B-cell lymphoma: a valuable tool to improve diagnostic yield of vitreous aspirates. Blood 2015;126:76–9.

68. Chan CC, Buggage RR, Nussenblatt RB. Intraocular lymphoma. Curr Opin Ophthalmol 2002;13:411–8.

69. Mohile NA, Deangelis LM, Abrey LE. The utility of body FDG PET in staging primary central nervous system lymphoma. Neuro Oncol 2008;10:223–8.

70. Ferreri AJ, Blay JY, Reni M, et al. Prognostic scoring system for primary CNS lymphomas: the International Extranodal Lymphoma Study Group experience. J Clin Oncol 2003;21:266–72.

71. Abrey LE, Ben-Porat L, Panageas KS, et al. Primary central nervous system lymphoma: the Memorial Sloan-Kettering Cancer Center prognostic model. J Clin Oncol 2006;24:5711–5.

72. DeAngelis LM, Yahalom J, Heinemann MH, et al. Primary CNS lymphoma: combined treatment with chemotherapy and radiotherapy. Neurology 1990;40:80–6.

73. Bataille B, Delwail V, Menet E, et al. Primary intracerebral malignant lymphoma: report of 248 cases. J Neurosurg 2000;92:261–6.

74. Weller M, Martus P, Roth P, et al. Surgery for primary CNS lymphoma? Challenging a paradigm. Neuro Oncol 2012;14:1481–4.

75. Nelson DF, Martz KL, Bonner H, et al. Non-Hodgkin's lymphoma of the brain: can high dose, large volume radiation therapy improve survival? Report on a prospective trial by the Radiation Therapy Oncology Group (RTOG): RTOG 8315. Int J Radiat Oncol Biol Phys 1992;23:9–17.

76. Abrey LE, DeAngelis LM, Yahalom J. Long-term survival in primary CNS lymphoma. J Clin Oncol 1998;16:859–63.

77. Correa DD, Rocco-Donovan M, DeAngelis LM, et al. Prospective cognitive follow-up in primary CNS lymphoma patients treated with chemotherapy and reduced-dose radiotherapy. J Neurooncol 2009;91:315–21.

78. Sun A, Bae K, Gore EM, et al. Phase III trial of prophylactic cranial irradiation compared with observation in patients with locally advanced non-small-cell lung cancer: neurocognitive and quality-of-life analysis. J Clin Oncol 2011;29: 279–86.

79. Morris PG, Correa DD, Yahalom J, et al. Rituximab, methotrexate, procarbazine, and vincristine followed by consolidation reduced-dose whole-brain radiotherapy and cytarabine in newly diagnosed primary CNS lymphoma: final results and long-term outcome. J Clin Oncol 2013;31:3971–9.

80. Blay JY, Conroy T, Chevreau C, et al. High-dose methotrexate for the treatment of primary cerebral lymphomas: analysis of survival and late neurologic toxicity in a retrospective series. J Clin Oncol 1998;16:864–71.

81. Glantz MJ, Cole BF, Recht L, et al. High-dose intravenous methotrexate for patients with nonleukemic leptomeningeal cancer: is intrathecal chemotherapy necessary? J Clin Oncol 1998;16:1561–7.

82. Khan RB, Shi W, Thaler HT, et al. Is intrathecal methotrexate necessary in the treatment of primary CNS lymphoma? J Neurooncol 2002;58:175–8.

83. Schwartz S, Borner K, Müller K, et al. Glucarpidase (carboxypeptidase g2) intervention in adult and elderly cancer patients with renal dysfunction and delayed methotrexate elimination after high-dose methotrexate therapy. Oncologist 2007;12:1299–308.

84. DeAngelis LM, Seiferheld W, Schold SC, et al. Combination chemotherapy and radiotherapy for primary central nervous system lymphoma: Radiation Therapy Oncology Group Study 93-10. J Clin Oncol 2002;20:4643–8.

85. DeAngelis LM, Yahalom J, Thaler HT, et al. Combined modality therapy for primary CNS lymphoma. J Clin Oncol 1992;10:635–43.

86. Glass J, Gruber ML, Cher L, et al. Preirradiation methotrexate chemotherapy of primary central nervous system lymphoma: long-term outcome. J Neurosurg 1994;81:188–95.

87. Ferreri AJ, Reni M, Foppoli M, et al. High-dose cytarabine plus high-dose methotrexate versus high-dose methotrexate alone in patients with primary CNS lymphoma: a randomised phase 2 trial. Lancet 2009;374(9700):1512–20.

88. Thiel E, Korfel A, Martus P, et al. High-dose methotrexate with or without whole brain radiotherapy for primary CNS lymphoma (G-PCNSL-SG-1): a phase 3, randomised, non-inferiority trial. Lancet Oncol 2010;11:1036–47.

89. Abrey LE, Childs BH, Paleologos N, et al. High-dose chemotherapy with stem cell rescue as initial therapy for anaplastic oligodendroglioma. J Neurooncol 2003;65:127–34.

90. Soussain C, Suzan F, Hoang-Xuan K, et al. Results of intensive chemotherapy followed by hematopoietic stem-cell rescue in 22 patients with refractory or recurrent primary CNS lymphoma or intraocular lymphoma. J Clin Oncol 2001; 19:742–9.

91. Ott RJ, Brada M, Flower MA, et al. Measurements of blood-brain barrier permeability in patients undergoing radiotherapy and chemotherapy for primary cerebral lymphoma. Eur J Cancer 1991;27:1356–61.

92. Reni M, Ferreri AJ, Landoni C, et al. Salvage therapy with temozolomide in an immunocompetent patient with primary brain lymphoma. J Natl Cancer Inst 2000;92:575–6.

93. Reni M, Zaja F, Mason W, et al. Temozolomide as salvage treatment in primary brain lymphomas. Br J Cancer 2007;96:864–7.

94. Wong ET, Tishler R, Barron L, et al. Immunochemotherapy with rituximab and temozolomide for central nervous system lymphomas. Cancer 2004;101:139–45.

95. Osoba D, Brada M, Yung WK, et al. Health-related quality of life in patients with anaplastic astrocytoma during treatment with temozolomide. Eur J Cancer 2000; 36:1788–95.

96. Osoba D, Brada M, Yung WK, et al. Health-related quality of life in patients treated with temozolomide versus procarbazine for recurrent glioblastoma multiforme. J Clin Oncol 2000;18:1481–91.

97. Damon LE, Johnson JL, Niedzwiecki D, et al. Immunochemotherapy and autologous stem-cell transplantation for untreated patients with mantle-cell lymphoma: CALGB 59909. J Clin Oncol 2009;27:6101–8.

98. Damon L, Damon LE, Gaensler K, et al. Impact of intensive PBSC mobilization therapy on outcomes following auto-SCT for non-Hodgkin's lymphoma. Bone Marrow Transplant 2008;42:649–57.

99. Linker CA, Owzar K, Powell B, et al. Auto-SCT for AML in second remission: CALGB study 9620. Bone Marrow Transplant 2009;44:353–9.

100. Wilson WH, Bryant G, Bates S, et al. EPOCH chemotherapy: toxicity and efficacy in relapsed and refractory non-Hodgkin's lymphoma. J Clin Oncol 1993; 11:1573–82.

101. Wilson WH, Dunleavy K, Pittaluga S, et al. Phase II study of dose-adjusted EPOCH and rituximab in untreated diffuse large B-cell lymphoma with analysis of germinal center and post-germinal center biomarkers. J Clin Oncol 2008;26: 2717–24.

102. Relling MV, Mahmoud HH, Pui CH, et al. Etoposide achieves potentially cytotoxic concentrations in CSF of children with acute lymphoblastic leukemia. J Clin Oncol 1996;14:399–404.

103. Boehme V, Zeynalova S, Kloess M, et al. Incidence and risk factors of central nervous system recurrence in aggressive lymphoma–a survey of 1693 patients treated in protocols of the German High-Grade Non-Hodgkin's Lymphoma Study Group (DSHNHL). Ann Oncol 2007;18:149–57.

104. Batchelor TT, Grossman SA, Mikkelsen T, et al. Rituximab monotherapy for patients with recurrent primary CNS lymphoma. Neurology 2011;76:929–30.

105. Omuro A, Correa DD, DeAngelis LM, et al. R-MPV followed by high-dose chemotherapy with TBC and autologous stem-cell transplant for newly diagnosed primary CNS lymphoma. Blood 2015;125:1403–10.

106. Omuro A, Chinot O, Taillandier L, et al. Methotrexate and temozolomide versus methotrexate, procarbazine, vincristine, and cytarabine for primary CNS lymphoma in an elderly population: an intergroup ANOCEF-GOELAMS randomised phase 2 trial. Lancet Haematol 2015;2:e251–9.

107. Correa DD, Shi W, Abrey LE, et al. Cognitive functions in primary CNS lymphoma after single or combined modality regimens. Neuro Oncol 2012;14:101–8.

108. Soussain C, Hoang-Xuan K, Taillandier L, et al. Intensive chemotherapy followed by hematopoietic stem-cell rescue for refractory and recurrent primary CNS and intraocular lymphoma: Societe Francaise de Greffe de Moelle Osseuse-Therapie Cellulaire. J Clin Oncol 2008;26:2512–8.

109. Cote GM, Hochberg EP, Muzikansky A, et al. Autologous stem cell transplantation with thiotepa, busulfan, and cyclophosphamide (TBC) conditioning in patients with CNS involvement by non-Hodgkin lymphoma. Biol Blood Marrow Transplant 2012;18:76–83.

110. Falzetti F, Di Ianni M, Ballanti S, et al. High-dose thiotepa, etoposide and carboplatin as conditioning regimen for autologous stem cell transplantation in patients with high-risk non-Hodgkin lymphoma. Clin Exp Med 2012;12:165–71.

111. Alvarnas JC, Negrin RS, Horning SJ, et al. High-dose therapy with hematopoietic cell transplantation for patients with central nervous system involvement by non-Hodgkin's lymphoma. Biol Blood Marrow Transplant 2000;6:352–8.

112. Raizer JJ, Rademaker A, Evens AM, et al. Pemetrexed in the treatment of relapsed/refractory primary central nervous system lymphoma. Cancer 2012;118:3743–8.

113. Feugier P, Virion JM, Tilly H, et al. Incidence and risk factors for central nervous system occurrence in elderly patients with diffuse large-B-cell lymphoma: Influence of rituximab. Ann Oncol 2004;15:129–33.

114. Tai WM, Chung J, Tang PL, et al. Central nervous system (CNS) relapse in diffuse large B cell lymphoma (DLBCL): pre- and post-rituximab. Ann Hematol 2011;90:809–18.

115. Yamamoto W, Tomita N, Watanabe R, et al. Central nervous system involvement in diffuse large B-cell lymphoma. Eur J Haematol 2010;85:6–10.

116. Rubenstein JL, Li J, Chen L, et al. Multicenter phase 1 trial of intraventricular immunochemotherapy in recurrent CNS lymphoma. Blood 2013;121:745–51.

117. Kadoch C, Li J, Wong VS, et al. Complement activation and intraventricular rituximab distribution in recurrent central nervous system lymphoma. Clin Cancer Res 2014;20:1029–41.

118. Shah GD, Yahalom J, Correa DD, et al. Combined immunochemotherapy with reduced whole-brain radiotherapy for newly diagnosed primary CNS lymphoma. J Clin Oncol 2007;25:4730–5.

119. Berenbom A, Davila HM, Lin HS, et al. Treatment outcomes for primary intraocular lymphoma: implications for external beam radiotherapy. Eye (Lond) 2007; 21:1198–201.
120. Kitzmann AS, Pulido JS, Mohney BG, et al. Intraocular use of rituximab. Eye (Lond) 2007;21:1524–7.
121. Itty S, Pulido JS. Rituximab for intraocular lymphoma. Retina 2009;29:129–32.
122. Chan CC, Rubenstein JL, Coupland SE, et al. Primary vitreoretinal lymphoma: a report from an International Primary Central Nervous System Lymphoma Collaborative Group symposium. Oncologist 2011;16:1589–99.
123. Batchelor TT, Kolak G, Ciordia R, et al. High-dose methotrexate for intraocular lymphoma. Clin Cancer Res 2003;9:711–5.
124. Jahnke K, Thiel E, Bechrakis NE, et al. Ifosfamide or trofosfamide in patients with intraocular lymphoma. J Neurooncol 2009;93:213–7.
125. Cheah CY, Milgrom S, Chihara D, et al. Intensive chemoimmunotherapy and bilateral globe irradiation as initial therapy for primary intraocular lymphoma. Neuro Oncol 2016;18:575–81.
126. Stefanovic A, Davis J, Murray T, et al. Treatment of isolated primary intraocular lymphoma with high-dose methotrexate-based chemotherapy and binocular radiation therapy: a single-institution experience. Br J Haematol 2010;151:103–6.
127. Jacomet C, Girard PM, Lebrette MG, et al. Intravenous methotrexate for primary central nervous system non-Hodgkin's lymphoma in AIDS. AIDS 1997;11: 1725–30.
128. Elstrom RL, Andreadis C, Aqui NA, et al. Treatment of PTLD with rituximab or chemotherapy. Am J Transplant 2006;6:569–76.
129. van de Glind G, de Graaf S, Klein C, et al. Intrathecal rituximab treatment for pediatric post-transplant lymphoproliferative disorder of the central nervous system. Pediatr Blood Cancer 2008;50:886–8.
130. Wang CC, Carnevale J, Rubenstein JL. Progress in central nervous system lymphomas. Br J Haematol 2014;166:311–25.
131. Hagner PR, Man HW, Fontanillo C, et al. CC-122, a pleiotropic pathway modifier, mimics an interferon response and has antitumor activity in DLBCL. Blood 2015; 126:779–89.
132. Ponzoni M, Issa S, Batchelor TT, et al. Beyond high-dose methotrexate and brain radiotherapy: novel targets and agents for primary CNS lymphoma. Ann Oncol 2014;25.316–22.
133. Fraser E, Gruenberg K, Rubenstein JL. New approaches in primary central nervous system lymphoma. Chin Clin Oncol 2015;4:11.

Transformed Lymphoma

Mary Ann Anderson, MBBS, FRACP, FRCPA[a,b],*,
Piers Blombery, MBBS, FRACP, FRCPA[c], John F. Seymour, MBBS, FRACP, PhD[c,d]

KEYWORDS

- Indolent lymphoma • Transformed lymphoma • Genetic drivers

KEY POINTS

- Transformation is a common occurrence among patients with indolent lymphoma and often carries a poor prognosis.
- Traditionally transformed lymphoma has been considered difficult to treat and associated with poor prognosis.
- Increasing knowledge of the genetic drivers of this event is leading to new therapeutic approaches.

INTRODUCTION

Transformed lymphoma is a complex syndrome that encompasses an array of different underlying low-grade lymphoproliferative conditions transforming into more aggressive disease as manifest by morphologic, clinical, and genetic features. Traditionally, transformed lymphoma has been considered difficult to treat and associated with poor prognosis. However, over the last decade, advances in chemoimmunotherapy have led to new options for affected patients and better outcomes. In more recent years, utilization of knowledge surrounding the genetic changes driving the process of transformation is leading to the development and application of novel targeted therapies. Such therapies are typically not associated with the same toxicities that have accompanied high-dose chemotherapy and stem cell transplantation (SCT) and, therefore, are often suitable for use in patients who have multiple comorbidities or are of advanced age. However, there is an ongoing unmet need for novel therapies among some patients with transformed lymphoma because many of the genetic aberrations seen converge on currently untargetable pathways, such as CDKN2A, MYC, or loss of TP53.

[a] Cancer and Haematology Division, Walter and Eliza Hall Institute of Medical Research, 1G Royal Parade, Parkville 3050, Australia; [b] Department of Clinical Hematology and Bone Marrow Transplantation, The Royal Melbourne Hospital, Parkville 3050, Australia; [c] Department of Haematology, Peter MacCallum Cancer Centre, Parkville 3050, Australia; [d] Faculty of Medicine, Dentistry and Health Sciences, The University of Melbourne, Parkville, Australia
* Corresponding author. Cancer and Haematology Division, Walter and Eliza Hall Institute of Medical Research, Parkville 3050, Australia.
E-mail address: manderson@wehi.edu.au

Hematol Oncol Clin N Am 30 (2016) 1317–1332
http://dx.doi.org/10.1016/j.hoc.2016.07.012
0889-8588/16/© 2016 Elsevier Inc. All rights reserved.

This article focuses on 2 of the more common scenarios: (1) the transformation of chronic lymphocytic leukemia (CLL) to diffuse large B-cell lymphoma (DLBCL), a process known as a Richter transformation (RT); and (2) the transformation of follicular lymphoma (FL) into DLBCL. For completeness, a variety of other less common situations in which transformation is recognized are described.

RICHTER TRANSFORMATION
Predisposing Factors for Richter Transformation Among Chronic Lymphocytic Leukemia Patients: Clinical and Genetic

RT is defined as the transformation of CLL into an aggressive lymphoma, most commonly DLBCL. Cumulatively, over the natural history of patients' course with CLL, RT occurs in between 5% to 20% of cases[1] and is a well-recognized and feared complication due to its poor prognosis (when compared with de novo DLBCL or CLL alone). Importantly, this inferior prognosis seems only to apply to cases in which the DLBCL is clonally related to the underlying CLL (eg, by demonstrating a shared immunoglobulin variable heavy chain [IGVH] usage). DLBCL arising in patients with CLL in whom there is not a clonal relationship to the preceding CLL (up to 20% of cases) has been reported to have a more favorable outcome.[2]

Rossi and colleagues[3] followed 185 CLL subjects from the time of CLL diagnosis to more accurately define the incidence and risk factors for RT. In this cohort, 17 subjects were diagnosed with an RT with an actuarial incidence of 13.6% and 16.2% at 5 and 10 years, respectively, with no further cases diagnosed beyond 82.5 months.[3] Among those subjects who developed RT, the median time to RT was 23 months from the diagnosis of CLL. In univariate analysis, lymph node bulk ($\geq$3 cm), higher numbers of nodal groups involved ($\geq$3), elevated serum levels of lactate dehydrogenase (LDH), diffuse bone marrow involvement, and more advanced Binet stage were all associated with a greater risk for transformation.[3] However, on multivariate analysis, only lymph node bulk remained independently associated with risk of transformation.[3] Other traditional clinical prognostic markers were not found to be associated with greater risk for transformation, including advanced age, poor performance status, Rai stage, cytopenias, lymphocyte count, splenomegaly, percentage bone marrow infiltration, and β_2-microglobulin (β_2M).[3] Importantly for therapeutic purposes, fludarabine exposure was not significantly associated with an increased risk of transformation.[3]

Numerous pathologic and genetic features have been associated with an increased risk of RT. The most potent of these seem to be (1) an unmutated IGVH, (2) the presence of NOTCH1 mutations, and (3) stereotypy of the B-cell receptor. IGVH 4–39 usage has also been associated with an increased risk of RT (particularly when occurring in cases with a NOTCH1 mutation).[4] Other features that have been associated with an increased risk of RT include CD38 expression, ZAP-70 expression, high-risk fluorescence in situ hybridization (FISH) lesions (eg, deletion 17p, deletion 11q), and trisomy 12 (**Box 1**).

Presentation of Richter Transformation: Clinical and Genetic Landscape at Transformation

Recognition of RT can be challenging. In advanced cases, patients can present with a fulminant illness characterized by florid B symptoms (including fatigue, reduced energy, reduction in performance status, significant unintentional weight loss, fevers, night sweats, malaise) and rapidly increasing lymphadenopathy and splenomegaly. In other cases, however, the presentation can be more subtle and even not recognized by less vigilant clinicians without a proactive approach to looking for the condition on lymph node biopsy or PET.[6,7]

Box 1
Clinical, immunophenotypic and genetic risk factors predisposing for Richter transformation among chronic lymphocytic leukemia patients

Clinical

Lymph node bulk ≥3 cm
  Univariate and multivariate[3]

≥3 nodal groups
  Univariate[3]

Elevated LDH
  Univariate[3]

Diffuse marrow involvement
  Univariate[3]

Advanced Binet stage
  Univariate[3,5]

Immunophenotypic

High CD38 expression

High ZAP-70 expression

Genetic

Unmutated IGVH[4]

NOTCH1[4]

Stereotypy of B-cell receptor[2,4]

IGVH 4–39 usage especially with NOTCH1 mutation[4]

Deletion 17p

Deletion 11q

Trisomy 12

Typical features of patients with newly diagnosed RT were reported in 1 study of 39 subjects with RT.[8] In this study, the clinical features at diagnosis included B symptoms (59%), progressive lymphadenopathy (64%), extranodal disease (41%), and elevated LDH (82%),[8] These features have been consistently noted in case series of RT since the late 1970s; other features reported include hepatosplenomegaly.[9]

Genomic analysis of paired samples suggests that, in most cases, the aggressive clone in RT directly evolves from the original CLL clone through acquisition of additional genetic lesions (linear evolution).[10] These genetic lesions converge on dysregulation of cell cycle control and activation of MYC. There are 2 predominant pathways through which this cell cycle/MYC dysregulation may occur:

1   Aberrancies of TP53, CDKN2A/B, and MYC: Acquired abnormalities in TP53 (either mutation or copy number loss) are a hallmark of CLL with poor prognosis. Although TP53 abnormalities can clearly exist within the CLL compartment without overt RT, TP53 abnormalities are acquired around the time of transformation in a proportion of patients.[2] In contrast, abnormalities in CDKN2A/B (typically copy number changes) are almost never observed in the CLL compartment and seem to be an RT-specific phenomenon.[11] In addition, abnormalities in MYC (either translocations, copy number amplifications, or mutations) tend to coexist with TP53/CDKN2A/B abnormalities and, in most cases, seem to occur around the time of transformation.[2]

2. Trisomy 12/NOTCH1 mutations. The presence of trisomy 12 and mutations that truncate the PEST domain of NOTCH1 result in a fertile ground for the development of RT. Unlike MYC/CDKN2A/B aberrancies, trisomy 12 and NOTCH1 mutations precede the development of RT in most cases (often by many years).[12] Notably, up-regulation of cell cycle–associated genes by gene expression profiling has been observed in trisomy 12 and NOTCH1-mutated CLL.[13] In addition, NOTCH1 signaling has been observed to induce MYC expression in T-acute lymphoblastic leukemia.[14]

The resultant clonally related DLBCL in RT is genetically distinct from both de novo DLBCL and clonally-unrelated DLBCL that arises concurrently in patients with CLL. RT is almost always of nongerminal center type when classified by immunohistochemistry.[2] Despite this, it does not display the typical mutational profile of an activated B-cell–subtype DLBCL.[2,10] The significantly inferior prognosis when compared with de novo DLBCL and the genetic differences, justify its consideration as a distinct entity.

Natural History and Prognosis of Richter Transformation

The median survival reported in the literature after the diagnosis of RT varies from 8 months[1] to 16.5 months[3]; however, the event of RT is universally considered to convey a far inferior prognosis than would be expected among the group of CLL patients as a whole. The variability in prognosis may in part relate to institutional and clinician-specific approaches to active surveillance for the condition, such as early lymph node biopsy potentially introducing lead-time basis into many estimates of survival.

A retrospective study of 148 patients with proven RT treated at the MD Anderson Cancer Center identified the following clinical and laboratory features as risk factors for adverse outcome in RT: poor performance status, elevated LDH, thrombocytopenia, bulky lymphadenopathy ($\geq$5 cm), and more than 2 prior lines of therapy.[15] The investigators found that the more of these adverse prognostic factors were present, the worse the survival. Using these prognostic factors the investigators developed a scoring system in which patients with zero to 1 risk factors had a median survival of 1.1 years, whereas those with 3 risk factors had a median survival of 0.33 years.[15]

More systematic elucidation of the genetic features predicting for outcome in confirmed cases of RT is important, given the range of survival reported in the disease, to better target therapy to more precise prognostic information.

Therapeutic Options for Richter Transformation

Tsimberidou and colleagues,[15] retrospectively report on the outcomes of 148 RT patients managed at the MD Anderson Cancer Center of whom 130 received active disease-directed treatment. The therapies used varied widely but included nucleoside-analog–based purine (18%); alternating fractionated cyclophosphamide, vincristine, doxorubicin, and dexamethasone with high-dose methotrexate and cytarabine (hyper-CVAD) and variants (16%); cyclophosphamide, adriamycin, vincristine and prednisolone (CHOP)-like therapy (8%); and other therapies (19%), including cytarabine, ifosfamide, and etoposide.[15] Notably, approximately 60% of these patients were managed in the pre-rituximab (R) era,[15] potentially limiting the applicability of these findings in the current therapeutic environment. Among patients treated with chemotherapy alone, 11% achieved a complete remission (CR) and 66% had no response to therapy. The outcomes were only slightly better among the immunochemotherapy cohort, with 13% achieving CR and 63% having no response.[15] Among this group of patients with RT, 20 received SCT. Patients receiving SCT were treated with a variety of regimens, including chemotherapy and chemoimmunotherapy, and most patients did not obtain a CR before transplant. For the patients who went into allograft while in CR or PR, the 3 year survival was approximately 75%, in contrast to 27% among the patients who achieved CR or PR with initial therapy but did not proceed to allograft and 21% among the patients who underwent transplant with relapsed or refractory RT.[15] Indeed, receipt of an allogeneic stem cell transplant was independently associated with prolonged survival in RT.[15] This suggests that the specific initial therapy is less important than the ability to achieve disease response and proceed to allograft as consolidation.

Notably, the chemotherapeutic regimens used in the MD Anderson cohort were relatively intensive and many patients presenting with RT are unfit for such regimens, and given that the median age at diagnosis of CLL is 72 years, most patients developing RT will unfortunately not be eligible for allogeneic SCT. The patients who did not receive allograft had a poor prognosis, highlighting the urgent clinical need for novel agents to manage this disease with less toxicity and greater efficacy.

One of the challenges in evaluating novel therapies in RT is that in many studies specifically exclude transformed lymphoma, including RT, meaning that there is limited evidence available. However, extrapolating from early phase data on Burton tyrosine kinase inhibitor (BTKi) ibrutinib, 7 out of 11 subjects whose CLL progressed on this agent developed RT.[16] Because many of these events occurred early in the study, it has been hypothesized that they represent residual nonresponsive disease that was present at study entry. In contrast, the BCL2 inhibitor venetoclax has been tested in phase I studies among 7 subjects with RT with an overall response rate (ORR) of 43%.[17]

Chronic Lymphocytic Leukemia Transformed to Prolymphocytic Leukemia

B prolymphocytic leukemia (B-PLL) is a monoclonal B cell neoplasm in which greater than 55% of the circulating malignant cells in the peripheral blood are prolymphocytes (large lymphocytes with prominent nucleolus). The disease can arise de novo or in the context of pre-existing CLL in which the prolymphocytes can be shown to be genetically transformed with clonal differentiation from the underlying CLL.[18] Transformed B-PLL is immuno-phenotypically distinct from both de novo B-PLL and the underlying CLL. A possible genetic contributor to prolymphocytic transformation of CLL was the observation of high levels of activation-induced cytidine deaminase and aberrant somatic hypermutation in patient samples with transformed disease.[19]

Although there is a spectrum of disease with prolymphocytes ranging from 55% to 100% of the circulating malignant cells, increasing circulating prolymphocyte percentage in CLL is often accompanied by worsening clinical symptoms requiring therapy.[18] Similarly to CLL that undergoes RT to DLBCL, transformation to B-PLL represents a change in the clinical behavior of the CLL to a disease that is less chemotherapy responsive and carries an inferior prognosis.[20]

Chronic Lymphocytic Leukemia Transformed to Hodgkin Lymphoma

Transformation of CLL to Hodgkin lymphoma is well described but much less common than the more typical RT to DLBCL, with only 86 cases described in the literature as of 2012.[21] This phenomenon is predominantly seen in older men and usually occurs within 5 years of the original CLL diagnosis.[21] Like RT to DLBCL, the occurrence of HL in patients with CLL portends a poor prognosis. However, it is not as profoundly adverse as DLBCL RT, with a mean survival of only 2.1 years, despite treatment in most cases with multiagent chemotherapy, such as adriamycin, bleomycin, vinblastine, and dacarbazine (AVBD).[11] However other case series have shown inferior survival with 50% cumulative survival at 12 months reported.[22] Survival is even worse among patients whose CLL has previously been treated with fludarabine-containing regimens (mean survival of only 0.7 years).[21]

As with most cases of transformed lymphoma, Hodgkin lymphoma arising in the setting of CLL has been shown to be clonally related to the underlying CLL. Sequencing of IGVH in microdissected Reed Sternberg cells has demonstrated that the Hodgkin lymphoma is clonally identical to the underlying CLL[23] in some cases. Although subject numbers remain limited, 1 study has found that most cases of CLL transformed to HL, and have evidence of Epstein Barr virus infection and unmutated IGVH.[23]

TRANSFORMED FOLLICULAR LYMPHOMA
Incidence and Risk Factors for Transformation in Follicular Lymphoma

Transformation of FL (typically to DLBCL) is a clinicopathological diagnosis characterized by histologic change in the lymphoma from small centrocyte cells with a follicular growth pattern to that of a disordered large cell growth pattern.[24] The definition implies that the DLBCL is clonally related to the FL. Accompanying transformation, the lymphoma typically develops the clinical behavior of an aggressive lymphoma-producing B symptoms, rapid enlargement of lymph nodes, and evidence of rapid cell turnover (eg, elevated LDH).

The reported incidence of transformed FL (t-FL) in the literature varies widely but is thought to be approximately 2% to 3% per year, implying that the cumulative incidence increases with duration of FL.[25] Some groups, however, report a plateau in the incidence of transformation beyond 15 to 20 years.[25] Disappointingly, this incidence seems unaltered in the post-R era,[26] suggesting that the risk of transformation is an inherent characteristic of the natural history of FL and not altered by more potent therapeutic intervention, at least those currently applied. Furthermore, the outcomes of early therapeutic intervention studies on the incidence of transformation have been contradictory. Some studies suggest benefit in terms of the risk transformation among patients whose FL was treated early and aggressively to maximize disease control.[26–29] Other studies, however, have demonstrated that the chemotherapy regimen used (eg, chlorambucil versus multiagent CHOP) and the degree of response to therapy (eg, partial remission [PR] versus CR) have no effect on the risk of transformation.[30]

A variety of risk factors have been associated with the development of transformed disease in FL on either univariate or multivariate analysis. Frequently, reported risk factors include elevated LDH,[26,27,30] advanced age,[26,27] high Follicular Lymphoma International Prognostic Index (FLIPI) or International Prognostic Index (IPI),[26,27,30] grade 3 FL histology,[27,30] cytopenias,[27] extranodal disease,[29] more than 3 nodal areas involved,[30] and elevated $\beta_2 M$[30] (**Box 2**).

Several putative genetic markers have been identified as predisposing for transformation in FL. In 1 study of 21 subjects who progressed to DLBCL and 16 subjects who did not, 4 out of 5 of the subjects who transformed harbored a TP53 mutation compared with none of the subjects who did not transform,[31] suggesting that TP53 mutations are a risk factor for transformation in FL. Another study identified FL subjects who harbored BCL6 translocations as at significantly increased risk of transformation[32] (see **Box 2**). Importantly, in view of its high incidence in FL (27%), EZH2 mutations do not seem to predict for t-FL[33] and, among patients with high FLIPI, may even be protective against transformation.[34]

Box 2
Clinical and genetic risk factors predisposing for transformation among follicular lymphoma patients

Clinical

Elevated LDH[26,27,30]

Advanced age[26,27]

High FLIPI score[26,27,30]

Grade 3 histology[27,30]

Cytopenias[27]

Extranodal disease[29]

$\geq$3 nodal areas[30]

Elevated $\beta_2 M$[30]

Genetic

TP53 mutation[31]

BCL6 translocations[32]

Presentation of Transformed Disease: Clinical and Genetic Landscape at Transformation

The gold standard for the diagnosis of transformation in FL is a biopsy demonstrating DLBCL in a patient with a previously confirmed diagnosis of FL. Clinically, the disease presents with a change in the tempo of disease progression. Characteristic clinical features may include new onset of hypercalcemia, new involvement of extranodal sites, rapid discordant lymph node growth, B symptoms, declining performance status, progressive cytopenias, and an elevated LDH.[25,26] Many patients with transformed disease will demonstrate greater fluorodeoxyglucose (FDG) uptake on PET scan compared with patients with FL alone.[35,36] In a study of 38 subjects with transformation from low-grade to high-grade lymphoma a maximum standardized uptake value (SUV_{max}) greater than 14 had a sensitivity for transformation of 93.9% and a specificity of 95.3%, whereas an SUV_{max} greater than 17 had a 100% positive predictive value for transformation.[37] In this same study, none of the subjects with SUV_{max} less than 11.7 had transformed disease.[37]

Transformation of FL (in most cases) occurs as a result of the aggressive clone arising from a common progenitor cell (CPC). This CPC is hypothesized to be the ancestral clone from which both the low-grade and high-grade components are derived (divergent evolution)[38] (Fig. 1). This is in contrast to the predominantly linear evolution that is observed in RT in CLL. The pattern of divergent evolution seen in t-FL is consistent with emerging data that suggest that, even in the indolent phase, FL harbors an unexpectedly high-degree of clonal complexity.[39] Another difference between RT and t-FL is that the gene expression profile and molecular lesions seen in t-FL are most similar to that seen in de novo germinal center B (GCB) diffuse large B-cell lymphoma as opposed to the nongerminal center subtype that predominates in RT.[40]

Despite the differences in the evolutionary and cell-of-origin classification, there is significant similarity between underlying genetic lesions seen in t-FL and RT, namely aberrations of TP53, MYC, and CDKN2A/B. Cell cycle dysregulation as a result of copy number loss (or copy number neutral loss of heterozygosity) of CDKN2A/B seems to be a relatively specific event occurring almost exclusively in the transformed

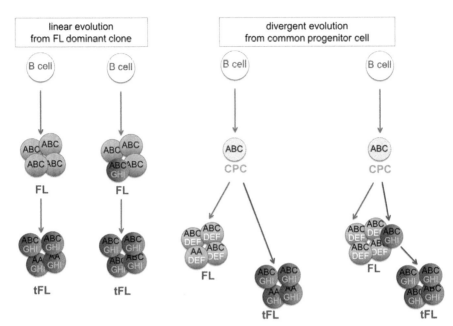

Fig. 1. Linear and divergent clonal evolution in FL. During the genetic evolution of FL to transformed disease multiple genetic subfamilies arise from the CPCs that lead to disease recurrence at different sites, and eventually transformation. ABC, DEF, GHI refer to genetic subfamilies arising during the evolution of FL. (*From* Pasqualucci L, Khiabanian H, Fangazio M, et al. Genetics of follicular lymphoma transformation. Cell Rep 2014;6:132; with permission.)

stage of disease and not in FL.[40] Dysregulation of MYC in t-FL may be the result of translocations or high level copy number gains.[40] Finally, TP53 function may be lost in t-FL through either copy number change, mutation or copy number neutral loss of heterozygosity.[40,41] As noted previously, TP53 dysfunction predicts for both the development of t-FL[31] and, as in most cancers, when present is a marker of more aggressive disease. Other genetic changes that have been observed accompanying transformation include amplification of REL (2p16), BCL6 (3q27-q29), and BCL2 (18q21).[42]

Natural History and Prognosis of Transformed-Follicular Lymphoma

Historically, the prognosis of t-FL has been quite poor. A retrospective study of 88 subjects with t-FL demonstrated a median overall survival (OS) from the time of transformation of only 1.2 years in the pre-R era.[27] As is the case in de novo DLBCL, the introduction of R to multiagent chemotherapy backbones (eg, CHOP) has been shown to significantly improve the progression-free survival (PFS) and OS of t-FL such that, in a more contemporary cohort of 34 transformed subjects, of whom 16 received R-CHOP and 13 received non-R containing combination chemotherapy, the addition of R increased the 3-year PFS to 78% versus 15% (P<.00001).[43]

Factors associated with inferior survival included second or subsequent presentation with DLBCL,[27] early versus late transformation from the time of diagnosis of FL,[26] more extensive disease,[44] higher LDH,[27] prior exposure to chemoimmunotherapy for FL,[45] achievement of PR as opposed to CR,[44] and worse performance status.[27] The National Comprehensive Cancer Network (NCCN) has established a

DLBCL-specific IPI (NCCN-IPI) that scores a patient's risk based on age, LDH, Ann Arbor stage, performance status, and extranodal disease.[46] This scoring system is particularly powerful because it has recently been validated in patients with transformed disease as well as the de novo population.[47]

Therapeutic Options at Transformation

As discussed previously, the role of combination chemoimmunotherapy is well established to improve survival in t-FL.[26,27,43] However, several questions regarding the optimal management of these patients remain under active investigation; in particular, (1) the role of consolidation autograft or allograft and (2) novel therapies in this high-risk group.

In the pre-R era, many studies of autologous SCT (ASCT) as consolidation therapy for t-FL were limited by small numbers of subjects, retrospective rather than prospective data, lack of randomized controlled trials, mixed histology, and highly selected subject cohorts. However, most demonstrated an improvement in survival with consolidation autograft[27] over combination chemotherapy alone, with reported survival ranging from 3-year PFS of 40%,[48] and 5-year PFS of 30% to 56%.[49–52] In the post-R era, the outcomes of autograft consolidation studies have varied. Some studies suggested improved outcomes with autograft over chemoimmunotherapy alone for t-FL[53] and others showed no overall benefit from autograft.[54] Again, however, interpretation is limited by small sample sizes and nonrandomized, often retrospective, data. In the face of these contradictory data, the authors' recommendation is for autograft in those in whom the transformed disease cannot be encompassed in a tolerable radiation field that would allow consolidative RT, and in whom predicted mortality from an autograft is less than 5%.

As with the autograft data, most of the evidence for allograft in t-FL comes from retrospective series, predominantly among subjects who have relapsed after autograft. Although some studies show improved outcomes with allograft, most report significant treatment-related mortality (TRM). A study of 172 subjects variously treated with allograft (13%), autograft (56%), or R-containing combination chemotherapy (31%) for t-FL demonstrated no improvement in outcome for allograft compared with autograft and at the cost of significantly greater toxicity.[53] Given the high rate of TRM across multiple studies for allograft in this group of patients,[54,55] the role of reduced-intensity conditioning regimens have been explored with some success in terms of more favorable toxicity profiles.[5,56] Currently the authors recommend allograft for

- Young patients with a predicted TRM of less than 15%
- Those who do not achieve a CR with their induction regimen
- Those with recurrent transformed disease after a prior autograft.

Clinical trials with novel agents often specifically exclude subjects with t-FL to ensure homogeny of data. Additionally, heterogeneity of disease in terms of evolution of FL to DLBCL at different sites via nonlinear transformation means that there are often multiple subpopulations of both FL and DLBCL present within any given individual.[40,57,58] This makes finding distinct genetic aberrations that may be susceptible to targeted novel agents challenging. Unfortunately, this also means there is a paucity of literature pertaining to use of novel approaches in this population.

Small studies (between 7 and 14 subjects) of the radioimmunotherapeutic agents yttrium (Y^{90}) ibritumomab, and iodine (I^{131}) tositumomab have been performed in t-FL, showing response rates between 56% and 79%, with a median duration of response ranging from 13.9–41.0 months.[59–62] However, these were likely relatively highly selected patients, given the requirement for minimal marrow involvement, and these agents are no longer commercially available.

Other investigators have studied the role of small molecules in the management of t-FL. Single agent lenalidomide, an immune-modulatory agent, has been tested specifically in 23 subjects with transformed FL and shown to have an ORR of 57% with a median duration of response of 12.8 months.[63] Venetoclax (ABT-199), a BCL2 selective inhibitor, has been tested in FL, DLBCL, and transformed disease in which it has been associated with ORRs of 38%, 18%, and 43%, respectively.[64] A study of alisertib, a selective aurora A kinase inhibitor, in 5 subjects with t-FL had an ORR of 2 out of 5 subjects.[65] In a study of ibrutinib combined with bendamustine in subjects with transformed disease, efficacy was limited although numbers remain small.[66] More promisingly, however, in another study that included relapsed and refractory FL and DLBCL subjects, single-agent ibrutinib was associated with an ORR of 60%.[67]

Although outcomes have improved in t-FL, especially with the introduction of R-based chemoimmunotherapy, the paucity of large randomized studies in this not uncommon group of patients is a major limitation. Although autograft has an established role in terms of prolonged survival, the role of allograft and novel therapies remains unclear, highlighting the need for better quality data to drive practice going forward.

Transformed Lymphoplasmacytic Lymphoma

The incidence of lymphoplasmacytic lymphoma (LPL) transforming to DLBCL has been reported as high as 13%.[68] Although the diagnoses of LPL and DLBCL may occasionally occur simultaneously, the DLBCL is typically diagnosed after a period of more indolent disease, with a median time to diagnosis in 1 series of 44 months from the diagnosis of LPL.[68] Clinically, the development of DLBCL in the setting of LPL is characterized by a change in behavior with a reduction in performance status, increasing cytopenias, organomegaly, rapid increase in lymphadenopathy, and rising LDH.[68] Such patients typically follow a fulminant course with poor response to therapy and short OS, with 73% of patients dead from disease within 10 months of transformation.[68] It is recommended that this be managed as per transformed FL, with a greater tendency to consolidate with a high-dose therapy procedure in eligible patients.

Unfortunately, there are no clinicopathological features of LPL that predict for the risk of transformation to DLBCL.[68] Common to other forms of transformation, the 2 diseases seem to be clonally related with identical immunoglobulin light chain expression in the LPL and DLBCL cells.[68] Compared with cases of pure LPL, patients with transformation to DLBCL demonstrate markedly abnormal and complex karyotypes.[68]

LESS COMMON TRANSFORMATION SCENARIOS
Blastic Transformation of Mantle Cell Lymphoma

Blastoid variant of mantle cell lymphoma (MCL) is a histologically defined entity that can arise de novo or in the context of pre-existing morphologically typical MCL. Blastoid MCL is identified microscopically by malignant cells with rounder nuclei and more dispersed chromatin, often with nucleoli.[69] Blastoid MCL often has a high proliferation index compared with typical MCL.[70] Blastoid variant of MCL has an inferior outcome to standard MCL with a median survival of 18 months compared with 50 months among those with typical histology.[71] The development of blastoid morphology in patients with typical MCL often portends a change in clinical behavior to a more aggressive course, and greater propensity for central nervous system infiltration.[72]

MCL is characterized by cyclin D1 overexpression due to juxtaposition with the immunoglobulin heavy chain (IGH) locus. This is detected with conventional cytogenetics by t(11;14). Although 8q24 abnormalities with overexpression of c-MYC are rare in MCL, they have been reported in blastoid variants at increased frequency, including as part of a complex karyotype containing t(11;14) as well as t(8;14) or t(2;8). Such cases typically involve a leukemic phase of the disease.[73]

Transformed Splenic Marginal Zone Lymphoma

Splenic marginal zone lymphoma (SMZL) is another typically indolent lymphoma, which can transform into DLBCL. The change in histology from SMZL to DLBCL is accompanied by a change in the clinical characteristics of the disease from an indolent to an aggressive lymphoma. The DLBCL can occur at the time of diagnosis of the SMZL and may also occur many years after initial diagnosis.[74] Polymerase chain reaction studies of the IGH gene confirm that the 2 diseases are clonally related.[74]

SUMMARY

Transformed lymphoma remains a key challenge in the field, presenting as it does in a myriad of guises and being predominantly a disease of aging whereby high-dose therapies are often contraindicated. However, with the evolution of genetic tools for interrogating the genome of lymphoma, the predisposing genetic features of low-grade processes that may lead to transformation are becoming clearer. Additionally a comprehensive picture of the key molecular drivers of transformation is emerging. This knowledge is critical to improvement in patient outcomes in the future by (1) identifying and targeting low-grade processes early in the disease when risk factors for transformation are present and (2) manipulating the genetic drivers of transformation for safer and more effective therapies.

REFERENCES

1. Tsimberidou AM, Keating MJ. Richter syndrome: biology, incidence, and therapeutic strategies. Cancer 2005;103:216–28.
2. Rossi D, Spina V, Deambrogi C, et al. The genetics of Richter syndrome reveals disease heterogeneity and predicts survival after transformation. Blood 2011;117: 3391–401.
3. Rossi D, Cerri M, Capello D, et al. Biological and clinical risk factors of chronic lymphocytic leukaemia transformation to Richter syndrome. Br J Haematol 2008;142:202–15.
4. Rossi D, Rasi S, Spina V, et al. Different impact of NOTCH1 and SF3B1 mutations on the risk of chronic lymphocytic leukemia transformation to Richter syndrome. Br J Haematol 2012;158:426–9.
5. Thomson KJ, Morris EC, Bloor A, et al. Favorable long-term survival after reduced-intensity allogeneic transplantation for multiple-relapse aggressive non-Hodgkin's lymphoma. J Clin Oncol 2009;27:426–32.
6. Papajik T, Myslivecek M, Urbanova R, et al. 2-[18F]fluoro-2-deoxy-D-glucose positron emission tomography/computed tomography examination in patients with chronic lymphocytic leukemia may reveal Richter transformation. Leuk Lymphoma 2014;55:314–9.
7. Mauro FR, Chauvie S, Paoloni F, et al. Diagnostic and prognostic role of PET/CT in patients with chronic lymphocytic leukemia and progressive disease. Leukemia 2015;29:1360–5.

8. Robertson LE, Pugh W, O'Brien S, et al. Richter's syndrome: a report on 39 patients. J Clin Oncol 1993;11:1985–9.

9. Foucar K, Rydell RE. Richter's syndrome in chronic lymphocytic leukemia. Cancer 1980;46:118–34.

10. Fabbri G, Khiabanian H, Holmes AB, et al. Genetic lesions associated with chronic lymphocytic leukemia transformation to Richter syndrome. J Exp Med 2013;210:2273–88.

11. Chigrinova E, Rinaldi A, Kwee I, et al. Two main genetic pathways lead to the transformation of chronic lymphocytic leukemia to Richter syndrome. Blood 2013;122:2673–82.

12. Fabbri G, Rasi S, Rossi D, et al. Analysis of the chronic lymphocytic leukemia coding genome: role of NOTCH1 mutational activation. J Exp Med 2011;208: 1389–401.

13. Del Giudice I, Rossi D, Chiaretti S, et al. NOTCH1 mutations in +12 chronic lymphocytic leukemia (CLL) confer an unfavorable prognosis, induce a distinctive transcriptional profiling and refine the intermediate prognosis of +12 CLL. Haematologica 2012;97:437–41.

14. Palomero T, Lim WK, Odom DT, et al. NOTCH1 directly regulates c-MYC and activates a feed-forward-loop transcriptional network promoting leukemic cell growth. Proc Natl Acad Sci U S A 2006;103:18261–6.

15. Tsimberidou AM, O'Brien S, Khouri I, et al. Clinical outcomes and prognostic factors in patients with Richter's syndrome treated with chemotherapy or chemoimmunotherapy with or without stem-cell transplantation. J Clin Oncol 2006;24: 2343–51.

16. Byrd JC, Furman RR, Coutre SE, et al. Targeting BTK with ibrutinib in relapsed chronic lymphocytic leukemia. N Engl J Med 2013;369:32–42.

17. Gerecitano JF, Roberts AW, Seymour JF, et al. A phase 1 study of venetoclax (ABT-199/GDC-0199) monotherapy in patients with relapsed/refractory non-Hodgkin lymphoma. Blood 2015;126:254.

18. Ghani AM, Krause JR, Brody JP. Prolymphocytic transformation of chronic lymphocytic leukemia. A report of three cases and review of the literature. Cancer 1986;57:75–80.

19. Reiniger L, Bodor C, Bognar A, et al. Richter's and prolymphocytic transformation of chronic lymphocytic leukemia are associated with high mRNA expression of activation-induced cytidine deaminase and aberrant somatic hypermutation. Leukemia 2006;20:1089–95.

20. Melo JV, Catovsky D, Galton DA. The relationship between chronic lymphocytic leukaemia and prolymphocytic leukaemia. II. Patterns of evolution of 'prolymphocytoid' transformation. Br J Haematol 1986;64:77–86.

21. Bockorny B, Codreanu I, Dasanu CA. Hodgkin lymphoma as Richter transformation in chronic lymphocytic leukaemia: a retrospective analysis of world literature. Br J Haematol 2012;156:50–66.

22. Brecher M, Banks PM. Hodgkin's disease variant of Richter's syndrome. Report of eight cases. Am J Clin Pathol 1990;93:333–9.

23. Mao Z, Quintanilla-Martinez L, Raffeld M, et al. IgVH mutational status and clonality analysis of Richter's transformation: diffuse large B-cell lymphoma and Hodgkin lymphoma in association with B-cell chronic lymphocytic leukemia (B-CLL) represent 2 different pathways of disease evolution. Am J Surg Pathol 2007;31:1605–14.

24. Casulo C, Burack WR, Friedberg JW. Transformed follicular non-Hodgkin lymphoma. Blood 2015;125:40–7.

25. Al-Tourah AJ, Gill KK, Chhanabhai M, et al. Population-based analysis of incidence and outcome of transformed non-Hodgkin's lymphoma. J Clin Oncol 2008;26:5165–9.

26. Link BK, Maurer MJ, Nowakowski GS, et al. Rates and outcomes of follicular lymphoma transformation in the immunochemotherapy era: a report from the University of Iowa/MayoClinic Specialized Program of Research Excellence Molecular Epidemiology Resource. J Clin Oncol 2013;31:3272–8.

27. Montoto S, Davies AJ, Matthews J, et al. Risk and clinical implications of transformation of follicular lymphoma to diffuse large B-cell lymphoma. J Clin Oncol 2007; 25:2426–33.

28. Horning SJ, Rosenberg SA. The natural history of initially untreated low-grade non-Hodgkin's lymphomas. N Engl J Med 1984;311:1471–5.

29. Conconi A, Ponzio C, Lobetti-Bodoni C, et al. Incidence, risk factors and outcome of histological transformation in follicular lymphoma. Br J Haematol 2012;157: 188–96.

30. Gine E, Montoto S, Bosch F, et al. The Follicular Lymphoma International Prognostic Index (FLIPI) and the histological subtype are the most important factors to predict histological transformation in follicular lymphoma. Ann Oncol 2006; 17:1539–45.

31. Lo Coco F, Gaidano G, Louie DC, et al. p53 mutations are associated with histologic transformation of follicular lymphoma. Blood 1993;82:2289–95.

32. Akasaka T, Lossos IS, Levy R. BCL6 gene translocation in follicular lymphoma: a harbinger of eventual transformation to diffuse aggressive lymphoma. Blood 2003;102:1443–8.

33. Bodor C, Grossmann V, Popov N, et al. EZH2 mutations are frequent and represent an early event in follicular lymphoma. Blood 2013;122:3165–8.

34. Pastore A, Jurinovic V, Kridel R, et al. Integration of gene mutations in risk prognostication for patients receiving first-line immunochemotherapy for follicular lymphoma: a retrospective analysis of a prospective clinical trial and validation in a population-based registry. Lancet Oncol 2015;16:1111–22.

35. Karam M, Novak L, Cyriac J, et al. Role of fluorine-18 fluoro-deoxyglucose positron emission tomography scan in the evaluation and follow-up of patients with low-grade lymphomas. Cancer 2006;107:175–83.

36. Noy A, Schoder H, Gonen M, et al. The majority of transformed lymphomas have high standardized uptake values (SUVs) on positron emission tomography (PET) scanning similar to diffuse large B-cell lymphoma (DLBCL). Ann Oncol 2009;20: 508–12.

37. Bodet-Milin C, Kraeber-Bodere F, Moreau P, et al. Investigation of FDG-PET/CT imaging to guide biopsies in the detection of histological transformation of indolent lymphoma. Haematologica 2008;93:471–2.

38. Okosun J, Bodor C, Wang J, et al. Integrated genomic analysis identifies recurrent mutations and evolution patterns driving the initiation and progression of follicular lymphoma. Nat Genet 2014;46:176–81.

39. Carlotti E, Wrench D, Rosignoli G, et al. High throughput sequencing analysis of the immunoglobulin heavy chain gene from flow-sorted B cell sub-populations define the dynamics of follicular lymphoma clonal evolution. PLoS One 2015; 10:e0134833.

40. Pasqualucci L, Khiabanian H, Fangazio M, et al. Genetics of follicular lymphoma transformation. Cell Rep 2014;6:130–40.

41. Fitzgibbon J, Iqbal S, Davies A, et al. Genome-wide detection of recurring sites of uniparental disomy in follicular and transformed follicular lymphoma. Leukemia 2007;21:1514–20.

42. Martinez Climent JA, Alizadeh AA, Segraves R, et al. Transformation of follicular lymphoma to diffuse large cell lymphoma is associated with a heterogeneous set of DNA copy number and gene expression alterations. Blood 2003;101: 3109–17.

43. Bains P, Al Tourah A, Campbell BA, et al. Incidence of transformation to aggressive lymphoma in limited-stage follicular lymphoma treated with radiotherapy. Ann Oncol 2013;24:428–32.

44. Yuen AR, Kamel OW, Halpern J, et al. Long-term survival after histologic transformation of low-grade follicular lymphoma. J Clin Oncol 1995;13:1726–33.

45. Ban-Hoefen M, Vanderplas A, Crosby-Thompson AL, et al. Transformed non-Hodgkin lymphoma in the rituximab era: analysis of the NCCN outcomes database. Br J Haematol 2013;163:487–95.

46. Zhou Z, Sehn LH, Rademaker AW, et al. An enhanced International Prognostic Index (NCCN-IPI) for patients with diffuse large B-cell lymphoma treated in the rituximab era. Blood 2014;123:837–42.

47. Spiegel JY, Cheung MC, Guirguis HR, et al. Validation of the NCC-IPI in both de novo and transformed diffuse large B cell lymphoma. Leuk Lymphoma 2016;1–4.

48. Hamadani M, Benson DM Jr, Lin TS, et al. High-dose therapy and autologous stem cell transplantation for follicular lymphoma undergoing transformation to diffuse large B-cell lymphoma. Eur J Haematol 2008;81:425–31.

49. Williams CD, Harrison CN, Lister TA, et al. High-dose therapy and autologous stem-cell support for chemosensitive transformed low-grade follicular non-Hodgkin's lymphoma: a case-matched study from the European Bone Marrow Transplant Registry. J Clin Oncol 2001;19:727–35.

50. Chen CI, Crump M, Tsang R, et al. Autotransplants for histologically transformed follicular non-Hodgkin's lymphoma. Br J Haematol 2001;113:202–8.

51. Friedberg JW, Neuberg D, Gribben JG, et al. Autologous bone marrow transplantation after histologic transformation of indolent B cell malignancies. Biol Blood Marrow Transplant 1999;5:262–8.

52. Sabloff M, Atkins HL, Bence-Bruckler I, et al. A 15-year analysis of early and late autologous hematopoietic stem cell transplant in relapsed, aggressive, transformed, and nontransformed follicular lymphoma. Biol Blood Marrow Transplant 2007;13:956–64.

53. Villa D, Crump M, Panzarella T, et al. Autologous and allogeneic stem-cell transplantation for transformed follicular lymphoma: a report of the Canadian blood and marrow transplant group. J Clin Oncol 2013;31:1164–71.

54. Wirk B, Fenske TS, Hamadani M, et al. Outcomes of hematopoietic cell transplantation for diffuse large B cell lymphoma transformed from follicular lymphoma. Biol Blood Marrow Transplant 2014;20:951–9.

55. Doocey RT, Toze CL, Connors JM, et al. Allogeneic haematopoietic stem-cell transplantation for relapsed and refractory aggressive histology non-Hodgkin lymphoma. Br J Haematol 2005;131:223–30.

56. Clavert A, Le Gouill S, Brissot E, et al. Reduced-intensity conditioning allogeneic stem cell transplant for relapsed or transformed aggressive B-cell non-Hodgkin lymphoma. Leuk Lymphoma 2010;51:1502–8.

57. Wartenberg M, Vasil P, zum Bueschenfelde CM, et al. Somatic hypermutation analysis in follicular lymphoma provides evidence suggesting bidirectional cell

migration between lymph node and bone marrow during disease progression and relapse. Haematologica 2013;98:1433–41.

58. Carlotti E, Wrench D, Matthews J, et al. Transformation of follicular lymphoma to diffuse large B-cell lymphoma may occur by divergent evolution from a common progenitor cell or by direct evolution from the follicular lymphoma clone. Blood 2009;113:3553–7.

59. Kaminski MS, Zelenetz AD, Press OW, et al. Pivotal study of iodine I 131 tositumomab for chemotherapy-refractory low-grade or transformed low-grade B-cell non-Hodgkin's lymphomas. J Clin Oncol 2001;19:3918–28.

60. Vose JM, Wahl RL, Saleh M, et al. Multicenter phase II study of iodine-131 tositumomab for chemotherapy-relapsed/refractory low-grade and transformed low-grade B-cell non-Hodgkin's lymphomas. J Clin Oncol 2000;18:1316–23.

61. Davies AJ, Rohatiner AZ, Howell S, et al. Tositumomab and iodine I 131 tositumomab for recurrent indolent and transformed B-cell non-Hodgkin's lymphoma. J Clin Oncol 2004;22:1469–79.

62. Witzig TE, Flinn IW, Gordon LI, et al. Treatment with ibritumomab tiuxetan radioimmunotherapy in patients with rituximab-refractory follicular non-Hodgkin's lymphoma. J Clin Oncol 2002;20:3262–9.

63. Czuczman MS, Vose JM, Witzig TE, et al. The differential effect of lenalidomide monotherapy in patients with relapsed or refractory transformed non-Hodgkin lymphoma of distinct histological origin. Br J Haematol 2011;154:477–81.

64. Gerecitano JF, Roberts AW, Seymour JF, et al. A phase 1 study of Venetoclax (ABT-199/GDC-0199) monotherapy in patients with relapsed/refractory non-Hodgkin lymphoma. New Orleands (LA): American Society of Haematology; 2015.

65. Friedberg JW, Mahadevan D, Cebula E, et al. Phase II study of alisertib, a selective Aurora A kinase inhibitor, in relapsed and refractory aggressive B- and T-cell non-Hodgkin lymphomas. J Clin Oncol 2014;32:44–50.

66. Blum KA, Christian B, Flynn JM, et al. A phase I trial of the Bruton's tyrosine kinase (BTK) inhibitor, ibrutinib (PCI-32765), in combination with rituximab (R) and bendamustine in patients with relapsed/refractory non-Hodgkin's lymphoma (NHL). Blood 2012;120:1643.

67. Advani RH, Buggy JJ, Sharman JP, et al. Bruton tyrosine kinase inhibitor ibrutinib (PCI-32765) has significant activity in patients with relapsed/refractory B-cell malignancies. J Clin Oncol 2013;31:88–94.

68. Lin P, Mansoor A, Bueso-Ramos C, et al. Diffuse large B-cell lymphoma occurring in patients with lymphoplasmacytic lymphoma/Waldenstrom macroglobulinemia. Clinicopathologic features of 12 cases. Am J Clin Pathol 2003;120:246–53.

69. Bea S, Ribas M, Hernandez JM, et al. Increased number of chromosomal imbalances and high-level DNA amplifications in mantle cell lymphoma are associated with blastoid variants. Blood 1999;93:4365–74.

70. Ott G, Kalla J, Ott MM, et al. Blastoid variants of mantle cell lymphoma: frequent bcl-1 rearrangements at the major translocation cluster region and tetraploid chromosome clones. Blood 1997;89:1421–9.

71. Bosch F, Lopez-Guillermo A, Campo E, et al. Mantle cell lymphoma: presenting features, response to therapy, and prognostic factors. Cancer 1998;82:567–75.

72. Cheah CY, George A, Gine E, et al. Central nervous system involvement in mantle cell lymphoma: clinical features, prognostic factors and outcomes from the European Mantle Cell Lymphoma Network. Ann Oncol 2013;24:2119–23.

73. Hao S, Sanger W, Onciu M, et al. Mantle cell lymphoma with 8q24 chromosomal abnormalities: a report of 5 cases with blastoid features. Mod Pathol 2002;15: 1266–72.

74. Camacho FI, Mollejo M, Mateo MS, et al. Progression to large B-cell lymphoma in splenic marginal zone lymphoma: a description of a series of 12 cases. Am J Surg Pathol 2001;25:1268–76.

Update on Burkitt Lymphoma

 CrossMark

Kieron Dunleavy, MD[a],*, Richard F. Little, MD[b], Wyndham H. Wilson, MD, PhD[a]

KEYWORDS

- Burkitt lymphoma • MYC • TCF3 • CCND3 • ID3 • Risk-adapted • Endemic
- Sporadic

KEY POINTS

- While Burkitt lymphoma (BL) is highly curable with short duration, intensive therapies in children these are poorly tolerated in middle-aged and older adults and immunosuppressed patients.
- Some novel less intensive approaches that maintain high cure rates while significantly decreasing treatment-related toxicity compared with traditional strategies are promising.
- There have been great strides in the molecular elucidation of BL that have provided several new targets for novel drug development in the disease.

INTRODUCTION

Burkitt lymphoma (BL), first described by Denis Burkitt in African children over 50 years ago, is a rare and highly aggressive B-cell lymphoma.[1] In Burkitt's initial paper, he reported unusual jaw tumors associated with a specific distribution pattern of anatomic sites in a group of 38 Ugandan children. This endemic variant, which was the first to be described, occurs in equatorial Africa and some other specific regions of the world, peaks in incidence in 4- to 7-year–old children, and has a predilection for males (**Table 1**). Two other epidemiologic variants are recognized. Sporadic BL typically affects children and young adults, presents worldwide, and is the most common variant in the Western world. Immunodeficiency-associated BL occurs in association with human immunodeficiency virus (HIV) infection and is approximately 1000 times more common in HIV-infected individuals compared with HIV-negative counterparts. Over recent years, the understanding of the biology of BL has advanced significantly with the identification of novel mutations that cooperate with *MYC*, and there has also

The authors have no conflicts of interest.
[a] Lymphoid Malignancies Branch, Center for Cancer Research, National Cancer Institute, Bethesda, MD 20892, USA; [b] HIV and Stem Cell Therapeutics, Cancer Therapeutic Evaluation Program (CTEP), National Cancer Institute, Bethesda, MD 20892, USA
* Corresponding author. Lymphoid Malignancies Branch, Building 10, Room 12N4114, 10 Center Drive, Bethesda, MD 20892.
E-mail address: dunleavk@mail.nih.gov

Hematol Oncol Clin N Am 30 (2016) 1333–1343
http://dx.doi.org/10.1016/j.hoc.2016.07.009
0889-8588/16/Published by Elsevier Inc.

hemonc.theclinics.com

Table 1
Comparison of endemic, sporadic, and human immunodeficiency virus-associated Burkitt lymphoma

	Endemic	Sporadic	HIV-Associated
Epidemiology	Equatorial Africa and Papua, New Guinea Geographic association with malaria	Worldwide	Worldwide
Incidence	5–10 cases per 100,000 population	2–3 cases per million population	6 per 1000 AIDS cases
Age and Gender	Malignancy of childhood	Malignancy of childhood and young adults	Malignancy of adults
	Peak Incidence: 4–7 y Male:female ratio of 2: 1	Median age: 30 y Male:female ratio of 2–3:1	Median age: 44 y Associated with higher CD4 counts >100/mm^3
EBV association	100%	25%–40%	25%–40%
Genomics	MYC mutation 100%; ID3 and/or TCF3 mutations 40%; CCND mutations 1.8%	MYC mutation 100%; ID3 and/or TCF3 mutations 70%; CCND mutations 38%	MYC mutation 100%; ID3 and/or TCF3 mutations 67%; CCND mutations 67%
Clinical Presentation	Jaw and facial bones in approximately 50%; Also involves mesentery and gonads Increased risk of CNS dissemination	Abdomen most common presentation often involving the ileo-cecal region Other extranodal sites include bone marrow, ovaries, kidneys, and breasts Increased risk of CNS dissemination	Nodal presentation most common with occasional bone marrow Increased risk of CNS dissemination

been therapeutic progress with the development of less toxic strategies that maintain the high cure rates of historical high-dose, intensive strategies.

PATHOBIOLOGY OF BURKITT LYMPHOMA

The pathobiology of BL is unique and distinct from that of other aggressive B-cell lymphomas. BL is characterized by an extremely high proliferation fraction and a high fraction of apoptosis, and this accounts for its starry sky appearance at low magnification under the microscope. The cells are intermediate in size, have little pleomorphism, and contain basophilic cytoplasm that contains small vacuoles and characteristically round nuclei with little variation in size and shape. The nuclear chromatin is granular and contains small nucleoli with frequent mitoses. Biologically, BL is derived from a germinal center B cell, and the cells are positive for CD10, BCL6, CD20, CD79a, and CD45. The cells are negative for terminal deoxynucleotidyl transferase (TdT) as well as BCL2. The growth fraction as measured by Ki67 staining approaches 100%. Epstein-Barr virus (EBV) is virtually always detected in endemic BL and is present in 25% to 40% of sporadic and immunodeficiency-associated cases.[2] Typically, latency type 1 is observed with restricted EBV nuclear antigen 1 (EBNA1) expression, and there is evidence for EBV's oncogenic role.[3–5] In endemic BL, EBV has been shown to contribute to genomic instability, and interestingly, cases are also linked to malaria prevalence. The incidence is highest in people with high titers of *Plasmodium falciparum*.[6–10]

Virtually all cases of BL harbor a *MYC* translocation—usually at 8q24—and leading to deregulation of the *MYC* gene.[11] In over 80% of cases, the translocation partner is the immunoglobulin heavy chain locus on chromosome 14; in the remaining cases, κ and λ light chain loci on chromosomes 2 and 22 are involved. *MYC* breakpoints can vary in their location between sporadic and endemic cases, suggesting that there may be some distinct pathogenetic mechanisms at play depending on the epidemiologic variant.[12,13] Recently, RNA sequencing (RNA-seq) studies have demonstrated that other genes in addition to *MYC* are frequently mutated in sporadic BL cases.[14–16] In approximately 70% of cases, there are mutations in *TCF3* or its negative regulator *ID3*, which encodes a protein that blocks *TCF3* action. Thirty-eight percent of sporadic cases harbor a mutation in *CCND3*, which is activated by *TCF3* and encodes cyclin D3, which promotes cell cycle progression. *TCF3* and/or *ID3* mutations are found in 67% and 40% of HIV-associated and endemic cases, respectively, and the ongoing Burkitt lymphoma Genome Sequencing Project (BLGSP) aims to further characterize the genomics of these different variants (https://ocg.cancer.gov/programs/cgci/projects/burkitt-lymphoma). Gene expression profiling studies have revealed that BL cases have a distinct molecular signature that is derived from a germinal center B-cell.[17,18] There is high expression of c-*MYC* target genes as well as germinal center-associated B-cell genes. Low expression of MHC class 1 molecules and NF-kappa B target genes is characteristic. In these molecular studies, a subset of aggressive B-cell lymphomas was identified that were diagnosed as diffuse large B-cell lymphoma (DLBCL) by current classification criteria but by gene expression, clearly fell into the BL category. Given that BL does not respond well to CHOP-based treatments, this distinction by molecular profiling is important, and gene expression profiling may be useful in rare cases that would otherwise be diagnosed as DLBCL. Additionally, there are cases with a profile intermediate between that of DLBCL and BL; these cases typically harbor *MYC* and have a poor outcome with CHOP-based regimens.

Recently, lymphomas that have intermediate morphologic features between DLBCL and BL (B-cell lymphoma, unclassifiable, with features intermediate between DLBCL and BL) have been identified. Many of these were previously classified as Burkitt-like lymphoma. Although they are distinct from BL, they share many genetic and clinical features with the former, although there is no preferential predilection for the ileo-cecal region or jaws.

CLINICAL PRESENTATION AND WORK-UP

The clinical presentation of BL is variable and depends on the epidemiologic variant and other factors. In endemic BL, patients commonly present with jaw and other facial disease, and other extranodal sites of involvement include the ileum and cecum, gonads, kidneys, and breasts. The ileo-cecal area is the most common site of disease involvement in sporadic BL, and unlike endemic BL jaw involvement, is very rare. In immunodeficiency-associated BL, involvement of the ileum and cecum, lymph nodes, and bone marrow is commonly observed. Central nervous system (CNS) disease may occur at presentation with all variants, particularly when there is advanced-stage disease, and leptomeningeal rather than parenchymal brain involvement is typically seen. Patients often present with advanced-stage and bulky disease caused by the short doubling time of the tumor. It is common for patients to develop tumor lysis syndrome (TLS) after the institution of therapy, and this needs to be anticipated.

It is critical that the histologic diagnosis is made by a hematopathologist with expertise in the diagnosis of lymphoma, as it may be challenging in some cases to distinguish BL from other aggressive B-cell lymphomas. Laboratory tests should include routine hematology and biochemistry panels to include lactate dehydrogenase (LDH) and uric acid, and testing for HIV and hepatitis B should be performed routinely. Staging should include computed tomography imaging with or without positron emission tomography, and a bone marrow biopsy is essential. A lumbar puncture with cerebrospinal fluid (CSF) analysis by cytology and flow cytometry should also be performed.

THERAPEUTIC APPROACH TO BURKITT LYMPHOMA

BL is a systemic disease that requires chemotherapy for all disease stages. In early development of therapeutic strategies for BL, the high proliferation rate of the tumor and the risk of kinetic failures in between cycles of therapy were deemed to be key to overcome, and therefore early strategies, modeled on approaches in acute lymphoblastic leukemia (ALL), employed short-duration, dose-intensive, multiagent regimens. Standard approaches today typically include multiple chemotherapy agents administered in alternating cycles. These agents are administered in a variety of combinations and schedules, indicating the empiric nature of the combinations. One of the greatest challenges with standard BL therapy is toxicity, and although children and young adults can tolerate standard aggressive approaches, this is not the case with older or immunosuppressed adults.[19] Although risk-adaptive therapy (ie, administering less toxic therapy to patients with lower-risk disease) has been somewhat helpful, there is a need to improve BL therapeutics and develop less toxic approaches while maintaining the high cure rates associated with standard regimens.[20] The risks of tumor lysis syndrome (TLS) and propensity for CNS dissemination in BL are also important therapeutic considerations when selecting up-front therapy. To reduce TLS, which can produce life-threatening renal failure and electrolyte imbalances, many regimens employ a prephase, whereby relatively low-dose cyclophosphamide and prednisone are administered. This strategy has been incorporated into the regimens of several groups. The high risk of CNS involvement is typically addressed by the use of high-dose intravenous methotrexate and cytarabine, both of which have CNS penetration, as well as intrathecal administration of these agents. An important advance over the years has been to eliminate whole-brain radiation for prophylaxis, which has significantly reduced CNS toxicity. Interestingly, a study published by the French, American, British/lymphomes malin B (FAB/LMB) demonstrated that patients with early stage BL had a high cure rate and low rate of CNS relapse without the use of intrathecal chemotherapy.[21]

TREATMENT OF BURKITT LYMPHOMA

Given the rarity of BL and the paucity of clinical trials, the optimal therapeutic approach is controversial, particularly in adults in whom toxicity is a significant challenge with many regimens. As BL is a common lymphoma in children, many of the approaches that are commonly used in adults today were initially developed in pediatric populations (**Table 2**).

The French Societe Francaise d'Oncologie Pediatrique (SOFP) group developed an early risk-adapted strategy in children with BL and L3 ALL (LMB89) where treatment

Table 2
Selected regimens for Burkitt lymphoma

Regimen	Patient Number	Histology	Median Age, y (Range)	Stage (%)	CR (%)	EFS (%)	OS (%)
LMB 89[22]	561	Burkitt B-ALL	8 (0.17–18)	III–IV 79%	97%	92% @ 5 y	92% @ 5 y
Modified LMB[23]	72	Burkitt B-ALL	33 (18–76)	III–IV 67%	72%	65% @ 2 y	70% @ 2 y
BFM 90[24]	413	Burkitt B-ALL	9 (1.2–17.9)	III–IV 60%	N/A	89% @ 6 y	14 deaths
CODOX-M/IVAC[25]	21 children 20 adult	Burkitt B-ALL	12 (3–17) 25 (18–59)	III–IV 78%	95%	85% (children) and 100% (adults) @ 2 y	2 deaths
CODOX-M/IVAC[20]	52	Burkitt	35 (15–60)	III–IV 61%	77%	65% @ 2 y	73% @ 2 y
Hyper-CVAD[26]	26	Burkitt/B-ALL	58 (17–79)	N/A	81%	61% @ 3 y for DFS	49% @ 3 y
R-Hyper-CVAD[27]	31	Burkitt/B-ALL	46 (17–77)	N/A	86%	80% @ 3 y	89% at 3 y
GMALL-B-ALL/NHL 2002[29]	363	Burkitt B-ALL	42 (16–85)	III–IV 71%	88%	PFS 75% @ 5 y	80% @ 5 y
DA-EPOCH-R[31]	19	Burkitt	25 (15–88)	III–IV 58%	N/A	FFP 95% @ 7 y	100% @ 7 y
SC-EPOCH-RR[31]	11	Burkitt HIV+	44 (24–60)	III–IV 82%	N/A	FFP 100% @ 6 y	90% @ 6 y
AMC 048[35]	34	Burkitt HIV+	42 (19–55)	III–IV 74%	N/A	PFS 69% @ 1 y	69% @ 2 y
RA-DA-EPOCH-R[32]	88	Burkitt HIV– + HIV+	46 (18–78)	III–IV 64%	N/A	PFS 84% @ 2 y	86% @ 2 y

was based on tumor burden and early response to chemotherapy.[22] Three risk groups (groups A, B and C) were defined, with group A receiving induction only; group B receiving pre-phase, induction, consolidation, and limited maintenance; and group C receiving extended maintenance and cranial irradiation if CNS disease was present. If a CR was not achieved in groups B and C after the third or fourth induction–consolidation course, patients underwent autologous transplant. This strategy was highly successful in pediatric patients with 5-year event-free and overall survivals of 92%. This led to the testing of the strategy in adults with minor modifications and in 72 adult patients who had a median age of 33 years - mostly with advanced disease; event-free survival (EFS) and overall survival (OS) at 2 years were 65% and 70%, respectively.[23] Toxicity was a significant problem for advanced stage patients due to treatment intensity, and treatment-related mortality was significant. The Berlin-Frankfurt-Munster (BFM) group developed an approach that was based on short, intensive cycles and over the course of several protocols led to a reduction in the number of cycles based on risk stratification. The BFM 90 protocol continued to further refine the risk stratification and to improve the outcome of patients who had an incomplete initial response with further treatment intensification. Among 266 pediatric patients with BL regimen, the overall EFS was 89% at 6 years.[24]

In the 1980s, CODOX-M/IVAC (cyclophosphamide, doxorubicin, vincristine, methotrexate/ifosfamide, cytarabine and etoposide) was developed at the National Cancer Institute (NCI), and patients were risk-stratified according to clinical presentation and LDH level.[25] Patients with a single extra-abdominal mass less than 10 cm or completely resected abdominal disease with a normal lactate dehydrogenase (LDH) were considered low risk, and all other patients were designated high risk. Low-risk patients received 3 cycles of CODOX-M, and high-risk patients received 4 cycles of alternating CODOX-M with IVAC. In 41 patients, including 20 adults with a median age of 25 years, the EFS was 92% at 2 years. Hematological toxicities were significant, and sepsis occurred in 22% of cycles. Other groups have confirmed the efficacy of this regimen, albeit with lower survival rates. Mead and colleagues[20] reported the outcome of 52 adult patients with a median age of 35 years. The overall EFS was 65% at 2 years and 83% and 59%, respectively, for the low-risk and high-risk arms. The Hyper-hyperfractionated cyclophosphamide, vincristine, doxorubicin and dexamethasone (CVAD) regimen was based on a modification of a regimen developed by Murphy and colleagues[26,27] for pediatric L3 ALL. In this regimen, hyperfractionated cyclophosphamide, vincristine, doxorubicin, and dexamethasone were alternated with methotrexate and cytarabine for a total of 8 cycles. In a study of 26 patients with BL and B-ALL (acute lymphoblastic lymphoma), the 3-year OS was 49%.[26] Later, a study looked at combining the regimen with rituximab and in a study of 31 similar population patients, the 3-year OS was 89%.[27]

Although there is little known about the clinical outcome of B-cell lymphoma unclassifiable with features intermediate between DLBCL and BL, many of these harbor an MYC rearrangement and are associated with a clinically aggressive presentation. The authors therefore favor a more aggressive approach than standard R-CHOP such as DA-EPOCH-R, with the caveat that there is a paucity of experience treating these diseases.

MOVING BEYOND STANDARD APPROACHES

Although current standard treatments are effective in children and younger patients with BL, toxicity of the regimens used for advanced stage disease is high, particularly in adults and immunosuppressed patients, and treatment-related mortality is excessive.[19] Therefore, new strategies are needed to improve the therapeutic index of treatment and to increase efficacy. The success of rituximab in diffuse large B-cell lymphoma has prompted its testing in BL and in a recent preliminary analysis of a randomized study in 257 adults where patients received an LMBA regimen with or without rituximab, there was a significant EFS and OS advantage in the rituximab arm (76% vs 64% and 82% vs 71%, respectively).[28] In single-arm studies, when rituximab has been incorporated into standard intensive BL regimens, survival end points improved compared with historical nonrituximab-containing regimens.[29]

Dose-adjusted EPOCH-R (etoposide, prednisone, vincristine, cyclophosphamide, doxorubicin, and rituximab) is an intermediate-intensity regimen that was tested in BL, due to its high efficacy in the GCB subtype of DLBCL, and the hypothesis that the high sensitivity of BL cells to genotoxic stress makes prolonged exposure time an important therapeutic strategy for maximizing tumor cell kill.[30,31] The regimen consists of 3 continuously infused drugs over 96 hours based on the demonstration from in vitro studies that enhanced tumor cell kill occurred with prolonged low-concentration drug exposure as compared to brief high-concentration exposure. In an initial study testing the strategy in 30 adult patients with sporadic and immunodeficiency-associated BL, with long median follow-up times, the freedom from progression was over 90%. Based on these single-center results, a multicenter study is currently underway where low-risk patients (all of: stage I or II disease, normal LDH, ECOG performance status of 0–1, and mass size <7 cm) receive 3 cycles of therapy, and high-risk (all other) patients receive 6 cycles of therapy. Low-risk patients receive 2 doses of rituximab on each cycle and do not receive intrathecal prophylaxis; high-risk patients receive 1 dose of rituximab on all 6 cycles and intrathecal prophylaxis with methotrexate from cycle 3 to 6. In a recently presented preliminary report of 88 patients on this multicenter study, progression-free survival (PFS) was 100% and 81% in low-risk and high-risk groups, respectively at 25 months follow-up, and age or HIV status did not portend on survival.[32] Importantly, toxicity was low with this approach compared with traditional BL platforms, and few patients developed tumor lysis syndrome. An analysis of the role of prophylactic intrathecal methotrexate, especially in high-risk patients, is underway. In addition, 13% of patients in this preliminary analysis had CNS disease and received an aggressive schedule of intrathecal methotrexate from cycle 1, and an analysis of this subset is also underway.[31]

MANAGEMENT OF RELAPSED BURKITT LYMPHOMA

The salvage treatment of relapse or refractory BL is usually unsuccessful. Early stage patients who relapse after having received limited treatment, however, may still be curable, whereas advanced-stage patients who have received intensive treatment or are primary induction failures are rarely curable. A retrospective review from the European Group for Blood and Marrow Transplantation (EBMT) reported an OS of 37% at 3 years for patients with a chemosensitive relapse but only 7% for those with resistant disease following autologous stem-cell transplantation (SCT).[33] In BL, there are no data that allogeneic transplant is beneficial in the relapsed setting, but this has not been well studied given the rarity of this disease and the high cure rates with up-front therapy.

HUMAN IMMUNODEFICIENCY VIRUS-ASSOCIATED BURKITT LYMPHOMA

BL comprises up to 20% of HIV-associated lymphomas and typically occurs at a high median CD4 count. Although some retrospective studies suggested that there had not been an improvement in the outcome of patients with BL in the antiretroviral era (as there has been with DLBCL), recent studies report good results for this population and dispute this.[31,34,35] The clinical presentation of BL in the setting of HIV infection is similar to sporadic BL and is variably associated with EBV. BL highlights the necessity to balance treatment efficacy and toxicity in patients with HIV infection. Standard BL regimens are generally considered too toxic for patients with HIV-associated BL; therefore less toxic modifications of approaches like CODOX-M/IVAC-R have been investigated with some success. A recent study from the AIDS Malignancy Consortium looked at the outcome of 27 patients who received modified CODOX-M/IVAC-rituximab and reported a 1 year PFS of 69%.[35] DA-EPOCH-R is well tolerated in the setting of HIV and has been associated with excellent outcomes; it is currently being investigated in a multicenter study in which outcomes are as good as in the HIV negative setting.[32] With these approaches, patients with HIV-associated BL should have an excellent outcome and similar survival to HIV-negative counterparts.

TREATMENT RECOMMENDATIONS IN BURKITT LYMPHOMA

For young adults with BL, standard regimens like CODOX-M/IVAC, although toxic, are tolerated, and outcomes are generally excellent. For older adults and immunosuppressed individuals, these approaches are not well tolerated, and alternative, less toxic strategies should be strongly considered. DA-EPOCH-R is well tolerated in all age groups, and a single-center study demonstrates high efficacy of this approach in BL. Based on this and early promising multicenter results of risk-adapted DA-EPOCH-R, this approach should be considered in adults of all ages. Randomized studies now show that rituximab is beneficial in BL, so this should be a standard part of therapy. CNS prophylaxis therapy should be given outside of a clinical trial, but extrapolating from pediatric literature, patients with very low-risk disease have a close to zero risk of CNS dissemination; intrathecal therapy is likely avoidable in this group, and this is currently being studied.

FUTURE DIRECTIONS AND SUMMARY

Although the outcome of young patients with BL is excellent with aggressive therapies, treatment-related toxicity remains a big challenge in BL therapeutics, especially for older adults, and future strategies should attempt to reduce toxicity while maintaining high cure rates. Many promising agents are in development for BL that include specific inhibitors of MYC. Small molecule inhibitors of the bromodomain and extraterminal (BET) domain proteins such as JQ1 and I-BET 151 are exciting to consider with respect to targeting MYC.[36] Recent studies have shown that BET and histone deacetylase (HDAC) inhibitors have synergistic activity in MYC-induced murine lymphoma, suggesting a rationale for the testing of promising combinations of these classes.[37,38] Other potential therapeutic targets that may be important in MYC-overexpressing cancers include human mitochondrial peptide deformylase (HsPDF) and the mitochondrial sirtuin SIRT 4.[39,40] Other than targeting MYC, recent advances have identified several new genes and pathways that cooperate with MYC. TCF3 and ID3, for example, are found in 70% of sporadic BL cases and are rarely seen in DLBCL. In addition, the CCND3 gene, which is activated by TCF3 and interacts with CDK6, is mutated in a high proportion of BL cases. These findings present a rationale for testing novel agents in this disease such as classes of PI3 kinase inhibitors and inhibitors of CDK6. Recently, immunotherapy strategies such as gene-modified T cells expressing chimeric antigen receptors (CARs) have demonstrated great promise in B-cell malignancies and are particularly effective in childhood ALL, suggesting a role in BL that is biologically similar to ALL.[41] Overall, as novel strategies and agents are developed in BL, they offer the possibility of less reliance on toxic agents than is the case today.

REFERENCES

1. Burkitt D. A sarcoma involving the jaws in African children. Br J Surg 1958; 46(197):218–23.
2. Kelly GL, Rickinson AB. Burkitt lymphoma: revisiting the pathogenesis of a virus-associated malignancy. Hematology Am Soc Hematol Educ Program 2007;277–84.
3. Heslop HE. Biology and treatment of Epstein-Barr virus-associated non-Hodgkin lymphomas. Hematology Am Soc Hematol Educ Program 2005;260–6.
4. Shimizu N, Tanabe-Tochikura A, Kuroiwa Y, et al. Isolation of Epstein-Barr virus (EBV)-negative cell clones from the EBV-positive Burkitt's lymphoma (BL) line Akata: malignant phenotypes of BL cells are dependent on EBV. J Virol 1994; 68(9):6069–73.
5. Komano J, Sugiura M, Takada K. Epstein-Barr virus contributes to the malignant phenotype and to apoptosis resistance in Burkitt's lymphoma cell line Akata. J Virol 1998;72(11):9150–6.
6. Kamranvar SA, Gruhne B, Szeles A, et al. Epstein-Barr virus promotes genomic instability in Burkitt's lymphoma. Oncogene 2007;26(35):5115–23.
7. Kelly GL, Milner AE, Baldwin GS, et al. Three restricted forms of Epstein-Barr virus latency counteracting apoptosis in c-myc-expressing Burkitt lymphoma cells. Proc Natl Acad Sci U S A 2006;103(40):14935–40.
8. Robbiani DF, Deroubaix S, Feldhahn N, et al. Plasmodium infection promotes genomic instability and AID-dependent B cell lymphoma. Cell 2015;162(4): 727–37.
9. Rochford R, Cannon MJ, Moormann AM. Endemic Burkitt's lymphoma: a polymicrobial disease? Nat Rev Microbiol 2005;3(2):182–7.
10. Chene A, Donati D, Orem J, et al. Endemic Burkitt's lymphoma as a polymicrobial disease: new insights on the interaction between *Plasmodium falciparum* and Epstein-Barr virus. Semin Cancer Biol 2009;19(6):411–20.
11. Dalla-Favera R, Bregni M, Erikson J, et al. Human c-myc onc gene is located on the region of chromosome 8 that is translocated in Burkitt lymphoma cells. Proc Natl Acad Sci U S A 1982;79(24):7824–7.
12. Lenze D, Leoncini L, Hummel M, et al. The different epidemiologic subtypes of Burkitt lymphoma share a homogenous micro RNA profile distinct from diffuse large B-cell lymphoma. Leukemia 2011;25(12):1869–76.
13. Piccaluga PP, De Falco G, Kustagi M, et al. Gene expression analysis uncovers similarity and differences among Burkitt lymphoma subtypes. Blood 2011; 117(13):3596–608.
14. Schmitz R, Young RM, Ceribelli M, et al. Burkitt lymphoma pathogenesis and therapeutic targets from structural and functional genomics. Nature 2012;490(7418): 116–20.
15. Love C, Sun Z, Jima D, et al. The genetic landscape of mutations in Burkitt lymphoma. Nat Genet 2012;44(12):1321–5.
16. Richter J, Schlesner M, Hoffmann S, et al. Recurrent mutation of the ID3 gene in Burkitt lymphoma identified by integrated genome, exome and transcriptome sequencing. Nat Genet 2012;44(12):1316–20.
17. Dave SS, Fu K, Wright GW, et al. Molecular diagnosis of Burkitt's lymphoma. N Engl J Med 2006;354(23):2431–42.
18. Hummel M, Bentink S, Berger H, et al. A biologic definition of Burkitt's lymphoma from transcriptional and genomic profiling. N Engl J Med 2006;354(23):2419–30.

19. Corazzelli G, Frigeri F, Russo F, et al. RD-CODOX-M/IVAC with rituximab and intrathecal liposomal cytarabine in adult Burkitt lymphoma and 'unclassifiable' highly aggressive B-cell lymphoma. Br J Haematol 2012;156(2):234–44.

20. Mead GM, Barrans SL, Qian W, et al. A prospective clinicopathologic study of dose-modified CODOX-M/IVAC in patients with sporadic Burkitt lymphoma defined using cytogenetic and immunophenotypic criteria (MRC/NCRI LY10 trial). Blood 2008;112(6):2248–60.

21. Gerrard M, Cairo MS, Weston C, et al. Excellent survival following two courses of COPAD chemotherapy in children and adolescents with resected localized B-cell non-Hodgkin's lymphoma: results of the FAB/LMB 96 international study. Br J Haematol 2008;141(6):840–7.

22. Patte C, Auperin A, Michon J, et al. The Societe Francaise d'Oncologie Pediatrique LMB89 protocol: highly effective multiagent chemotherapy tailored to the tumor burden and initial response in 561 unselected children with B-cell lymphomas and L3 leukemia. Blood 2001;97(11):3370–9.

23. Divine M, Casassus P, Koscielny S, et al. Burkitt lymphoma in adults: a prospective study of 72 patients treated with an adapted pediatric LMB protocol. Ann Oncol 2005;16(12):1928–35.

24. Reiter A, Schrappe M, Tiemann M, et al. Improved treatment results in childhood B-cell neoplasms with tailored intensification of therapy: a report of the Berlin-Frankfurt-Munster Group Trial NHL-BFM 90. Blood 1999;94(10):3294–306.

25. Magrath I, Adde M, Shad A, et al. Adults and children with small non-cleaved-cell lymphoma have a similar excellent outcome when treated with the same chemotherapy regimen. J Clin Oncol 1996;14(3):925–34.

26. Thomas DA, Cortes J, O'Brien S, et al. Hyper-CVAD program in Burkitt's-type adult acute lymphoblastic leukemia. J Clin Oncol 1999;17(8):2461–70.

27. Thomas DA, Faderl S, O'Brien S, et al. Chemoimmunotherapy with hyper-CVAD plus rituximab for the treatment of adult Burkitt and Burkitt-type lymphoma or acute lymphoblastic leukemia. Cancer 2006;106(7):1569–80.

28. Ribrag V, Koscielny S, Bouabdallah K, et al. Addition of rituximab improves outcome of HIV negative patients with randomized lymphoma treated with the LMBA protocol: results of the randomized intergroup (GRAALL-LYSA) LMBA02 protocol [abstract]. Blood 2012;120(21):685.

29. Hoelzer D, Walewski J, Dohner H, et al. Improved outcome of adult Burkitt lymphoma/leukemia with rituximab and chemotherapy: report of a large prospective multicenter trial. Blood 2014;124(26):3870–9.

30. Wilson WH, Dunleavy K, Pittaluga S, et al. Phase II study of dose-adjusted EPOCH and rituximab in untreated diffuse large B-cell lymphoma with analysis of germinal center and post-germinal center biomarkers. J Clin Oncol 2008;26(16):2717–24.

31. Dunleavy K, Pittaluga S, Shovlin M, et al. Low-intensity therapy in adults with Burkitt's lymphoma. N Engl J Med 2013;369(20):1915–25.

32. Dunleavy K, Noy A, Abramson J, et al. Risk-adapted therapy in adults with burkitt lymphoma: preliminary report of a multicenter prospective phase II study of DA-EPOCH-R [abstract]. Blood 2015;126(23):342.

33. Sweetenham JW, Pearce R, Taghipour G, et al. Adult Burkitt's and Burkitt-like non-Hodgkin's lymphoma—outcome for patients treated with high-dose therapy and autologous stem-cell transplantation in first remission or at relapse: results from the European Group for Blood and Marrow Transplantation. J Clin Oncol 1996;14(9):2465–72.

34. Little RF, Pittaluga S, Grant N, et al. Highly effective treatment of acquired immunodeficiency syndrome-related lymphoma with dose-adjusted EPOCH: impact of antiretroviral therapy suspension and tumor biology. Blood 2003;101(12):4653–9.

35. Noy A, Lee JY, Cesarman E, et al. AMC 048: modified CODOX-M/IVAC-rituximab is safe and effective for HIV-associated Burkitt lymphoma. Blood 2015;126(2): 160–6.

36. Tolani B, Gopalakrishnan R, Punj V, et al. Targeting Myc in KSHV-associated primary effusion lymphoma with BET bromodomain inhibitors. Oncogene 2014;33: 2928–37.

37. Trabucco SE, Gerstein RM, Evens AM, et al. Inhibition of bromodomain proteins for the treatment of human diffuse large B-cell lymphoma. Clin Cancer Res 2015; 21:113–22.

38. Bhadury J, Nilsson LM, Veppil Muralidharan S, et al. BET and HDAC inhibitors induce similar genes and biological effects and synergize to kill in Myc-induced murine lymphoma. Proc Natl Acad Sci U S A 2014;111(26):E2721–30.

39. Sheth A, Escobar-Alvarez S, Gardner J, et al. Inhibition of human mitochondrial peptide deformylase causes apoptosis in c-myc-overexpressing hematopoietic cancers. Cell Death Dis 2014;5:e1152.

40. Jeong SM, Lee A, Lee J, et al. SIRT4 protein suppresses tumor formation in genetic models of Myc-induced B cell lymphoma. J Biol Chem 2014;289(7): 4135–44.

41. Kochenderfer JN, Dudley ME, Kassim SH, et al. Chemotherapy-refractory diffuse large B-cell lymphoma and indolent B-cell malignancies can be effectively treated with autologous T cells expressing an anti-CD19 chimeric antigen receptor. J Clin Oncol 2015;33(6):540–9.

Mantle Cell Lymphoma

Is It Time for a New Treatment Paradigm?

Andre Goy, MD

KEYWORDS

- Mantle cell • Stem cell transplantation • Maintenance • MRD • Novel therapies
- Bortezomib • Ibrutinib • Lenalidomide

KEY POINTS

- Mantle cell lymphoma (MCL) outcome has improved thanks to the achievement of deeper remission (complete remission [CR] and molecular CR), which translates into much longer progression-free survival (>5 years) and greater overall survival (OS).
- Maintenance rituximab in responders (post-R-CHOP [rituximab plus cyclophosphamide, doxorubicin, vincristine, and prednisolone] and post-high-dose therapies–autologous stem cell transplantation) improves duration of response and might improve OS in some cases.
- Novel therapies (bortezomib, lenalidomide, ibrutinib) which have shown durable responses in the relapsed/refractory setting, including in chemorefractory patients, offer an opportunity to build up on current regimens as either combination and/or maintenance strategies, while also offering hope for non-chemotherapy-based options, particularly in elderly MCL patients.
- Integrating biologicals into current regimens will likely improve quality and durability of response in both combination and maintenance settings.
- Biologicals-only combinations might help develop non-chemotherapy-based options, particularly in elderly MCL patients.
- A shift in the MCL paradigm is definitely seen. Finally, a greater awareness of biological heterogeneity might serve to stratify patients better in the clinic.

BACKGROUND

The field of mantle cell lymphoma (MCL) has changed dramatically since its recognition as a separate entity more than 30 years ago. The concept of mantle-zone lymphoma first introduced in 1982 by Weisenburger and colleagues[1] was confirmed by the International Lymphoma Study Group in 1992 and refined in the Revised European-American Lymphoma and World Health Organization classification in 1994.[2] MCL recognition was based on its distinct morphologic and molecular features (hallmark t(11;14) translocation),[3,4] but also its immunophenotype and distinct clinical course, with much poorer outcome among "indolent lymphomas."

Disclosure: Submitted separately.
John Theurer Cancer Center, Hackensack University Medical Center, Hackensack, NJ, USA
E-mail address: agoy@hackensackUMC.org

Hematol Oncol Clin N Am 30 (2016) 1345–1370
http://dx.doi.org/10.1016/j.hoc.2016.07.014
0889-8588/16/© 2016 Elsevier Inc. All rights reserved.

MCL represents 6% to 10% of non-Hodgkin lymphomas with a median age at diagnosis in the mid to late 60s and a clear predominance in men (ratio 3:1). Some data suggest a possible increase in MCL incidence over the last two decades, albeit likely reflecting improved diagnostics. Although most MCL cases are thought to derive from an antigen-naive pre-germinal center B cell, there is definite evidence of cases with restricted immunoglobulin gene repertoire (particularly IGHV3-21 and IGHV4-34 genes), which together with precise somatic hypermutation patterns suggest a role for chronic antigenic stimulation. Moderate associations with MCL risk have been reported for *Borrelia burgdorferi* infection,[5] lifestyle-related factors, family history of hematopoietic malignancies, or genetic susceptibility (interleukin-10 and tumor necrosis factor genes),[6] while others suggest molecularly defined antigenic specificity for B-cell receptor (BCR) in some series.[7]

The t(11;14)(q13;q32) translocation that juxtaposes the proto-oncogene *CCND1* at 11q13 to the immunoglobulin heavy chain complex (*IGH*) at chromosome 14q32 is considered the primary oncogenic mechanism (although not sufficient) for the development of MCL. This translocation forces the constitutive overexpression of cyclin D1, which can also be expressed (at a much lower level) by other B-cell lymphomas and is typically not detected in normal B lymphocytes. The overexpression of cyclin D1 leads to deregulation of the cell cycle at the G_1/S phase transition: cyclin D1 binding to CDK4/6 activates the transcription factor E2F by phosphorylating its inhibitor, retinoblastoma 1 (RB1) and further promotes cyclin E/CDK2 activation, which triggers entry into the S phase of the cell cycle. Several secondary genomic alterations targeting genes involved in key molecular pathways have been reported as involved in MCL pathogenesis and/or its aggressive clinical course. Together these genetic alterations affect important pathways such as INK4A/CDK4/RB1 and ARF/MDM2/p53 (cell cycle/survival), PI3K/AKT/mTOR (cell growth/survival), ataxia telangiectasia mutated (*ATM*) gene at 11q22-23 (genetic stability), mutations or deletions of *TP53*/*RB* or deregulation of checkpoint kinases *CHK1* and *CHK2* (DNA damage response), amplifications/overexpression of *BCL2* (cell death/fate), or constitutive activation of nuclear factor κB (cell survival).[8] Many of these genomic alterations as well as complex karyotypes have also definite prognostic value in MCL.[9] SOX11 (neuronal transcription factor of the high-mobility group) expression is typically associated with minimal somatic hypermutation and genetic instability and with worse outcome. On the opposite, SOX11-negative variants are typically associated with indolent behavior; such cases (10%–15% of MCL) present with high white blood cell count, splenomegaly, no or minimal nodal disease (ie, mimicking chronic lymphocytic leukemia [CLL] but negative for both CD23 and CD200). These cases derive from postgerminal center B cells, show hypermutated *IGHV*, low/no karyotype complexity, and longer survival with prolonged stable clinical course. Rarely, some of these indolent (SOX11-negative) MCL may "transform" into aggressive disease usually associated with 17p/*TP53* alterations.

The classical immunophenotype of MCL reflects a mature B-cell lymphoma (positive for CD19, CD20, CD22, CD79a, PAX5, and FMC7) with coexpression of CD5. MCL cells also show typically immunoglobulin M/D positivity with more frequent lambda expression over kappa (ratio 1:13) and are negative for CD23, CD10, CD200, and BCL6.[10] The diagnosis is confirmed through cyclin D1 overexpression and/or by the presence of t(11;14) translocation, more frequently seen by fluorescence *in situ* hybridization than cytogenetics.[11] A small subset of truly *cyclin D1*-negative MCL (5%–10%) will show overexpression of *cyclin D2* or *D3*[12] predominantly through alternative translocations with immunoglobulin light chain genes.[13] SOX11 expression has been reported as a tool to help diagnose such cyclin D1-negative MCL,[14] which otherwise cannot be distinguished by gene-expression profiling (GEP), and carry similar clinical characteristics and outcome and therefore should be treated accordingly.[15]

Typically, MCL patients present with advanced stage disease (>80% Ann Arbor stage IV), although B symptoms are found in less than one-third of patients. One remarkable feature of MCL is the almost constant extranodal involvement, including gastrointestinal tract,[16] liver, and spleen, but also bone marrow and peripheral blood (flow peripheral blood lymphocyte positive in >90% cases).[17] Recent reports suggest that central nervous system (CNS) involvement might be underestimated in MCL, although its incidence at baseline remains low (<1%), whereas CNS involvement can occur in up to 15% to 20% at 5 years, particularly in patients with high-risk disease, high Ki-67, and/or blastoid variants and carries then regardless a dismal prognosis.[18–20]

Although treatment strategies in MCL have been very diverse, the persistent disappointing outcome led to explore novel approaches early on, which have translated over time into an improvement of patient outcome from a median overall survival (OS) of 2.5 years in the late 1970s to 4.8 years in the mid 1990s and well over 5 to 7 years in the late 2000s.[21,22] Not surprisingly, this continued improvement is attributable to several factors from better supportive care to the use of dose-intensive (DIT)/high-dose therapies (HDT), which have clearly led to much longer progression-free survival (PFS) intervals, and the development of promising novel therapies for a disease that commonly shows chemoresistance in the relapse setting.[23] Nevertheless, there remains nowadays a wide heterogeneity in the management of MCL, with many different treatment approaches, which may be influenced by age, comorbidities, disease biology, as well as patient and physician preferences. This is reflected by the rather long list of potential regimens (>10 options) for initial treatment of MCL in the National Comprehensive Cancer Network current guidelines. In itself, such diverse management definitely represents a true challenge, including a greater heterogeneity in the relapse setting, but looking at the overall picture, patterns emerge that might help clarify treatment options and shed some light on emerging trends and shifting paradigm.

FROM "MORE IS BETTER" TO ESTABLISHING NEW STANDARDS IN THE DOSE-INTENSIVE THERAPY/HIGH-DOSE THERAPY SETTINGS

Based on the poor results of conventional chemotherapy regimens (CVP [cyclophosphamide, vincristine, and prednisolone], MCP [mitoxantrone, chlorambucil, and prednisolone], cyclophosphamide, doxorubicin, vincristine, and prednisolone [CHOP]) in MCL, a natural shift led to the use of HDT followed by autologous stem cell transplantation (ASCT) as consolidation in first remission. The initial favorable results of smaller phase II trials were confirmed by a large German phase III trial in which responding patients to CHOP chemotherapy were randomized between maintenance interferon (IFN-α) versus HDT-ASCT.[24] In that study, there was a significant improvement of both PFS and duration of response (DOR) in favor of the HDT-ASCT consolidation arm (but no difference in OS likely due to crossover design) (**Table 1**).

The next step was the addition of rituximab (Rtx) to established induction regimens for newly diagnosed MCL. In the ASCT setting, Rtx likely increased the transplantation eligible pool (improving response rate after induction) and helped as an *in vivo* purging before transplantation.[25] The benefit of Rtx was also confirmed in the MCL2 Nordic Lymphoma Group trial (R-MaxiCHOP alternating with R-High-dose cytarabine followed by ASCT), which recent update showed a median event-free survival (EFS) >7 years.[26] In this trial, patients were monitored for molecular relapse

Table 1
Selected trials as induction in dose-intensive therapy/high-dose therapy FIT versus non-dose-intensive therapy FIT patients with mantle cell lymphoma

Study for DIT-HDT-FIT Patients	Setting	No. of Patients	MIPI % (L/I/H)	ORR, %	CR, %	Med PFS	Med OS	Comments
R-CHOP-R-DHAP/ASCT Delarue 2013[113]	Ph II multicenter	60	55/32/13	100	96	6.9 y	5 y OS 75%	
R-Maxi-CHOP/HDAraC/ASCT (MCL NORDIC-2) (maint based on RQ PCR) Geisler 2008[114]	Ph II multicenter	160	51/26/23	96	54	7.5 y	10 y OS 64%	Mol relapses received additional R2 (not considered failures)
R-CHOP vs R-CHOP/R-DHAP/ASCT Hermine 2016[115]	Ph III multicenter	497	60/25/15	R-CHOP 90 R-CHOP/R-DHAP 95	83 82	Med TTF 9 y vs 3.9 y	Exp arm also > for OS	Earlier and deeper CR and mol CR in exp arm R-CHOP/R-DHAP
R-DHAP/ASCT/Maint R2 LeGouill 2014[116]	Ph III multicenter	299	53/27/19	NA	92	Med PFS 88% in maint arm vs 745 in Obs. arm		Maint q2 ms × 3 y MRD studies: pre-ASCT MRD status +++ impact on outcome R maint improves PFS regardless of MRD status pre-ASCT {Callanan, 2015 #118314}
R-Maxi-CHOP/HDAraC/90Y-ibritumomab-tiuxetan/ASCT (MCL NORDIC-3)[117]	Ph II multicenter	160	48/31/21	97	67	4 y EFS 62%	4 y OS 78%	RIT was given to non-CR pts after receiving similar induction than MCL2
R-HyperCVAD Romaguera 2010[118]	Ph II single center	97	47/29/18	97	87	Med TTF for <65 y 6.9 y	NR	Estimated 15-y FFS of 30% n ≤65 y {Chihara, 2016 #118285}
R-HyperCVAD Bernstein 2013[119]	Ph II multicenter	49	55/31/14	86	47	Med PFS 4.8 y 6.8 y		
R-HyperCVAD Merli 2011[120]	Ph II multicenter	63	60/33/7	83	72	5 y PFS 61%	5 y OS 73%	

Study for Non DIT-HDT =IT Patients (ie, Elderly)	Setting	No. of Patients	MIPI % (L/I/H)	ORR, %	CR, %	Med PFS	Med OS	Comments
R-CHOP alone Lenz 2005[121]	Ph II multicenter	62	NA	94	34	Med TTF 21 ms	NA	
R-CHOP/B-R Rummel 2013[122]	Ph III multicenter	274/275	NA	93	30	Med PFS 35 ms vs 22 ms for R-CHOP	No diff	
B-R vs R-CHOP/R-CVP Flinn 2014[123]	Ph III multicenter	36/38	NA	97/91	31/25	NA (but no diff)	NR	
R-CHOP vs FCR Kluin-Nelemans 2012[53]	Ph III multicenter	560	NA	86/78	34/40	Med TTF 26/28 ms	62/47 P = .005	More toxicity and POD in FCR arm In responders to R-CHOP, maint R improved DOR and OS
R-BAC Visco 2013[124]	Ph II multicenter	40	28/25/47	100	95	2 y PFS 95%	95%	Study had ½ untreated and ½ r/r MCL
R-CHOP/90Y-ibritumomab-tiuxetan RIT Smith 2012[125]	Ph II multicenter	56	NA	82	55	Med TTF 34 ms	5 y OS 73%	
R-CHOP-vs BTZ-R-CAP (-YM-3002) Robak 2015[126]	Ph III multicenter	487	30/39/31	89/92	42/53	Med PFS 14 ms vs 24 ms for VR-CAP P<.001		59% improvement PFS >CR rate >DOR of CR 18 ms vs 42 ms
B-R with maintenance randomization (MAINTAIN) Rummel 2016[52]	Ph II multicenter	122	16/45/37	85	27	Med PFS 64 ms overall	NR	PFS obs 55 ms vs 72 ms in maint R arm P = .22

(not considered failures), which would trigger additional Htx converting typically patients back into durable remission.

Several strategies, regrouped under DIT/HDT (see **Table 1**), have repeatedly confirmed an extension of the median PFS well over 5 years,[25,27,28] comparing to rituximab plus cyclophosphamide, doxorubicin, vincristine, and prednisolone (R-CHOP), which remains in the 14- to 18-months range. It became also clear through these DIT-HDT strategies that incorporating cytarabine as part of induction pre-ASCT was critical. The benefit of cytarabine, initially shown by a French group (R-CHOP-R-DHAP [rituximab plus dexamethasone, high-dose cytarabine, cisplatin]/ ASCT, leading to tripled complete remission [CR] rate and a median EFS of 83 ms),[29] was also a key conclusion of the NORDIC MCL2 trial mentioned above.[26] The benefit of high-dose cytarabine was definitely proven thanks to a large and remarkable (>400 patients) EU phase III trial comparing R-CHOP/R-DHAP (alternating × 6) followed by HDT (using AraC Melphalan and total body irradiation [TBI]) versus R-CHOP × 6 followed by HDT (using Cy-TBI).[28] The results showed superiority for the cytarabine-containing arm, in terms of time to treatment failure (TTTF), the primary endpoint, with a 30% reduction in the risk of progression but also superior OS ([NR] vs 82 ms, p .045); note, this advantage was seen across all MCL International Prognostic Index (MIPI) subgroups. These results were attributed to the quality of the response seen in the high-dose cytarabine arm with much earlier and higher CR rate than with R-CHOP, which translated into longer duration of first response and better outcome. In addition, built-in MRD studies in this study revealed the profound impact on outcome of achieving negative MRD status (ie, a molecular CR), which has now been shown to predict outcome across the board in several studies and will likely become a future key endpoint in MCL.[30] In the randomized EU MCL trial, the molecular CR rate post induction was 83% in the cytarabine arm versus 51% in the control arm (p<.0001), confirming again the cytarabine arm superiority while translating into a new standard for DIT-HDT in MCL frontline therapy.[31]

The induction for Nordic regimen MCL2 is not very different from R-HyperCVAD (hyperfractionated cyclophosphamide, vincristine, doxorubicin, and dexamethasone; alternating with methotrexate and high-dose cytarabine), another dose-intensive regimen frequently used in MCL patients 65 years or younger with MCL. The initial experience with R-HyperCVAD (97 patients; 1/3 >65 years old)[32] showed a CR rate of 87% and a 3-year failure-free survival (FFS) of 73% in the 65 years and younger group, consistent with the results seen with ASCT consolidation. In a recent update with 15-year follow-up,[33] the median OS exceeded 10 years for all patients, whereas about one-third of the 65 years and younger group were still in their first remission. Although the efficacy of R-HyperCVAD has been recognized in the multicenter setting,[34-36] it is definitely associated with significant toxicity, including secondary MDS (although in smaller numbers than after HDT/ASCT),[32] feeding the debate of benefit of intensive therapies in MCL. On the other hand, an abbreviated version (4 cycles) of R-HyperCVAD regimen has been used as induction pre-ASCT leading to very impressive results.[37] On the other hand, based on the high CR (and molecular CR rate) seen with these high dose cytarabine containing regimens, one can logically wonder if HDT-ACST consolidation upfront is still needed. This issue is currently being addressed through the ongoing TRIANGLE study in Europe, which aims at introducing ibrutinib in the frontline setting, including a randomization of HDT-ASCT versus maintenance ibrutinib post induction. Another EU large (299 patients) phase 3 trial (LyMA) looked at R-DHAP x 4 cycles (and if not at least in PR, patients could receive 4 cycles of R-CHOP) followed by HDT-ASCT in untreated MCL (<66 years). Patients were randomized post-ASCT for observation versus Rtx maintenance (375 mg/m^2 every 2 months for 3 years). The CR/CRu rates before and after ASCT were 81% and 92%, respectively. At the last follow-up, the median EFS (primary endpoint) was not reached, and at 2 years was 93% in the Rtx arm versus 81% in the observation arm (hazard ratio 2.1). The study included again remarkable multicenter serial quantitative polymerase chain reaction (PCR) monitoring showing that pre-ASCT MRD status in both bone marrow (BM) and peripheral blood PB was a strong predictor of PFS in younger MCL patients.[38] Early monitoring post-ASCT could help guide future MRD-based risk-adapted treatment. Interestingly, Rtx maintenance improved the PFS (ie, reduced the risk of recurrence) even in patients who were MRD negative post completion of induction-ASCT phase, suggesting potentially rare residual circulating or "tissue-resident" MCL cells.

The emergence of bendamustine in the management of elderly patients offered another opportunity as induction in younger patients as well. A randomized study of B-R (bendamustine + rituximab) against R-HyperCVAD in transplant-eligible patients was closed prematurely (53/160 patients accrued) due to unexpected (and surprising) failure of stem cell collection in the R-HyperCVAD arm. Of note in this trial, the CR rate post-R-HyperCVAD was very low (31%) versus 70% to 85% in other reported series. Nevertheless, results were encouraging with a 2-year PFS for R-Hyper-CVAD and B-R arms of 87% and 88%, respectively. In addition, in a subset of patients with MRD data available, results suggested that B-R can lead to deep remission with high-molecular CR rate.[39] Although this needs to be validated in larger trials, B-R is also being looked at in combination with cytarabine (B-R/R-AraC induction) before ASCT with also preliminary but intriguing results.[40] On the other hand, recent data suggest that cytarabine alone–based regimens might not be sufficient as frontline therapy for MCL.[41]

If no one would argue about the progress accomplished through DIT/HDT over standard therapy, such strategies are not always usable in MCL patients, given the median age at diagnosis in the mid to late 60s, although comorbidities, not just age, should be the critical factors for treatment decisions, as selected patients greater than 65 years can enjoy similar outcome as younger patients even with HDT-ASCT.[42] However, such patients are typically excluded from studies, and it becomes then important to look at real world data outside clinical trials, where, unfortunately, overall the outcome of MCL has not really changed since the mid 1990s according to US registry data.[43] However, even in that setting, interestingly, the impact of DIT/HDT has been verified. A large Scandinavian study of more than 1300 patients[22] confirmed the positive impact of both Rtx-containing regimen and ASCT consolidation on MCL patients' OS. In the United States, data from the SEER database comparing R-CHOP versus R-Hyper-CVAD or R-CHOP/R-HyperCVAD/ASCT confirmed in our experience,[44] that R-CHOP leads to clearly inferior outcome than DIT-HDT strategies, both for PFS and for OS when comparing pooled DIT/HDT versus R-CHOP alone.

IN SUMMARY

- DIT/HDT strategies lead to a much higher CR rate, in the range of 55%–80% pre-ACST and going up to 85% to 90% post-ACST (vs 30%–35% range for R-CHOP or 35%–45% for B-R alone), which not surprisingly translates into much more durable remission and disease-free intervals leading to OS advantage.
- Furthermore, induction regimens that incorporate Rtx and high-dose cytarabine lead to a very high rate of early molecular CR that is emerging as likely a critical endpoint and is currently being validated in ongoing MCL trials.

- Although there are limited data yet to compare with DIT, small phase II studies support further exploration of potentially less toxic regimens such as B-R or B-R + cytarabine as induction as well as in younger patients.
- To build on the success of DIT/HDT, ongoing studies are also looking at a combinations with novel agents together or as maintenance/consolidation post-HDT. Preliminary results of bortezomib as consolidation or maintenance post-HDT-ASCT (CALGB) suggests improved outcome compared with historical controls.[45] Meanwhile, the benefit of maintenance Rtx was also shown after HDT as mentioned in the LyMa trial above, significantly reducing the risk of relapse and prolonging PFS.[46] Although there was no OS advantage in the maintenance arm in that study, a combination of Rtx plus other biologicals might further improve the outcome post induction in MCL and is the subject of several ongoing clinical trials, including after HDT-ASCT.

PATIENTS NOT ELIGIBLE FOR DOSE-INTENSIVE THERAPY/HIGH-DOSE THERAPY APPROACHES: BUILDING UP ON NEW BACKBONES, AND IMPACT OF MAINTENANCE INSTEAD OF CONSOLIDATION WITH HIGH-DOSE THERAPIES/AUTOLOGOUS STEM CELL TRANSPLANTATION

Given the median age at diagnosis (in some series up to 70 years), alternative approaches to DIT/HDT are needed. When added to CHOP, Rtx clearly increased overall response rate (ORR), CR rate, and TTTF but had no significant impact on PFS (25% at 2 years) or OS compared with CHOP alone.[47] Although BR has been reported superior to R-CHOP (med PFS 22 vs 35 ms, $p = .004$) in the MCL subset (92 patients) from the STiL trial,[48] the attempted confirmatory BRIGHT trial in the United States was not suggestive of superiority of BR over R-CHOP (except for CR rate, although control arm had pooled R-CHOP-R-COP [is CHOP without antracyclin]).[49] Fludarabine-containing regimens such as fludarabine, cyclophosphamide and rituximab (FCR) had shown durable remission in MCL[50] and was tested against R-CHOP in a large (560 patients) randomized trial in elderly MCL (>60 and/or not eligible for HDT). A second randomization in this trial looked at maintenance (until POD or toxicity) with Rtx versus IFN-α.[51] Although the CR rate was similar (40% with FCR vs 34% with R-CHOP), both progressive disease and toxicity were worse with FCR as well as OS (47% with FCR vs 62% with R-CHOP, $p = .005$). Interestingly, looking at maintenance impact, Rtx reduced the risk of progression or death by 45% (4 years remission, 58%, vs 29% with IFN-α; p< .01). In addition, in patients responding to R-CHOP, R2 maintenance significantly improved OS (4-year OS 87%, vs 63% with IFN-α; $P = .005$). Putting aside any caveat from selection (related to double randomization design), such results are not very different from HDT/ASCT seen in younger patients, suggesting that maintenance might provide similar benefit as consolidation with ACST in some cases. Although the maintenance benefit has been shown in both younger (post-ASCT) and elderly patients, this might depend on the context, particularly on the type of induction as shown recently with the MAINTAIN trial of maintenance Rtx versus observation after B-R induction in non-ASCT candidates of MCL patients.[52] Although this study might have been underpowered, similar results were seen in the EU trial FCR arm, where maintenance Rtx had no impact,[53] suggesting that lymphopenia commonly seen after either fludarabine or bendamustine might interfere with effector cells responsible for most of Rtx effect.

The emergence of novel agents in the relapsed/refractory setting with nonoverlapping toxicities with cytotoxics offered an opportunity for new combinations. The recent LYM3002 phase III trial compared 6 cycles of R-CHOP versus R-CAP + bortezomib

(1.3 mg/m^2 IV on days 1, 4, 8, and 11) in non-HDT/ASCT eligible newly diagnosed MCL patients (244 per arm),[54] aiming at PFS as primary endpoint. After a median follow-up of 40 months, results showed a relative improvement of 59% of median PFS (by independent radiologic review) from 14.4 months in the R-CHOP group to 24.7 months in the VR-CAP group (*p*<.001). Secondary end points were consistently improved in the VR-CAP group, including CR rate (42% vs 53%), median CR duration (18.0 months vs 42.1 months), median treatment-free interval (20.5 months vs 40.6 months), and 4-year OS rate (54% vs 64%). Rates of neutropenia and thrombocytopenia were higher in the VR-CAP group but manageable, setting a new standard and becoming the first US Food and Drug Administration (FDA) -approved frontline combination in MCL. Similarly, a modified R-HyperCVAD regimen (no methotrexate, no cytarabine, and built-in maintenance with 4 weekly doses of Rtx 375 mg/m^2 every 6 months for 2 years), to reduce toxicity, was initially piloted in previously untreated MCL[55] and then combined with bortezomib (Vc-R-CVAD). Results showed a very promising ORR of 90% and CR rate of 77% (vs 77% and 63%, respectively, in modified R-Hyper-CVAD without bortezomib), translating into a 3-year PFS of 63% and OS of 86%.[56] The benefit of this combination was confirmed in the extended Eastern Cooperative Oncology Group (ECOG)-1405 trial,[57] with interestingly similar results in patients who received maintenance Rtx or underwent ASCT consolidation, which was optionally offered in this trial.

Despite the lack of difference in OS of BR versus R-CHOP, its favorable short-term toxicity profile, particularly in the STiL trial, established a new backbone in MCL for combinations, such as BR plus bortezomib, which showed very promising results in phase II studies in the relapsed/refractory setting (83% ORR, 52% CR).[58] This concept is currently tested in the frontline setting in a large intergroup randomized US trial, which also integrates maintenance Rtx versus Rtx plus lenalidomide. The LYSA group recently presented impressive results with RiBVD (rituximab, bendamustine, bortezomib, and dexamethasone) in 74 frontline elderly MCL (no maintenance) with a 74% CR/CRu rate alongside measurable molecular remissions in peripheral blood (83%) and bone marrow (74%), translating into an estimated 24-month PFS and OS of 69% and 80%, respectively.[59] Other combinations with BR are ongoing, such as with ibrutinib (SHINE randomized phase III trial in frontline >65 years MCL completed, results pending) or with other biologicals such as lenalidomide, with promising CR rate (NORDIC MCL4 trial)[60] or temsirolimus,[61] in either combination or maintenance, including as part of the randomized evaluation between high-dose cytarabine containing regimen versus R-CHOP for elderly MCL patients. Finally, the addition of cytarabine to BR was reported in MCL patients 65 years of age or older; although a small series, results were impressive with 100% ORR (95% CR) and 95% 2-year PFS for previously untreated MCL (n = 20), and 80% ORR (74% CR) with a 70% 2-year PFS for relapsed/refractory (R/R) MCL (n = 20).[62] With more novel agents in the pipeline, in the future, studies will likely aim at continuing to build up on such platforms, with the goal and hope to reach early on deeper responses as in younger patients, a critical factor toward better long-term disease control.

IN SUMMARY

- Less toxic regimens offer new backbone for combination with biological agents such as in R-CHOP-Bortezomib (first FDA-approved new induction regimen), while studies using B-R combinations (bortezomib, lenalidomide, ibrutinib) are still ongoing. It is likely that the integration of biological agents to standard regimens will increase CR and molecular CR rates and help continue improve the outcome in non-DIT/HDT-eligible patients.

- Maintenance Rtx has improved PFS and OS in patients responding to R-CHOP. Interestingly, it is likely that the underlying regimen (through immunotoxicity/ effector cells) might affect the impact of maintenance Rtx (for example, after bendamustine or fludarabine). The next step in maintenance approaches include other biologicals (ibrutinib, lenalidomide) as single agent or combined with Rtx.
- MRD as in younger patients is emerging as likely the next endpoint in the management of MCL. Furthermore, integrating MRD monitoring after induction might help decide on indication and/or duration of maintenance Rtx, allowing one also to take into account costs and clinical benefits issues.
- As in younger patients, the goal should be to continue integrating biological agents to increase CR and molecular CR rates, as MRD becomes an endpoint.
- Chemotherapy-free alternatives: might be within reach (as shown in later discussion), although additional follow-up is needed particularly for response to standard therapies afterwards and/or salvage, in a disease with clearly a different course than CLL.

NOVEL THERAPIES ARE CHANGING THE LANDSCAPE: FROM PROVIDING REAL OPTIONS IN THE R/R SETTING (CHEMORESISTANT DISEASE), BUILDING ON EXISTING REGIMENS AND PROVIDING AN OPPORTUNITY FOR NEW NON CHEMOTHERAPY OPTIONS IN MANTLE CELL LYMPHOMA

Unfortunately, even with DIT/HDT strategies, a significant number of patients relapse over time and then experience only transient benefit from additional chemotherapy or even HDT-ASCT.[63] Non-myeloablative allogenic stem transplantation if feasible represents the only potentially curative option in that setting, with its inherent limitations: donor's availability, age, and chronic graft versus host disease (GVHD) (>50%).[64] Meanwhile, productive efforts have led to the approval of several novel therapies over the last 10 years: bortezomib (December 2006),[65,66] temsirolimus (EU only; August 2009),[67] lenalidomide (June 2013),[68] and ibrutinib (November 2013).[69] The results of the single-agent activity that led to the approval of each of those compounds are summarized in **Table 2**. Overall, the activity of several of these agents has been very impressive even in heavily pretreated and often chemorefractory patients as well as carrying p53mut and/or del17p in particular for ibrutinib. Although many of these responses were very durable, there is the emerging, although debated concern, that post ibrutinib patients progress very rapidly as seen in CLL as well, behaving often like Richter even without clear histological transformation.[70]

Beyond the combinations discussed previously aiming at integrating biological agents to improve the efficacy of chemoimmunotherapy regimens in MCL patients, they also offer the option to develop biologically based therapies. Starting with monoclonal antibodies (mAb), second-generation mAb such as ofatumumab, which had shown anecdotal but impressive response in R/R MCL,[71] was not as promising (1/12 patients achieved a PR) in a following phase II.[72] Ongoing studies are looking at other anti-CD20 mAb, such as obinutuzumab, or other targets, such as CD38 or CD74 among others. More importantly, each one of the new-targeted therapies approved and mentioned above has been added to Rtx with suggestion of clinical benefit. Ibrutinib and Rtx combination was tested in patients with r/r MCL with very promising results.[73] Ibrutinib was given in this study at 560 mg daily until progression or toxicity, whereas Rtx (375 mg/m^2) was given weekly $\times$ 4 for cycle 1 and on day 1 of cycles 3 to 8 and once every other cycle thereafter up to 2 years. The series, which

Table 2
Approved biological agents in r/r mantle cell lymphoma: Comparative activity

Agent	Design/Nb pts	ORR (%)	CR (%)	Med DOR (mo)	Med PFS (mo)	Med OS (mo)
Bortezomib PINNACLE	155	32	8	9.2	6.5	23.5
Temsirolimus	175/75 mg (54 pts/arm) vs investig choice (54 pts)	22 vs 6 vs 2	2 vs 0 vs 2	7.1 vs 3.6 vs N/A	4.8 vs 3.4 vs 1.9	12.8 vs 10.0 vs 9.7
Lenalidomide EMERGE	134	28	8	16.6	4.0	19.0
Ibrutinib	111	67	23	17.5	13	22
Ibrutinib vs Temsirolimus	139 vs 141	72/40	18 vs 1.4	NA	14.6 vs 6.2	NR vs 21.3

included a total of 50 patients with r/r MCL (median of 3 prior therapies; range 1–9), showed an ORR of 88%, including 44% CR. The I-R combination was well tolerated with mostly grade 1 to 2 toxicities (gastrointestinal, fatigue) and only a few cases of atrial fibrillation (12% patients) and bleeding (2%). Although the population was not as high risk (12% vs 49% high-risk MIPI in the single-agent ibrutinib series), the CR in the I-R study was twice the one observed with ibrutinib alone,[69] despite the theoretical underlying concern of decreased Rtx efficacy, based on a known off-target inhibition of ITK (interleukin-2-inducible kinase) in natural killer cells by ibrutinib.[74] The next logical step is to explore such chemotherapy-free combinations in the frontline setting, which is the subject of an ongoing randomized study in the UK looking at I-R versus B-R in elderly MCL, which might offer a first new non chemotherapy option for the management of elderly newly diagnosed MCL patients.

Similarly, lenalidomide was combined with Rtx in r/r MCL in a phase I-II study[75] with dose escalation of lenalidomide, whereas Rtx was given weekly × 4 for cycle 1 and then with every cycle afterward, this until progression, stem-cell transplantation, or severe toxicity. The MTD was defined at 20 mg qd 21/28 days for lenalidomide (related to myelotoxicity), setting the dosing for the expansion phase. Among the 44 patients in phase II, the ORR was 57% with 36% CR; these responses were durable (med DOR 18.9 ms), including in patients who had failed prior bortezomib. A similar combination in the frontline setting this time generated much interest recently.[76] Patients with appropriate renal function (clearance creatinine $\geq$ 60 m/mn) received treatment in 2 phases. During induction phase (about 1 year), lenalidomide was given at 20 mg daily (25 mg after cycle 2 if no toxicity) for 21/28 days × 12 cycles and combined with Rtx 375 mg/m^2 once weekly × 4 and then once every other cycle. Maintenance phase started with year 2, using a reduced dose of lenalidomide (15 mg daily) together with Rtx given with every other cycle, up to 36 cycles or until patient withdrawal, disease progression, or toxicity. A total of 38 MCL patients (median age 65 years) were enrolled from multiple centers with an even distribution of MIPI risk (1/3 low, 1/3 intermediate, 1/3 high risk). The most common grade 3 or 4 adverse events were neutropenia (50%), rash (29%), thrombocytopenia (13%), "tumor flare" (11%), anemia (11%), serum sickness (8%), and fatigue (8%). At a median follow-up of 30 months, the ORR was 92% with 64% CR, while 2-year PFS was estimated to be 85% and 2-year OS 97%. These results were very impressive, although they need further follow-up, while some have raised the question of potential risk of impairing stem cell collection after prolonged exposure to lenalidomide, potentially compromising subsequent use of HDT-ASCT. This data as well as other ongoing studies raise the possibility of future non chemotherapy options in MCL. However, the follow-up of these studies is rather short, and there is not yet any experience of response to standard therapies and/or salvage therapy in that setting. MCL is a disease that becomes easily chemoresistant over time, including after biological agents as shown by a median OS following cessation of ibrutinib of only 2.9 months,[77] leading one to remain cautious moving forward. In addition, responses improve over time (med time to CR for R2 combination was 11 ms), and regimen is planned for years (initially 3 extended then to 5 years), raising costs concerns not addressed at this point and which should be included when talking about shifting paradigm, particularly when adding or combining additional biologicals. Nevertheless, multiple other promising novel agents are currently in development in MCL, as summarized in **Table 3**. Beyond the new mAb mentioned above, new BCR targeting agents such as PIK3-δ inhibitors idelalisib[78] or TGR-1202[79,80] (promising results in combination with TG-1101 (ublituximab, new anti CD20 against distinct epitope), and ibrutinib), and finally, BCL-2 inhibitors with ABT-199 (venetoclax),[81] which showed impressive activity in heavily pretreated MCL patients. In addition, the recent, likely game-changing, developments in immunotherapy from checkpoint inhibitors, to BiTE antibodies and cell therapy with CAR-T cells, will definitely impact the management of MCL. Evidently, a growing number of studies are currently looking at multicombinations to further establish the concept of biological chemotherapy-free therapy in this disease. It will be important to see if those can lead to earlier and durable CR that might allow stopping therapy while maintaining clinical benefit.

HETEROGENEITY OF MANTLE CELL LYMPHOMA: CAN PROGNOSTIC FACTORS HELP STRATIFYING PATIENTS?

The heterogeneity of MCL has been recognized since its morphologic description with both histological (nodular, diffuse, mantle zone) and cytological variants (small cells, pleiomorphic, and blastoid) that can affect outcome. Clinically, the MIPI, obtained through a calculation based on age, ECOG performance status, lactate dehydrogenase, and total white blood cell counts, can help better stratify patients than International Prognostic Index or Follicular Lymphoma International Prognostic Index.[82] The simplified version of MIPI, which can segregate MCL patients into low- (med OS not reached), intermediate- (med OS, 51 months), and high-risk groups (med OS, 29 months), has been validated in both standard regimens and HDT settings[83] with a 5-year OS rate in MIPI low-, intermediate-, and high-risk groups of 83%, 63%, and 34%, respectively. GEP revealed early on the impact of proliferation signature on MCL outcome (median OS from <1 to >7 years) in patients treated with CHOP-based chemotherapy.[84] Ki-67 (or MIB1) has been used as a surrogate marker of proliferation (</≥30%), showing survival-related value independently of MIPI.[85] Although Ki67 has been integrated into the MIPI-b (MIPI-biological) (http://bloodref.com/lymphoid/lymphoma/mipib), this has not translated into truly stratifying patients upfront, yet in addition to issues related to quantification of Ki67 and its reproducibility.[86] Rare cases at baseline present with high Ki67, often carrying also *DEL17P/P53* mutation; both of these features consistent with blastoid variant are more commonly seen with successive relapses over time (clonal evolution). The recent years have shed increasing light on the molecular diversity of MCL: from SOX11 expression to the mutational landscape of MCL that contributes to pathogenesis and disease progression, including mutations in *ATM*, *P53*, *BIRC3*, *WHSC1*, and *NOTCH1* among others.[87,88] Several other prognostic variables have been reported in MCL, including β2-microglobulin, miRNAs,[89] and epigenetic signatures,[90] as well as complex karyotypes, whereas overall *p53* abnormalities are likely underestimated in MCL and translate into significantly worse outcome even after HDT-ASCT.[91] Recent data using Nanostring technology suggest a new validated MCL55 (16 genes/proliferation signature) assay usable on formaldehyde fixed-paraffin embedded biopsies,, which define groups of patients with MCL with significantly different OS independent of the MIPI.[92]

In conclusion, together multiple research and clinical aspects are together reshaping the paradigm in MCL, as summarized below and as shown in **Fig 1**.

- MCL carries a high degree of both clinical and biological diversity
- Indolent MCL (iMCL)
  - iMCL: represent 10%–15% of cases, are characterized by lymphocytosis, splenomegaly, no or minimal nodal disease, SOX11-ve, somatically mutated and genetically stable, and show prolonged stable course. Such cases should be treated expectantly; although similar to CLL, the development of alternative non chemotherapy options might offer an option to intervene earlier, notwithstanding it remains unclear yet if this would alter (improve or affect) the natural history of the disease.

Table 3
Novel therapies in mantle cell lymphoma

Target	Agent/Trial	Efficacy	Comments
Proteasome	Bortezomib	ORR 33% CR 8%[65,66] Med OR 16.8 ms VR-CAP (LYM-3001) B-R-BTZ ORR 83%, 2 y PFS 47%[58] R-hyperCVAD-BTZ	CR med DOR >27 ms subcutaneous significantly reduced risk of neuropathy[94] 59% increased PFS to >24 ms vs 14 ms w/R-CHOP[54] w/R2 vs R maintenance (Alliance, ongoing) Ph I, no issues[95] Ph II, completed P
	Carfilzomib	Maint post R-chemo or HDT-ASCT 1 MCL resp (CRu) in small ph II[96] Carfilzomib single-agent ongoing Carfilzomib + Len + R2 ongoing	CALGB maintenance PFS > historical controls[45]
IMiDs	Lenalidomide	Single-agent 25 mg qd 21/28 d ORR 28% CR 7%[68] Len + R2[73] ORR 57% 36% CR Len + R frontline ORR was 92% 61% CR Maintenance	Med DOR 16.6 ms All pts had failed prior BTZ Ongoing Post-BBR ongoing Post-HDT-ASCT ongoing
mTOR	Temsirolimus	ORR 38% 3% CR[97] Toxicity ++ BR + Temsirolimus in r/r MCL Tesmsirolimus + cladribine + Rtx as frontline therapy in MCL[99]	Approved in EU[67] 15 pts/ORR 93% 5 CR in MCL[98] ORR 94%; 53% CR Med PFS 18 ms
	Everolimus	ORR 8% no CR[100]	

Category	Agent	Detail	Notes
BTK	Ibutinib	ORR 68% CR 21%[69]	Med DOR 17.5 ms
		BR ± Ibrutinib SHINE in elderly MCL trial completed	
		Ib + R ORR 88% CR 44%[73]	
		Ib + Len + Rtx	
		Ib vs Temsirolimus in EU	Ongoing 280 pts Med PFS 14 ms vs 6 ms Med OS NR vs 21 ms ORR 72% vs 40% CR 18% vs 1.4% Med DOR NR vs 7 ms
	Acalabrutinib (ACP-196)	Ph II completed 134 pts	
PI3K	Idelalisib (PI3Kδ) inhibition	ORR 40%, 5% CR Median DOR was 2.7 ms[101]	P110α-mediated constitutive PI3K signaling limits the efficacy of p110δ-selective[102]
	Duvelisib	Dual inhibitor γ and δ	Ongoing
	Copanlisib	Dual inhibitor α and δ[103]	ORR 64% 2 CR, 5 PR in r/r MCL 1 CR in MCL
	TGR-1202	Ibrutinib, Ublituximab, TGR-1202 Triplet	Ongoing
Bcl2	Venetoclax (ABT-199)	7/8 responders[104]	Comb ongoing ABT-199 + Ibrutinib BR-ABT-199 ongoing 29/38 resp 10 CR
		BR-ABT-199 in r/r NHL[105]	
Cyclins	CDK 4/6 inhibitor palbociclib	Activity single agent based on SUV reduction[106]	Preclinical rationale for comb with ibrutinib (overcome resistance)/ BTZ, cr PI3K inhibition[107]
Epigenetics	Vorinostat	Modest clinical activity[108]	But strong preclinical data for combinations ongoing
New mAb	Obinutuzumab	Single-agent activity in r/r MCL[109]	Combinations ongoing w/chemo or ibrutinib or lenalidomide
	Ofatumumab	1 CR as single agent[110]	Combinations ongoing
	Ublituximab (TG-1101)	Glycoengineered anti-CD20	Comb w/ibrutinib ORR 83% CR 33%[111]
Immune-based therapies	Checkpoint inhibitors	Activity in several subtypes of NHL	Comb ongoing with nivolumab + ibrutinib ORR 71%[112]
	BiTE antibodies	Blinatumomab	
	CAR-T cells	ZUMA-2 trial	Ongoing

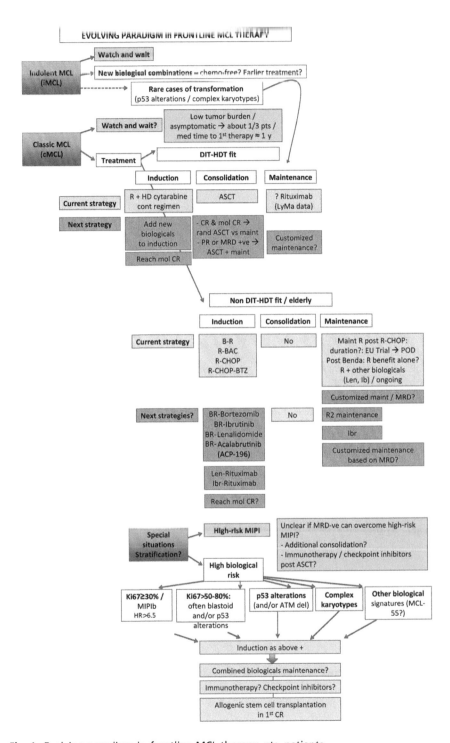

Fig. 1. Evolving paradigm in frontline MCL therapy. pts, patients.

- ○ Such cases of iMCL can "transform" over time through acquisition of p53 aberrations and/or complex karyotypes and then should be managed as aggressive variants.
- By opposition in classic MCL, Ki-67 and MIPI are the only 2 prognostic factors "available routinely."
  - ○ Both MIPI and Ki-67 should be combined (MIPI-b) because data suggest that low risk (MIPI-b <5.7) and intermediate risk (MIPI-b $\geq$ 5.70 but $\leq$6.50) do very well (75%–80% OS) at 8 years with dose-intensive strategies.[93] Interestingly, the outcome of such patients is not very different in "elderly protocols" reflecting the impact of improvement of induction regimens and superior salvage options (novel therapies), while it might be premature yet to decide on the impact of maintenance.
  - ○ On the other hand, high-risk MIPI and high-risk MIPI-b have definitely a worse outcome regardless of the strategy used (25%–35% at 8 years). It remains unclear how much reaching an MRD negative status in these patients impacts their outcome. Novel strategies with consolidation/maintenance using new biological combinations and/or immunotherapy approaches are ongoing.
  - ○ The next generation of trials will be to combine novel therapies with previous chemoimmunotherapy regimens to improve CR/mol CR rates in both younger and elderly patients, raising then the question of the need for ASCT consolidation versus maintenance or both.
- Patients with Ki-67 greater than 50% to 80%, blastoid variants, and/or p53 alterations (frequent overlap), or with complex karyotypes, should be considered for potential allogenic stem cell transplantation upfront.
- Overall, efforts should be continued toward clinical trials as well as education in the community to prevent a clear disparity of outcome across the board for all MCL patients, giving them the best opportunities they deserve in a field that is finally changing, thanks to their participation and trust in our endeavors.

REFERENCES

1. Weisenburger DD, Kim H, Rappaport H. Mantle-zone lymphoma: a follicular variant of intermediate lymphocytic lymphoma. Cancer 1982;49:1429–38.
2. Harris NL, Jaffe ES, Stein H, et al. A revised European-American classification of lymphoid neoplasms: a proposal from the International Lymphoma Study Group. Blood 1994;84:1361–92.
3. Tsujimoto Y, Finger LR, Yunis J, et al. Cloning of the chromosome breakpoint of neoplastic B cells with the t(14;18) chromosome translocation. Science 1984; 226:1097–9.
4. Williams ME, Swerdlow SH, Meeker TC. Chromosome t(11;14)(q13;q32) breakpoints in centrocytic lymphoma are highly localized at the bcl-1 major translocation cluster. Leukemia 1993;7:1437–40.
5. Schollkopf C, Melbye M, Munksgaard L, et al. Borrelia infection and risk of non-Hodgkin lymphoma. Blood 2008;111:5524–9.
6. Smedby KE, Sampson JN, Turner JJ, et al. Medical history, lifestyle, family history, and occupational risk factors for mantle cell lymphoma: the InterLymph Non-Hodgkin Lymphoma Subtypes Project. J Natl Cancer Inst Monogr 2014; 2014:76–86.
7. Thurner L, artmann S, Dieter Preuss K, et al. LRPAP1 is a frequent B-cell receptor antigen in mantle cell lymphoma (MCL). Blood 2015;126:2685.

8. Jares P, Colomer D, Campo E. Molecular pathogenesis of mantle cell lymphoma. J Clin Invest 2012;122:3416–23.

9. Espinet B, Salaverria I, Bea S, et al. Incidence and prognostic impact of secondary cytogenetic aberrations in a series of 145 patients with mantle cell lymphoma. Genes Chromosomes Cancer 2010;49:439–51.

10. Armitage JO. Management of mantle cell lymphoma. Oncology 1998;12:49–55.

11. Avet-Loiseau H, Garand R, Gaillard F, et al. Detection of t(11;14) using interphase molecular cytogenetics in mantle cell lymphoma and atypical chronic lymphocytic leukemia. Genes Chromosomes Cancer 1998;23:175–82.

12. Herens C, Lambert F, Quintanilla-Martinez L, et al. Cyclin D1-negative mantle cell lymphoma with cryptic t(12;14)(p13;q32) and cyclin D2 overexpression. Blood 2008;111:1745–6.

13. Wlodarska I, Dierickx D, Vanhentenrijk V, et al. Translocations targeting CCND2, CCND3, and MYCN do occur in t(11;14)-negative mantle cell lymphomas. Blood 2008;111:5683–90.

14. Mozos A, Royo C, Hartmann E, et al. SOX11 expression is highly specific for mantle cell lymphoma and identifies the cyclin D1-negative subtype. Haematologica 2009;94:1555–62.

15. Fu K, Weisenburger DD, Greiner TC, et al. Cyclin D1-negative mantle cell lymphoma: a clinicopathologic study based on gene expression profiling. Blood 2005;106:4315–21.

16. Romaguera JE, Medeiros LJ, Hagemeister FB, et al. Frequency of gastrointestinal involvement and its clinical significance in mantle cell lymphoma. Cancer 2003;97:586–91.

17. Ferrer A, Salaverria I, Bosch F, et al. Leukemic involvement is a common feature in mantle cell lymphoma. Cancer 2007;109:2473–80.

18. Ferrer A, Bosch F, Villamor N, et al. Central nervous system involvement in mantle cell lymphoma. Ann Oncol 2008;19:135–41.

19. Cheah CY, George A, Gine E, et al. Central nervous system involvement in mantle cell lymphoma: clinical features, prognostic factors and outcomes from the European Mantle Cell Lymphoma Network. Ann Oncol 2013;24:2119–23.

20. Chihara D, Asano N, Ohmachi K, et al. Ki-67 is a strong predictor of central nervous system relapse in patients with mantle cell lymphoma (MCL). Ann Oncol 2015;26(5):966–73. http://dx.doi.org/10.1093/annonc/mdv074.

21. Herrmann A, Hoster E, Zwingers T, et al. Improvement of overall survival in advanced stage mantle cell lymphoma. J Clin Oncol 2009;27:511–8.

22. Abrahamsson A, Albertsson-Lindblad A, Brown PN, et al. Real world data on primary treatment for mantle cell lymphoma: a Nordic Lymphoma Group observational study. Blood 2014;124:1288–95.

23. Skarbnik A, Goy A. Mantle cell lymphoma: state of the art. Clin Adv Hematol Oncol 2015;13(1):44–55.

24. Dreyling M, Lenz G, Hoster E, et al. Early consolidation by myeloablative radiochemotherapy followed by autologous stem cell transplantation in first remission significantly prolongs progression-free survival in mantle-cell lymphoma: results of a prospective randomized trial of the European MCL Network. Blood 2005; 105:2677–84.

25. Damon LE, Johnson JL, Niedzwiecki D, et al. Immunochemotherapy and autologous stem-cell transplantation for untreated patients with mantle-cell lymphoma: CALGB 59909. J Clin Oncol 2009;27:6101–8.

26. Geisler CH, Kolstad A, Laurell A, et al. Nordic MCL2 trial update: six-year follow-up after intensive immunochemotherapy for untreated mantle cell lymphoma

followed by BEAM or BEAC + autologous stem-cell support: still very long survival but late relapses do occur. Br J Haematol 2012;158:355–62.

27. Geisler CH, Kolstad A, Laurell A, et al. Long-term progression-free survival of mantle cell lymphoma after intensive front-line immunochemotherapy with in vivo-purged stem cell rescue: a nonrandomized phase 2 multicenter study by the Nordic Lymphoma Group. Blood 2008;112:2687–93.

28. Hermine O, Hoster E, Walewski J, et al. Alternating courses of 3x CHOP and 3x DHAP plus rituximab followed by a high dose ARA-C containing myeloablative regimen and autologous stem cell transplantation (ASCT) increases overall survival when compared to 6 courses of CHOP plus rituximab followed by myeloablative radiochemotherapy and ASCT in mantle cell lymphoma: final analysis of the MCL younger trial of the European Mantle Cell Lymphoma Network (MCL net). Blood 2012;120 [abstract: 151].

29. Delarue R, Haioun C, Ribrag V, et al. CHOP and DHAP plus rituximab followed by autologous stem cell transplantation in mantle cell lymphoma: a phase 2 study from the Groupe d'Etude des Lymphomes de l'Adulte. Blood 2013;121: 48–53.

30. Pott C, Macintyre E, Delfau-Larue M, et al. MRD eradication should be the therapeutic goal in mantle cell lymphoma and may enable tailored treatment approaches: results of the intergroup trials of the European MCL Network. Blood 2014;124 [abstract: 147].

31. Hermine O, Hoster E, Walewski J, et al. Addition of high-dose cytarabine to immunochemotherapy before autologous stem-cell transplantation in patients aged 65 years or younger with mantle cell lymphoma (MCL Younger): a randomised, open-label, phase 3 trial of the European Mantle Cell Lymphoma Network. European Mantle Cell Lymphoma Network. Lancet 2016;388(10044): 565–75. http://dx.doi.org/10.1016/S0140-6736(16)00739-X.

32. Romaguera JE, Fayad L, Rodriguez MA, et al. High rate of durable remissions after treatment of newly diagnosed aggressive mantle-cell lymphoma with rituximab plus hyper-CVAD alternating with rituximab plus high-dose methotrexate and cytarabine. J Clin Oncol 2005;23:7013–23.

33. Chihara D, Cheah CY, Westin JR, et al. Rituximab plus hyper-CVAD alternating with MTX/Ara-C in patients with newly diagnosed mantle cell lymphoma: 15-year follow-up of a phase II study from the MD Anderson Cancer Center. Br J Haematol 2016;172:80–8.

34. Bernstein SH, Epner E, Unger JM, et al. A phase II multicenter trial of hyper-CVAD MTX/Ara-C and rituximab in patients with previously untreated mantle cell lymphoma; SWOG 0213. Ann Oncol 2013;24:1587–93.

35. Merli F, Luminari S, Ilariucci F, et al. Rituximab plus HyperCVAD alternating with high dose cytarabine and methotrexate for the initial treatment of patients with mantle cell lymphoma, a multicentre trial from Gruppo Italiano Studio Linfomi. Br J Haematol 2012;156:346–53.

36. Chen R, Li H, Bernstein S, et al. Pre-transplant R-bendamustine induces high rates of minimal residual disease in MCL patients: updated results of S1106: US Intergroup Study of a Randomized Phase II Trial of R-HCVAD vs. R-bendamustine followed by autologous stem cell transplants for patients with mantle cell lymphoma. Blood 2015;126 [abstract: 518].

37. Till BG, Gooley TA, Crawford N, et al. Effect of remission status and induction chemotherapy regimen on outcome of autologous stem cell transplantation for mantle cell lymphoma. Leuk Lymphoma 2008;49:1062–73.

38. Callanan M, Delfau MH, Macintyre E, et al. Predictive Power of Early, Sequential MRD Monitoring in Peripheral Blood and Bone Marrow in Patients with Mantle Cell Lymphoma Following Autologous Stem Cell Transplantation with or without Rituximab Maintenance, Interim Results from the LyMa-MRD Project, Conducted on Behalf of the Lysa Group. Blood 2015;126:338.

39. Chen R, Hongli LI, Bernstein SH, et al. Pre-Transplant R-Bendamustine Induces High Rates of Minimal Residual Disease in MCL Patients: Updated Results of S1106: US Intergroup Study of a Randomized Phase II Trial of R-HCVAD Vs. R-Bendamustine Followed By Autologous Stem Cell Transplants for Patients with Mantle Cell Lymphoma. Blood 2015;126:518.

40. Armand P, Redd R, Bsat J, et al. A phase 2 study of Rituximab-Bendamustine and Rituximab-Cytarabine for transplant-eligible patients with mantle cell lymphoma. Br J Haematol 2016;173(1):89–95. http://dx.doi.org/10.1111/bjh.13929.

41. Laurell A, Kolstad A, Jerkeman M, et al. High dose cytarabine with rituximab is not enough in first-line treatment of mantle cell lymphoma with high proliferation: early closure of the Nordic Lymphoma Group MantleCell Lymphoma 5 trial. Leuk Lymphoma 2014;55(5):1206–8. http://dx.doi.org/10.3109/10428194.2013.825906.

42. Dahi PB, Tamari R, Devlin SM, et al. Favorable outcomes in elderly patients undergoing high-dose therapy and autologous stem cell transplantation for non-Hodgkin lymphoma. Biol Blood Marrow Transplant 2014;20:2004–9.

43. Chandran R, Gardiner SK, Simon M, et al. Survival trends in mantle cell lymphoma in the United States over sixteen years 1992-2007. Leuk Lymphoma 2012;53(8):1488–93.

44. Mato AR, Svoboda J, Feldman T, et al. Post-treatment (not interim) positron emission tomography-computed tomography scan status is highly predictive of outcome in mantle cell lymphoma patients treated with R-HyperCVAD. Cancer 2011;118(14):3565–70.

45. Kaplan LD, Jung S, Stock W, et al. Bortezomib maintenance (BM) versus consolidation (BC) following aggressive immunochemotherapy and autologous stem cell transplant (ASCT) for untreated mantle cell lymphoma (MCL): CALGB (ALLIANCE) 50403. Blood 2015;126 [abstract: 337].

46. Le Gouill S, Thieblemont C, Oberic L, et al. Rituximab maintenance versus wait and watch after four courses of R-DHAP followed by autologous stem cell transplantation in previously untreated young patients with mantle cell lymphoma. First interim analysis of the phase III prospective lyma trial, a Lysa Study. Blood 2014;124 [abstract: 146].

47. Lenz G, Dreyling M, Hoster E, et al. Immunochemotherapy with rituximab and cyclophosphamide, doxorubicin, vincristine, and prednisone significantly improves response and time to treatment failure, but not long-term outcome in patients with previously untreated mantle cell lymphoma: results of a prospective randomized trial of the German Low Grade Lymphoma Study Group (GLSG). J Clin Oncol 2005;23:1984–92.

48. Rummel MJ, Niederle N, Maschmeyer G, et al. Bendamustine plus rituximab versus CHOP plus rituximab as first-line treatment for patients with indolent and mantle-cell lymphomas: an open-label, multicentre, randomised, phase 3 non-inferiority trial. Lancet 2013;381:1203–10.

49. Flinn IW, van der Jagt R, Kahl BS, et al. Randomized trial of bendamustine-rituximab or R-CHOP/R-CVP in first-line treatment of indolent NHL or MCL: the BRIGHT study. Blood 2014;123:2944–52.

50. Eve HE, Linch D, Qian W, et al. Toxicity of fludarabine and cyclophosphamide with or without rituximab as initial therapy for patients with previously untreated

mantle cell lymphoma: results of a randomised phase II study. Leuk Lymphoma 2009;50:211–5.

51. Kluin-Nelemans HC, Hoster E, Hermine O, et al. Treatment of older patients with mantle-cell lymphoma. N Engl J Med 2012;367:520–31.

52. Rummel M, Knauf W, Goerner M, et al. Two years rituximab maintenance vs. observation after first-line treatment with bendamustine plus rituximab (B-R) in patients with mantle cell lymphoma: First results of a prospective, randomized, multicenter phase II study (a subgroup study of the StiL NHL7-2008 MAINTAIN trial). J Clin Oncol 2016;34(Suppl):Abstract 7503.

53. Kluin-Nelemans HC, Hoster E, Hermine O, et al. Treatment of Older Patients with Mantle-Cell Lymphoma. N Engl J Med 2012;367(6):520–31. http://dx.doi.org/10.1056/NEJMoa12009.

54. Robak T, Huang H, Jin J, et al. Bortezomib-based therapy for newly diagnosed mantle-cell lymphoma. N Engl J Med 2015;372:944–53.

55. Kahl BS, Longo WL, Eickhoff JC, et al. Maintenance rituximab following induction chemoimmunotherapy may prolong progression-free survival in mantle cell lymphoma: a pilot study from the Wisconsin Oncology Network. Ann Oncol 2006;17:1418–23.

56. Chang JE, Peterson C, Choi S, et al. VcR CVAD induction chemotherapy followed by maintenance rituximab in mantle cell lymphoma: a Wisconsin Oncology Network study. Br J Haematol 2011;155:190–7.

57. Chang JE, Li H, Smith MR, et al. Phase 2 study of VcR-CVAD with maintenance rituximab for untreated mantle cell lymphoma: an Eastern Cooperative Oncology Group study (E1405). Blood 2014;123:1665–73.

58. Friedberg JW, Vose JM, Kelly JL, et al. The combination of bendamustine, bortezomib, and rituximab for patients with relapsed/refractory indolent and mantle cell non-Hodgkin lymphoma. Blood 2011;117:2807–12.

59. Gressin R, Callanan M, Daguindau N, et al. The RIBVD regimen (rituximab IV, bendamustine IV, velcade SC, dexamethasone IV) offers a high complete response rate in elderly patients with untreated mantle cell lymphoma. Preliminary results of the lysa trial "Lymphome Du Manteau 2010 SA". Blood 2013; 122 [abstract: 370].

60. Albertsson-Lindblad A, Kolstad A, Laurell A, et al. Lenalidomide-bendamustine-rituximab in untreated mantle cell lymphoma > 65 years, the Nordic Lymphoma Group phase I+II trial NLG-MCL4. Blood 2016. [Epub ahead of print].

61. Hess G, Keller U, Scholz CW, et al. Safety and efficacy of Temsirolimus in combination with Bendamustine and Rituximab in relapsed mantle cell and follicular lymphoma. Leukemia 2015;29(8):1695–701.

62. Visco C, Finotto S, Zambello R, et al. Combination of rituximab, bendamustine, and cytarabine for patients with mantle-cell non-Hodgkin lymphoma ineligible for intensive regimens or autologous transplantation. J Clin Oncol 2013; 31(11):1442–9.

63. Robinson S, Dreger P, Caballero D, et al. The EBMT/EMCL consensus project on the role of autologous and allogeneic stem cell transplantation in mantle cell lymphoma. Leukemia 2015;29:464–73.

64. Vaughn JE, Sorror ML, Storer BE, et al. Long-term sustained disease control in patients with mantle cell lymphoma with or without active disease after treatment with allogeneic hematopoietic cell transplantation after nonmyeloablative conditioning. Cancer 2015;121:3709–16.

65. Goy A, Younes A, McLaughlin P, et al. Phase II study of proteasome inhibitor bortezomib in relapsed or refractory B-cell non-Hodgkin's lymphoma. J Clin Oncol 2005;23:667–75.

66. Fisher RI, Bernstein SH, Kahl BS, et al. Multicenter phase II study of bortezomib in patients with relapsed or refractory mantle cell lymphoma. J Clin Oncol 2006; 24:4867–74.

67. Hess G, Herbrecht R, Romaguera J, et al. Phase III study to evaluate temsirolimus compared with investigator's choice therapy for the treatment of relapsed or refractory mantle cell lymphoma. J Clin Oncol 2009;27:3822–9.

68. Goy A, Sinha R, Williams ME, et al. Single-agent lenalidomide in patients with mantle-cell lymphoma who relapsed or progressed after or were refractory to bortezomib: phase II MCL-001 (EMERGE) study. J Clin Oncol 2013;31(29): 3688–95.

69. Wang ML, Rule S, Martin P, et al. Targeting BTK with ibrutinib in relapsed or refractory mantle-cell lymphoma. N Engl J Med 2013;369:507–16.

70. Martin P, Maddocks K, Leonard JP, et al. Postibrutinib outcomes in patients with mantle cell lymphoma. Blood 2016;127(12):1559–63. http://dx.doi.org/10.1182/blood-2015-10-673145.

71. Hunstig F, Hammersen J, Kunert C, et al. Complete remission after treatment with single-agent ofatumumab in a patient with high-risk leukemic mantle-cell lymphoma. J Clin Oncol 2013;31(19):e312–5.

72. Furtado M, Dyer MJ, Johnson R, et al. Ofatumumab monotherapy in relapsed/refractory mantle cell lymphoma–a phase II trial. Br J Haematol 2014;165(4): 575–8.

73. Wang ML, Lee H, Chuang H, et al. Ibrutinib in combination with rituximab in relapsed or refractory mantle cell lymphoma: a single-centre, open-label, phase 2 trial. Lancet Oncol 2016;17:48–56.

74. Kohrt HE, Sagiv-Barfi I, Rafiq S, et al. Ibrutinib antagonizes rituximab-dependent NK cell-mediated cytotoxicity. Blood 2014;123:1957–60.

75. Wang M, Fayad L, Wagner-Bartak N, et al. Lenalidomide in combination with rituximab for patients with relapsed or refractory mantle-cell lymphoma: a phase 1/2 clinical trial. Lancet Oncol 2012;13:716–23.

76. Ruan J, Martin P, Shah B, et al. Lenalidomide plus rituximab as initial treatment for mantle cell lymphoma. N Engl J Med 2015;373:1835–44.

77. Martin P, Maddocks K, Leonard JP, et al. Post-ibrutinib outcomes in patients with mantle cell lymphoma. Blood 2016;127(12):1559–63.

78. Kahl BS, Spurgeon SE, Furman RR, et al. A phase 1 study of the PI3Kδ inhibitor idelalisib in patients with relapsed/refractory mantle cell lymphoma (MCL). Blood 2014;123(22):3398–405. http://dx.doi.org/10.1182/blood-2013-11-537555.

79. O'Brien S, Fowler N, Nastoupil N, et al. Safety and activity of the chemotherapy-free triplet of ublituximab, TGR-1202, and ibrutinib in relapsed B-cell malignancies. J Clin Oncol 2015;33(Suppl):Abstract 8501.

80. Fowler NH, Nastoupil LJ, Lunning MA, et al. Safety and activity of the chemotherapy-free triplet of ublituximab, TGR-1202, and ibrutinib in relapsed B-cell malignancies. J Clin Oncol 2015;33(Suppl):Abstract 8501.

81. Gerecitano JF, Roberts AW, Seymour JF, et al. A Phase 1 Study of Venetoclax (ABT-199 / GDC-0199) Monotherapy in Patients with Relapsed/Refractory Non-Hodgkin Lymphoma. Blood 2015;126:254.

82. Hoster E, Dreyling M, Klapper W, et al. A new prognostic index (MIPI) for patients with advanced-stage mantle cell lymphoma. Blood 2008;111:558–65.

83. Hoster E, Klapper W, Hermine O, et al. Confirmation of the mantle-cell lymphoma International Prognostic Index in randomized trials of the European Mantle-Cell Lymphoma Network. J Clin Oncol 2014;32:1338–46.
84. Rosenwald A, Wright G, Wiestner A, et al. The proliferation gene expression signature is a quantitative integrator of oncogenic events that predicts survival in mantle cell lymphoma. Cancer cell 2003;3:185–97.
85. Determann O, Hoster E, Ott G, et al. Ki-67 predicts outcome in advanced-stage mantle cell lymphoma patients treated with anti-CD20 immunochemotherapy: results from randomized trials of the European MCL Network and the German Low Grade Lymphoma Study Group. Blood 2008;111:2385–7.
86. Geisler CH, Kolstad A, Laurell A, et al. The Mantle Cell Lymphoma International Prognostic Index (MIPI) is superior to the International Prognostic Index (IPI) in predicting survival following intensive first-line immunochemotherapy and autologous stem cell transplantation (ASCT). Blood 2010;115:1530–3.
87. Hartmann EM, Campo E, Wright G, et al. Pathway discovery in mantle cell lymphoma by integrated analysis of high-resolution gene expression and copy number profiling. Blood 2010;116:953–61.
88. Bea S, Valdes-Mas R, Navarro A, et al. Landscape of somatic mutations and clonal evolution in mantle cell lymphoma. Proc Natl Acad Sci U S A 2013;110: 18250–5.
89. Iqbal J, Shen Y, Liu Y, et al. Genome-wide miRNA profiling of mantle cell lymphoma reveals a distinct subgroup with poor prognosis. Blood 2012;119: 4939–48.
90. Enjuanes A, Fernandez V, Hernandez L, et al. Identification of methylated genes associated with aggressive clinicopathological features in mantle cell lymphoma. PLoS One 2011;6:e19736.
91. Delfau-Larue MH, Klapper W, Berger F, et al. High-dose cytarabine does not overcome the adverse prognostic value of CDKN2A and TP53 deletions in mantle cell lymphoma. Blood 2015;126:604–11.
92. Scott DW, Abrisqueta P, Wright G, et al. Prognostic significance of the proliferation signature in mantle cell lymphoma measured using digital gene expression in formalin-fixed paraffin-embedded tissue biopsies. J Clin Oncol 2016; 34(Suppl):Abstract 7510.
93. Dreyling M, Ferrero S, Vogt N, et al. New paradigms in mantle cell lymphoma: is it time to risk-stratify treatment based on the proliferative signature? Clin Cancer Res 2014;20:5194–206.
94. Skarbnik A, MPH E, Lafeuille M, et al. Subcutaneous (SQ) bortezomib (BTZ) in patients (patients) with relapsed mantle cell lymphoma (MCL): retrospective, observational study of treatment patterns and outcomes in US community oncology practices. Blood 2014;124 [abstract: 1740].
95. Romaguera JE, Fayad LE, McLaughlin P, et al. Phase I trial of bortezomib in combination with rituximab-HyperCVAD alternating with rituximab, methotrexate and cytarabine for untreated aggressive mantle cell lymphoma. Br J Haematol 2010;151:47–53.
96. O'Connor OA, Stewart AK, Vallone M, et al. A phase 1 dose escalation study of the safety and pharmacokinetics of the novel proteasome inhibitor carfilzomib (PR-171) in patients with hematologic malignancies. Clin Cancer Res 2009;15: 7085–91.
97. Witzig TE, Geyer SM, Ghobrial I, et al. Phase II trial of single-agent temsirolimus (CCI-779) for relapsed mantle cell lymphoma. J Clin Oncol 2005;23:5347–56.

98. Hess G, Keller U, Scholz CW, et al. Safety and efficacy of Temsirolimus in combination with Bendamustine and Rituximab in relapsed mantle cell and follicular lymphoma. Leukemia 2015;29:1695–701.

99. Inwards DJ, Fishkin PA, LaPlant BR, et al. Phase I trial of rituximab, cladribine, and temsirolimus (RCT) for initial therapy of mantle cell lymphoma. Ann Oncol 2014;25:2020–4.

100. Wang M, Popplewell LL, Collins RH Jr, et al. Everolimus for patients with mantle cell lymphoma refractory to or intolerant of bortezomib: multicentre, single-arm, phase 2 study. Br J Haematol 2014;165:510–8.

101. Kahl BS, Spurgeon SE, Furman RR, et al. A phase 1 study of the PI3Kdelta inhibitor idelalisib in patients with relapsed/refractory mantle cell lymphoma (MCL). Blood 2014;123:3398–405.

102. Iyengar S, Clear A, Bodor C, et al. P110alpha-mediated constitutive PI3K signaling limits the efficacy of p110delta-selective inhibition in mantle cell lymphoma, particularly with multiple relapse. Blood 2013;121:2274–84.

103. Cunningham D, Zinzani P, Assouline S, et al. Results of the mantle cell lymphoma subset from a phase 2a study of copanlisib, a novel PI3K inhibitor, in patients with indolent and aggressive lymphoma. Blood 2015;126 [abstract: 3935].

104. Gerecitano J, Roberts A, Seymour J, et al. A phase 1 study of venetoclax (ABT-199/GDC-0199) monotherapy in patients with relapsed/refractory non-hodgkin lymphoma. Blood 2015;126 [abstract: 254].

105. Sven de Vos S, Swinnen L, Kozloff M, et al. A dose-escalation study of venetoclax (ABT-199/GDC-0199) in combination with bendamustine and rituximab in patients with relapsed or refractory non-Hodgkin's lymphoma. Blood 2015;126 [abstract: 255].

106. Leonard JP, LaCasce AS, Smith MR, et al. Selective CDK4/6 inhibition with tumor responses by PD0332991 in patients with mantle cell lymphoma. Blood 2012; 119:4597–607.

107. Chiron D, Di Liberto M, Martin P, et al. Cell-cycle reprogramming for PI3K inhibition overrides a relapse-specific C481S BTK mutation revealed by longitudinal functional genomics in mantle cell lymphoma. Cancer Discov 2014;4:1022–35.

108. Kirschbaum M, Frankel P, Popplewell L, et al. Phase II study of vorinostat for treatment of relapsed or refractory indolent non-Hodgkin's lymphoma and mantle cell lymphoma. J Clin Oncol 2011;29:1198–203.

109. Morschhauser FA, Cartron G, Thieblemont C, et al. Obinutuzumab (GA101) monotherapy in relapsed/refractory diffuse large b-cell lymphoma or mantle-cell lymphoma: results from the phase II GAUGUIN study. J Clin Oncol 2013; 31:2912–9.

110. Hunstig F, Hammersen J, Kunert C, et al. Complete remission after treatment with single-agent ofatumumab in a patient with high-risk leukemic mantle-cell lymphoma. J Clin Oncol 2013;31:e312–5.

111. Kolibaba K, Burke J, Brooks H, et al. Ublituximab (TG-1101), a novel glycoengineered anti-CD20 monoclonal antibody, in combination with ibrutinib is highly active in patients with relapsed and/or refractory mantle cell lymphoma; results of a phase II Trial. Blood 2015;126 [abstract: 3980].

112. Goebeler ME, Knop S, Viardot A, et al. Bispecific T-cell engager (BiTE) antibody construct blinatumomab for the treatment of patients with relapsed/refractory non-hodgkin lymphoma: final results from a phase I study. J Clin Oncol 2016; 34:1104–11.

113. Delarue R, Haioun C, Ribrag V, et al. CHOP and DHAP plus rituximab followed by autologous stem cell transplantation inmantle cell lymphoma: a phase 2

study from the Groupe d'Etude des Lymphomes de l'Adulte. Blood 2013;121(1): 48–53.

114. Geisler CH, Kolstad A, Laurell A, et al. Long-term progression-free survival of mantle cell lymphoma after intensive front-line immunochemotherapy with in vivo-purged stem cell rescue: a nonrandomized phase 2 multicenter study by the Nordic Lymphoma Group. Blood 2008;112(7):2687–93.

115. Hermine O, Hoster E, Walewski J, et al. Addition of high-dose cytarabine to immunochemotherapy before autologous stem-cell transplantation in patients aged 65 years or younger with mantle cell lymphoma (MCL Younger): a randomised, open-label, phase 3 trial of the European Mantle Cell Lymphoma Network. Lancet 2016;388(10044):565–75.

116. Le Gouill S, Thieblemont C, Oberic L, et al. Rituximab Maintenance Versus Wait and Watch after Four Courses of R-DHAP Followed By Autologous Stem Cell transplantation in Previously Untreated Young Patients with Mantle Cell Lymphoma: First Interim Analysis of the Phase III Prospective Lyma Trial, a Lysa Study. Blood 2014;124(21):Abstract #146.

117. Kolstad A, Laurell A, Jerkeman M, et al. Nordic MCL3 study: 90Y-ibritumomab-tiuxetan added to BEAM/C in non-CR patients before transplant in mantle cell lymphoma. Blood 2014;123(19):2953–9.

118. Romaguera JE, Fayad L, Rodriguez MA, et al. High rate of durable remissions after treatment of newly diagnosed aggressive mantle-cell lymphoma with rituximab plus hyper-CVAD alternating with rituximab plus high-dose methotrexate and cytarabine. J Clin Oncol 2005;23(28):7013–23.

119. Bernstein SH, Epner E, Unger JM, et al. A phase II multicenter trial of hyper-CVAD MTX/Ara-C and rituximab in patients with previously untreated mantle cell lymphoma; SWOG 0213. Ann Oncol 2013;24(6):1587–93.

120. Merli F, Luminari S, Ilariucci F, et al. Rituximab plus HyperCVAD alternating with high dose cytarabine and methotrexate for the initial treatment of patients with mantle cell lymphoma, a multicentre trial from Gruppo Italiano Studio Linfomi. Br J Haematol 2012;156(3):346–53.

121. Lenz G, Dreyling M, Hoster E, et al. Immunochemotherapy with rituximab and cyclophosphamide, doxorubicin, vincristine, and prednisone significantly improves response and time to treatment failure, but not long-term outcome in patients with previously untreated mantle cell lymphoma: results of a prospective randomized trial of the German Low Grade Lymphoma Study Group (GLSG). J Clin Oncol 2005;23(9):1984–92.

122. Rummel MJ, Niederle N, Maschmeyer G, et al. Bendamustine plus rituximab versus CHOP plus rituximab as first-line treatment for patients with indolent and mantle-cell lymphomas: an open-label, multicentre, randomised, phase 3 non-inferiority trial. Lancet 2013;381(9873):1203–10.

123. Flinn IW, van der Jagt R, Kahl BS, et al. Treatment of older patients with mantle-cell lymphoma. Blood 2014;123(19):2944–52.

124. Visco C, Finotto S, Zambello R, et al. Combination of rituximab, bendamustine, and cytarabine for patients with mantle-cell non-Hodgkin lymphoma ineligible for intensive regimens or autologous transplantation. J Clin Oncol 2013;1442–9.

125. Smith MR, Li H, Gordon L, et al. Phase II study of rituximab plus cyclophosphamide, doxorubicin, vincristine, and prednisone immunochemotherapy followed by yttrium-90-ibritumomab tiuxetan in untreated mantle-cell lymphoma: Eastern Cooperative Oncology Group Study E1499. J Clin Oncol 2012; 30(25):3119–26.

126. Rummel M, Knaut W, Goerner M, et al. Two years rituximab maintenance vs observation after first-line treatment with bendamustine plus rituximab (B-R) in patients with mantle cell lymphoma: First results of a prospective, randomized, multicenter phase II study (a subgroup study of the StiL NHL7 2008 MAINTAIN trial). J Clin Oncol 2016;34(Suppl):Abstract 7503.

Index

Note: Page numbers of article titles are in **boldface** type.

Hematol Oncol Clin N Am 30 (2016) 1371–1379
http://dx.doi.org/10.1016/S0889-8588(16)30144-7
0889-8588/16

.

Printed and bound by CPI Group (UK) Ltd, Croydon, CR0 4YY

03/10/2024

01040395-0006